The Complete

Yoga Tutor

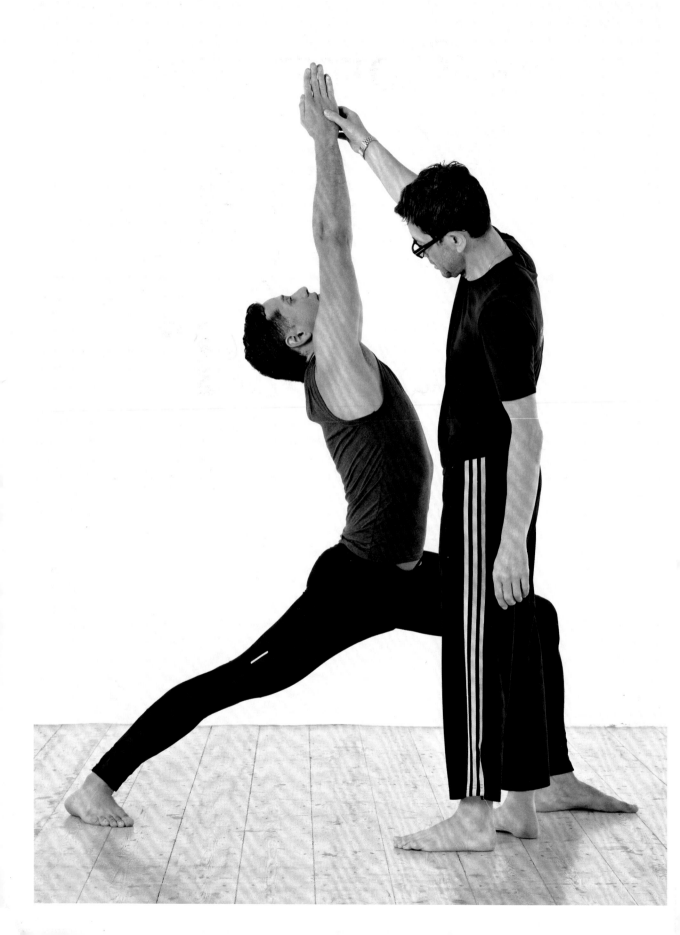

The Complete Yoga Tutor

*A structured course to achieve
professional expertise*

Mark Kan

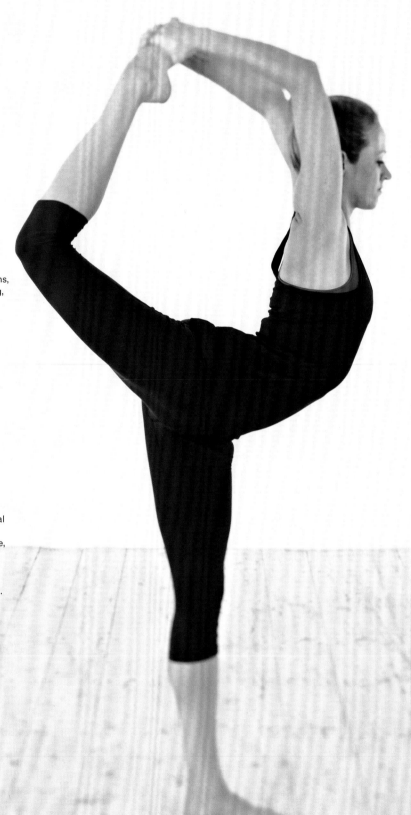

An Hachette UK Company
www.hachette.co.uk

First published in Great Britain in 2013 by Gaia,
a division of Octopus Publishing Group Ltd
Endeavour House, 189 Shaftesbury Avenue
London WC2H 8JY
www.octopusbooks.co.uk

ISBN 978-1-85675-330-2

A CIP catalogue record for this book is
available from the British Library

Printed and bound in China

10 9 8 7 6 5 4 3 2 1

All reasonable care has been taken in the
preparation of this book, but the information it
contains is not meant to take the place of medical
care under the direct supervision of a doctor.
Before making any changes in your health regime,
always consult a doctor. While all the practices
detailed in this book are completely safe if done
correctly, you must seek professional advice if
you are in any doubt about any medical condition.
Any application of the ideas and information
contained in this book is at the reader's sole
discretion and risk.

Contents

Foreword   7

Introduction   8

How to Use This Book   9

1 The History and Origins of Yoga   11

2 Yoga Anatomy   27

3 The Science of Yoga   57

4 *Asanas*   79

5 The Art of Breathing   215

6 Teaching Yoga   236

Glossary   250

Index   252

Acknowledgements   256

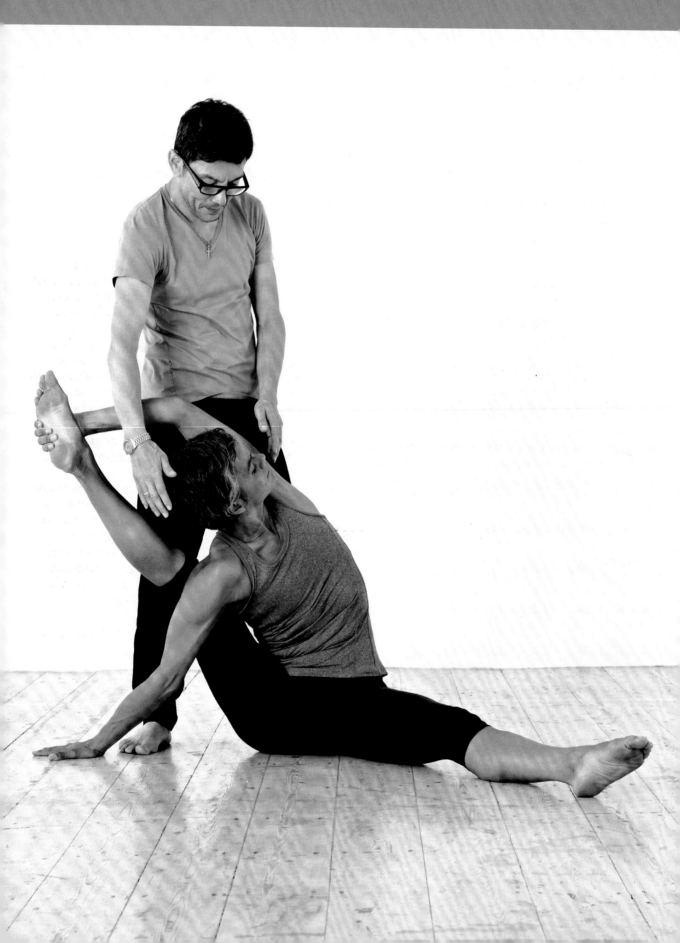

Foreword

Yoga is not a religion or a cult, but a set of divinely-realized techniques which, when practised correctly, within a short time help one to achieve radiant health, mental powers and, with the two first steps of yoga (*yama* and *nyama*), spiritual power.

Sri Dharma Mittra

Since the dawn of time, all living beings have possessed a strong, natural inclination towards comfort. Indeed, all beings love life and long to be physically comfortable. Over time, living beings evolved and eventually began to seek mental comfort also. A higher quest of psychic nature, the birth of the spiritual man, is the result of this process of ascending evolution. Obtaining inner peace is only possible when all doubts are gone – only knowledge can relieve all pain and suffering, turning darkness into light. This essential knowledge, stored in the Eternal Etheric Records, is easily obtained by high beings and, when people are fit to receive and thirsty for this knowledge, pure enlightened Divine Beings like Lord Buddha, Lord Jesus, Maharishi Patanjali, Paramahansa Yogananda and others volunteer to be born here among us to receive and share this profound knowledge. These saints and sages use their psychic abilities to access the knowledge always present in the Etheric Records at exactly the right time, in the right way and to the level of those fit to receive it. The knowledge is then collected on the physical plane in scrolls and books through various methods, and then manifests further as religion, philosophy and yoga, etc.

About 2,312 years ago, Maharishi Patanjali gathered and codified the divine esoteric knowledge that became known as yoga in his *Yoga Sutras*. Since then, countless numbers of yogis and yoga teachers have practised this discipline, constantly developing new methods and *asanas* (postures) to fit the times in which they lived. This process continues to this day.

The Ashtanga or eight-limbed yoga that Patanjali describes in the *Yoga Sutras* is not a religion, but a wonderful set of divine techniques that, if practised under the guidance of a knowledgeable teacher, allows the earnest practitioner to attain physical powers (radiant health), mental powers (psychic abilities) and spiritual powers (extremely subtle mental powers). I have devoted almost 50 years of my life to the practice of yoga. I realized and experienced some divine things under the guidance of my Guru-ji, Yogi Gupta, but since 1975 I have relied only on the True Guru within. Since 1967 I have been sharing Hatha and Raja yoga in a very simple, easy and straightforward way: I only recommend and teach the practices that will lead one in a short time to radiant health and mental powers, preparing one for self-knowledge. I am not Patanjali, but when the teacher is totally free from 'I' (ego) and 'mine' (attachment), one is free to borrow from the rich tradition and knowledge of the entire yoga system. This method of yoga is a shortcut to immortality.

About five years ago I first met Mark Kan when he became one of my students. It has been a great pleasure and has given me much satisfaction over the years since to watch his progress. The progress he has made is all due to obedience, and I am glad and happy that he has written this book. It will hopefully share some of this profound yogic knowledge with those that are seeking important answers and relief from pain and suffering.

May the best of all the blessings be bestowed upon you.

Dharma Mittra (Dharmananda)

Sri Dharma Mittra is director of the Dharma Yoga Center in New York City. A celebrated yogi, described by many as the teacher's teacher, he has been teaching in New York for over 50 years and is renowned for creating the Master Yoga Chart of 908 Postures. He teaches daily master classes and psychic development techniques at his New York temple.

Introduction

Yoga is like music. The rhythm of the body, the melody of the mind and the harmony of the soul create the symphony of life.

B. K. S. Iyengar

Today, yoga is a mainstream activity in Western culture. No longer regarded as an esoteric practice from the Asian subcontinent, postural yoga, more commonly known as *asana*, is practised in yoga studios, gyms and holistic centres in most cities, and has become one of the many ways in which we keep our bodies fit, toned and healthy.

Some might argue that this form of yoga bears scant resemblance to the original practices that emerged some two thousand years ago and has merely become another form of exercise, albeit with the kudos of its spiritual foundations. Whatever views we may hold, we will discover in this book that yoga has evolved to suit the needs of those cultures that have adopted its practices.

A Need for Change

Many of us find ourselves turning to yoga because we need something else – a greater purpose or a deeper meaning to life – or perhaps for physical reasons, to help us recover from injury or ailments. Either way, there is something we feel we need to change about ourselves. My own relationship with yoga began out of curiosity. I hadn't speculated on the idea of spiritual enlightenment, nor did I imagine it would lead to a greater examination of my internal and external worlds. Living in an era of increasing social and economic pressure can leave many of us feeling disenchanted and disconnected. Yoga provides us with a science of living that can bring a sense of wholeness and serenity and has no prerequisites that must be met before we embark on this path.

It is human nature to seek happiness and tranquillity, and to search for meaning in life. The disciplines, techniques and philosophy that underpin yoga can guide the seeker to a greater understanding of the nature of his or her being. Yoga is the art and science of self-care, self-development and self-realization. It has nothing to do with religion or nationality. It may have originated in India, but we don't need be Indian or Hindu to practise it. Non-divisive, it excludes no-one and is a universal path for all, a practical method developed for the purpose of bringing human beings to their highest levels of physical health, mental clarity and spiritual consciousness.

Yoga sets up no particular god or gods; neither does it deny the existence of God. Moreover, it is the science of all religion and, in practice, an applied science of the body and mind. The Sanskrit word *yoga* derives from the same root as the English *yoke,* and can thus have the meaning of union or identification. This identification or union, yoking or yoga with divinity is self-realization – the merging of the individual consciousness with the universal consciousness. This is the goal of yoga, to transcend the limits of our gross physical self and find our true nature through the awakening of the subtle or real self.

The practice and study of yoga offer us instruction and insight into every aspect of life – the physical, mental and spiritual, which harmonize and balance the body, mind and emotions, allowing the individual to arrive at a state of optimum dynamic health.

Age should not be an impediment to yoga practice. Physical and mental training through prescribed postures, breathing exercises and meditation can bring to all ages equanimity and freedom that might never otherwise be experienced. The body loses strength and flexibility only if we allow it to. My own guru, Sri Dharma Mittra, is living proof of the benefits a sustained regular practice can bring to the physical body. Now in his seventies, he is still master of postures that people less than half his age are unable to achieve.

Yoga is transformative, not only in changing how we see things, but in changing who we are: it challenges and transforms how we perceive our lives and our values, elevating us to new realms of wisdom through the unification of all aspects of our being. When you take up yoga you find that, starting with your physical body, you embark on an inward journey to discover the more subtle layers of your being and explore and analyse the inseparable relationship between nature and soul.

How to Use This Book

This book is a comprehensive manual for any aspiring yoga tutor, serious practitioner or teacher requiring specific information on *asanas* or other yoga practices.

In the first section, we will explore the real goal of yoga, its origins and the philosophy on which it was founded. This book gives a concise history of yoga's evolution, from the Tantric origins of the Pre-classical Period to Patanjali's eight-fold path, which signalled the emergence of the classical period that underpins modern yoga systems.

The Complete Yoga Tutor provides a framework for those who are interested in teaching yoga as a career and will also serve as a useful reference manual for qualified teachers. It provides a basic understanding of anatomy and physiology and how the body's systems are affected by yoga. At the heart of the book lies a fully illustrated section featuring over 50 yoga postures with step-by-step instructions on how to practise and demonstrate them safely, including the benefits of each pose, any contraindications and details of its biomechanical function. This section also includes yoga for pregnancy, for old age and for children.

A detailed section explains the science of yoga and ancient techniques developed to purify the physical and subtle bodies. The anatomy of the subtle body is explained: the five *prana*s, the five *kosha*s and the *chakra* and *nadi* systems and how they correspond with the physical body. The art of *pranayama* – breathing techniques – and an explanation of *mudhras* and *bandhas*, with photographs explaining how to apply them, complete this section.

The book concludes with information on teaching practice. For most new teachers, setting up their own studio may not be a viable option; teaching to small groups or one-to-one is the likely alternative. Advice is given on health and safety, teaching ethics and how to promote yourself as a yoga teacher.

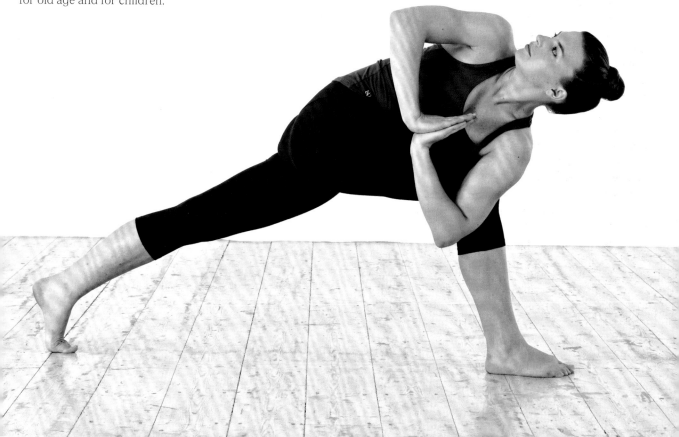

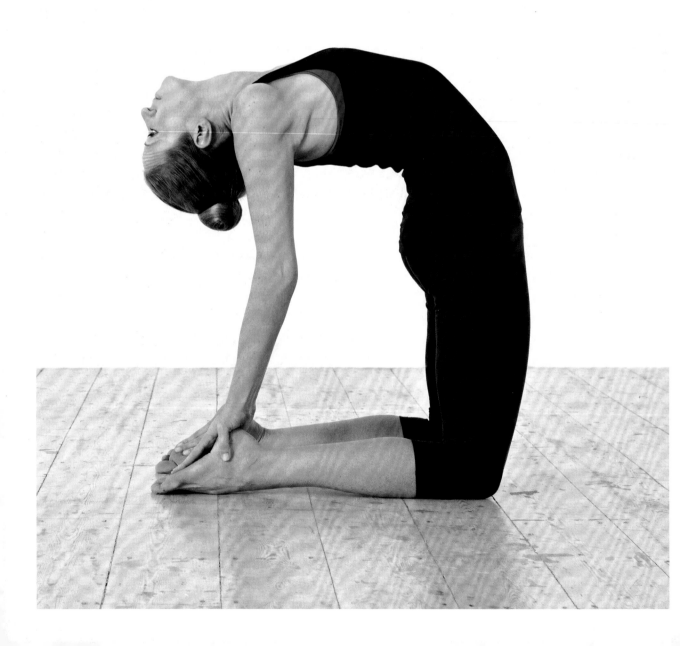

The History and Origins of Yoga

The Hatha yoga we practise today was developed as part of the Tantric civilization that existed in India more than ten thousand years ago. Two thousand years ago *asanas* consisted of a few seated poses, such as the Lotus, *Padmasana* and *Siddhasana*. The term *asana*, meaning seat, was derived from these poses. They have evolved and expanded over time so that now there is a myriad of postures that stretch, bend, twist and invert us, with the purpose of strengthening the body and increasing our flexibility, taking us on a journey from the physical to the more subtle realms of our being.

The Vedic or Pre-classical Period   12
Classical Yoga and Patanjali's *Yoga Sutras*   16
Yoga and the Post-classical Period   21
Yoga Today   25

The Vedic or Pre-classical Period

The earliest written evidence of yogic practice emerged at a time known as the Vedic period (4500–2500 BCE). The earliest archaeological evidence can be traced back about 4,500 years, to two sites in the Indus Valley.

The most signigicant of the many statues excavated by archaeologists in 1921 at two sites in the Indus Valley, Harappa and Mohenjo-daro (both in modern Pakistan), was a horned figure, seated in the cross-legged Lotus position and surrounded by wild animals. The Pashupati Seal, as it became known, is thought to be a prototype of Shiva, Lord of the Beasts.

The Harappan culture existed during what is referred to as the pre-Vedic age (6500–4500 BCE), before the Aryan civilization began to emerge in the Indus subcontinent. As this Indus Valley civilization died, so too did its language, and we can only speculate that these findings denote yoga positions, rather than habitual sitting positions of the time.

The Vedic Period

The Vedic or Pre-classical Period is the period within which the *Vedas*, the oldest record of Indian culture and the first textual references to yoga, emerged. It is also the period from which later religions and spiritual expressions evolved. Considered the most sacred of Hindu scriptures, the *Vedas* are described as *sruti*, which means their wisdom was only recited orally; they are therefore difficult to date, as it was some time before any textual evidence appeared. But most scholars agree that they date back to at least 1500–1200 BCE. *Veda* means 'knowledge', and the *Vedas* were among the first works to speculate on the interconnection between all things in

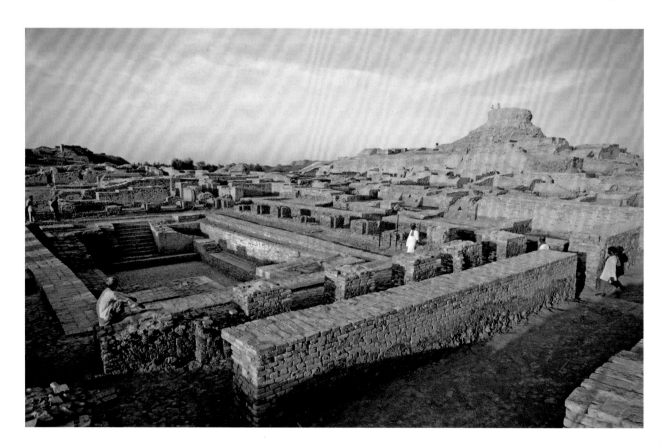

the known and unknown universe. They are said to have been revealed by God to the ancient masters of Vedic yoga, who were called *rishis* or 'seers'.

The main religion of that time was Brahmanism, wherein offerings were made to gods as a means of joining the material and spirit world. To perform the rituals, the sacrificers had to be able to focus their mind for prolonged periods of time. This inner focus, in order to transcend the limitations of the ordinary mind, is at the heart of yoga.

The *Vedas*

The *Vedas* are divided into four main parts: *Rig, Sama, Yajur* and *Atharva*, which comprise 1,180 sections in total.

The **Rig Veda** has 21 sections and is a collection of songs or hymns; it provides an insight into the social, religious, political and economic background of the Vedic civilization. The oldest book in any Indo-European language, it contains the earliest form of Sanskrit *mantras*, dating back to 1500–1000 BCE. The hymns praise a supreme power and offer thanks for victories and wealth, as well as prayers for worldly benefits such as health and protection.

Divided into 109 sections, the **Yajur Veda** is a collection of instructions on how to execute religious rites. It served as a guidebook for the priests who performed ceremonies while reciting prose prayers and sacrificial formulae.

The **Sama Veda** is a liturgical collection of melodies (*saman*), divided into 1,000 sections. Considered to be the original Indian music, this collection helped to train musicians and functioned as a hymnal for religious rites.

Divided into 50 sections, **Atharva Veda** is composed of hymns containing magic spells and incantations.

Each *Veda* is divided into four parts that are thought to correspond with the four stages of a man's life – the *Mantra Samhitas*, hymns; the *Brahmanas*, rituals; the *Aranyakas*, theologies; and of most importance to yoga, the *Upanishads*, philosophies.

The *Mantra Samhitas* are metrical poems comprising prayers and incantations addressed to various Vedic deities for attaining material prosperity here and happiness hereafter, while the *Brahmanas* were written in prose to explain the sacrificial practices. The *Aranyakas* or forest texts are intended to serve as objects of meditation for ascetics and deal with mysticism and symbolism.

Abandoned around 1900 BCE, Mohenjo-daro (meaning 'Mound of the Dead') was once was an important city in the Indus Valley civilization. The site was not rediscovered until the early 1920s.

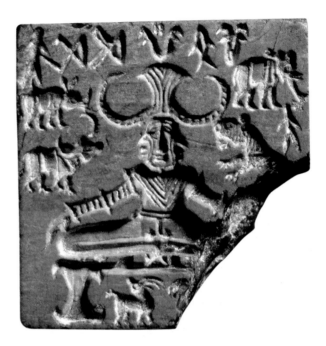

The Pashupati Seal was discovered at the Mohenjo-daro archaeological site. The cross-legged figure has been interpreted by some as a prototype of Shiva, and by others as a yogi.

Ascetics retreated into the forest to study the spiritual doctrines with their students, leading to less emphasis on the sacrificial rites that were still performed in the towns. The forest texts are transitional between the *Brahmanas* and the *Upanishads* in that they still discuss rites, but also contain early forms of the speculations and intellectual discussions that flowered in the *Upanishads*, which are Gnostic texts expounding hidden teachings about the ultimate unity of all things.

It is in the *Rig Veda*, the oldest Vedic text, that yoga is first mentioned and described as yoking or discipline, but there is no mention of any form of practice. Yoga isn't mentioned again until *Vratya Kanda*, the fifteenth book of the *Atharva Veda*, where it is referred to as a means of harnessing or yoking. Also, and of more significance, there is a reference to *pranayama*, breath control. But yoga really came into its own with the *Upanishads*.

The *Upanishads*

As the concluding portions of the *Vedas*, the *Upanishads* are also called the *Vedanta* or 'end of the Veda'. Deriving from the Sanskrit words *upa* (which means near), *ni* (down) and *shad* (to sit), *Upanishad* literally means 'sit down near' and it marks a period when students would learn the truths hidden in these mystic revelations

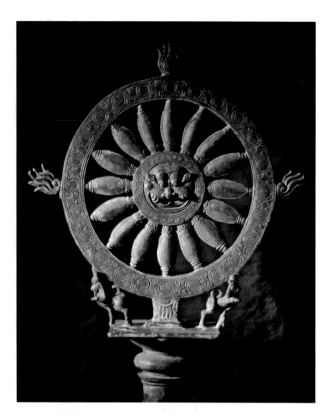

The Sanskrit word *samsara* means 'the running around'. In Indian philosophy, *samsara* denotes the never-ending cycle of birth, death and rebirth.

by sitting at the feet of their guru or teacher. These philosophical texts, which were passed down orally, contain the fundamental teachings central to the Hindu religion, as well as the essence of Vedic teachings that provide the main foundation of yoga philosophy today. There are more than 200 known *Upanishads*, but modern scholars recognize the first 13 as the principal texts.

The *Upanishads* reveal a gradual departure from the Brahmanic rituals of sacrifice towards an understanding of the higher truths of our existence. The gurus began to teach that the ego must be sacrificed in order to obtain liberation as opposed to the sacrifice of animals or offerings of crops in return for a peaceful and fruitful life. In the *Upanishads*, yoga is referred to as a path to achieve liberation from suffering through wisdom. Two yoga disciplines in particular emerged during this period – *Karma* yoga, the yoga of action, and *Jnana* yoga, the yoga of wisdom or discrimination.

Although the *Upanishads* concentrate on the cultivation of knowledge or *jnana* as a means of realizing *brahman* – the absolute truth – there are also references

to other techniques, called yoga, as espoused by the following tenets. The foremost, that your true nature – what we might refer to as the soul or *atman* – is the same as the nature of the universe, often referred to as universal consciousness, or *brahman*. Secondly, we are all subject to the cycle of birth, death and rebirth, *samsara*. Finally, your actions in this life determine the nature of your rebirth. In Vedic times this law of cause and effect, or *karma*, led to the belief that if you committed evil, you could find yourself reborn as an outcaste. However, through practices such as meditation and renunciation, the effects of *karma* could be reversed. In much later *Upanishads*, yoga became known as the path of renunciation, *sannyasa*.

The first reference to yoga is in the *Katha Upanishad*, where it is described as a means to transcend joy and sorrow and overcome death. In the *Svetasvatara Upanishad,* there is mention of the body being held in an upright posture while the mind is quietened by the control of the breath. The later *Maitri Upanishad*, from the second or third century BCE, includes references to yoga as unity of the breath and mind, and there are descriptions of a six-fold yoga path with practices to connect or yoke the universal *brahman* to the individual *atman* within all beings. This path comprises *pranayama*, controlling the breath; *pratyahara*, withdrawing the senses; *dhyana*, meditation; *dharana*, concentration; *tarka*, inquiry; and *samadhi,* final absorption in the self. Five of these limbs correspond with Patanjali's eight-fold path which emerged in the second century CE (see pages 18-18). In conclusion, the *Upanishads* provide us not with a systematic philosophy for the yoga system we know today, but with profound and mystical utterances.

The *Bhagavad Gita*

The most famous of all yoga texts that originated from the *Upanishads* is the *Bhagavad Gita* ('The Lord's Song'). Dated to about the fourth century BCE and considered to be the first yoga scripture, it is embedded in the *Mahabharata*, one of the longest epic poems in history, generally attributed to the Vedic sage Vyasa. The *Bhagavad Gita* tells the story of a civil war in ancient India between the sons of Kuru (the Kauravas) and the sons of Pandu (the Pandavas) and takes the form of a dialogue between Lord Krishna and Prince Arjuna on the battlefield of Kurukshetra.

Prince Yudhishthira, one of King Pandu's sons, loses the Pandavas' share in the kingdom in a rigged game of

In the framing story of the *Bhagavad Gita*, Prince Arjuna of the Pandavas seeks counsel from Krishna, serving as his charioteer and guide, on the battlefield of the Kurukshetra War.

dice. He and his four brothers, including Prince Arjuna, are banished for 13 years. At the end of their exile, they try to reclaim their share in the kingdom, which is now ruled by their blind uncle and his 100 sons. When their lawful claim is dismissed, the Pandavas declare war on the Kauravas. On the side of the Pandavas is God's incarnate, Krishna. Though a non-combatant, Krishna employs divine tactics to help Pandu's sons to victory. The Kauravas, although far more numerous, are defeated.

Krishna and Arjuna are friends and companions, but in a deeper sense they are one soul with two bodies, incomplete without the other. Arjuna represents the individual soul and Krishna the Supreme Soul that dwells in every heart. Arjuna's chariot represents the body, the blind king stands for the mind under the spell of ignorance and his many sons for man's evil tendencies. The battle is the perennial battle between good and evil. The overriding metaphor is of God and man, face to face and fully engaged in man's process of discovery of that which lies hidden in the innermost part of his heart.

Yoga in the *Bhagavad Gita*

The *Bhagavad Gita* lays out a three-fold path to yoga by which an aspirant can attain liberation. The first is the path of action or *Karma* yoga, in which one gives up the fruits of one's actions, but continues to be an agent in the world. Prince Arjuna struggles with his duties as a warrior to fight the forces of evil – 'in this case, the Kauravas, his own cousins. But, guided by Krishna, he is drawn into war with the intention of maintaining a higher moral order. The Kauravas are corrupt usurpers, while the peace-loving Pandavas have the welfare of the people at heart. Arjuna is willing to cast down his bow and relinquish his rights to the throne, but Lord Krishna instructs him otherwise, declaring that his yogic teaching transcends both pacifism and warmongering.

The second element is the path of devotion to the divine (*Bhakti* yoga). This is of primary importance in Krishna's teaching. Through love and devotion to Krishna, the devotee is granted liberation from suffering. Dedication to God is the inherent teaching of the *Gita* and all the other yoga systems described within it.

The third path is that of wisdom or *Jnana* (meditative) yoga, which liberates, through discrimination, the true nature of the self and the universe, and separates the real from the unreal. The *Gita* also describes a range of practices undertaken by yogis of the day, such as *pratyahara*, withdrawing the senses, and *pranayama*, controlling the breath. The *Gita* is the central text of the Hindu faith and is considered crucial to those wishing to experience yoga. Its central tenet is that one must endeavour to discharge one's duties sincerely, without regard for the outcome. 'Make every action an act of adoration to the Supreme Self or God.'

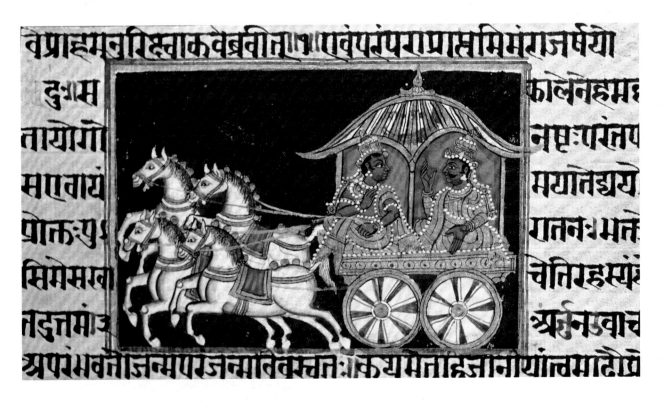

Classical Yoga and Patanjali's *Yoga Sutras*

Having some knowledge of the six main schools of Indian philosophy that came out of the Upanishadic period helps us understand how yoga has evolved. Although their views on some issues differed, all six believed in a universal law, concerning religious and metaphysical issues.

Mimamsa

The Mimamsa system is possibly the earliest of the six schools, founded by Jaimini around the fourth century BCE. As a fundamental component of the much later Vedanta, it had a profound influence on the development of Hinduism, providing rules for the interpretation of the *Vedas* and a philosophical justification for the observance of Vedic ritual. It also supported the view that the soul survives after death.

Vaisheshika

Founded around the second or third century CE by Kanada Kashyapa, Vaisheshika is a pluralistic realism, which explains the nature of the world with seven categories: substance, quality, action, universality, particularity, inherence and non-existence. According to this school, the will of God is the cause for creation. The Vaisheshika school merged with the Nyaya (see below) in the 11th century. Thereafter the combined school was referred to as Nyaya-Vaisheshika.

Nyaya

This school was founded around the same time as the Vaisheshika by Akshapada Gautama. Its key text is the *Nyaya Sutras*, primarily a theory of logic and argument. The major contribution of the Nyaya school lies in its working out the reasoning method of inference and the means of right knowledge.

Yoga

In the context of the six schools of Hindu philosophy, yoga came to be identified with the school of Patanjali, compiler of the *Yoga Sutras* (see page 18). This school is generally referred to as classical yoga and, as it shares the same metaphysics, is closely connected to Samkhya

(see below). Both are dualist philosophies, which teach that the transcendental self, *purusha*, is separate from the manifest world, *prakriti*. Whereas *purusha* is eternally unchanging, *prakriti* is in a constant state of flux and therefore leads to suffering.

Vedanta or Uttara Mimamsa

Shankara (c.eighth–ninth century CE) is credited as being the founder of this school. Vedanta means the conclusion (*anta*) of the *Vedas* and the name applies to the *Upanishads* and to the school that arose out of their study. Vedanta's three fundamental texts are the *Upanishads*, the *Brahma-sutras* (also called *Vedanta Sutras*) and the *Bhaghavad Gita*.

Samkhya

The Samkhya school of philosophy is believed to owe its existence to the sage Kapila. Around the middle of the Pre-classical Period, which gave rise to the *Upanishads*, this more radical metaphysical school was emerging, concerned with enumeration or ontology – the nature of being. Although closely aligned, Samkhya wasn't strictly a school of yogic thought. Whereas the yoga tradition was characterized by the belief that liberation could be achieved through meditation and renunciation, Samkhya applied the practices of *Jnana* yoga, using discrimination and reasoning to understand the nature of reality as well as renunciation as a vehicle to liberation.

This was not an entirely new concept, since renunciation or *sannyasa* featured in the earliest *Upanishads*. And, by the time Samkhyan philosophy began to emerge, the mainstream yoga tradition had already incorporated *Karma* and *Jnana* yoga into their practices, believing that renunciation itself was not enough to achieve true liberation. However, Samkhya achieved notoriety when it espoused the dualistic notion of two separate forms of reality or existence – *purusha*, pure consciousness, and *prakriti*, the world of matter, within which *purusha* is embedded. According to Samkhya, suffering occurs as a result of identification or attachment to body and mind and other aspects of the manifest world, *prakriti*, rather than their intrinsic essence, pure consciousness, *purusha*.

The Three *Gunas*

The Samkhyan concept of dualism was rejected by subsequent schools of yoga, but they recognized the theory, which explained the difference between the seer, *purusha*, and that which is seen, *prakriti*. Purusha, the real self, is beyond name, form and time and exists as pure consciousness.

However, *prakriti*, being the vehicle of *purusha*, is the basis of all activity by which our manifest world exists and functions. And while all phenomena in our cosmos are created by *prakriti*, it is the interplay of the primary forces of *sattva* (purity), *rajas* (action) and *tamas* (inertia) which forms the operating principle that governs *prakriti*. These three forces, also known as *gunas* or strands, are

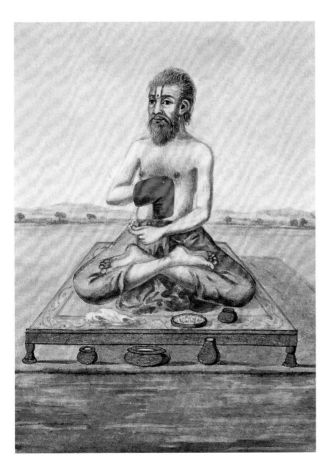

The concept of *prakriti* in Samkhya

Classical Samkhya recognizes 24 ingredients that form the matrix of *prakriti*, material existence. The first is **mahat**, which means great one, also referred to as *buddhi*. From the intelligence of *mahat* emerges **ahamkara** – I-ness or ego, which distinguishes between the subject and the object. This gives rise to the lower mind or **manas** and to the cognitive senses of sight, smell, taste, touch and hearing and the senses of action – speech, movement, grasping, excretion and reproduction. Underlying these elements are the subtle elements or **tanmatras** of sound, touch, form, taste and smell, which in turn produce the gross material elements or **maha bhutas** – earth, water, fire, air and ether.

interdependent and exist simultaneously, but fluctuate in degrees of dominance. Depending on their relative strength and concentration, they determine the nature of a being, its actions, attitude and its attachment to the world it lives in. They are responsible for our illusions and suffering on earth.

The purpose of describing the three qualities is not to encourage us to become sattvic or to eliminate the other forces – cultivation of *sattva* is not an end unto itself. *Sattva* is only the means to overcome *rajas* and *tamas*, in order to achieve self-realization through purity of mind and heart. One must transcend the *gunas* to attain immortality and freedom from birth, death, old age and sorrow.

The characteristics of the three *gunas* are as follows:
* **Sattva** is inherently pure and illuminating. It is regarded as the *guna* of the mind and the cognitive senses which connect us to the external world through our sensory organs – eyes, ears, nose, tongue and skin.
* **Rajas** is stimulating and mobile. The *guna* of the gross motor responses and physical experience, it dominates the senses of yearning. *Rajas* makes physical experience possible and controls the activity of the body – voice, hands, feet, anus and genitals.
* **Tamas** is inert and concealing, the *guna* of darkness and ignorance and inherently negative. This *guna* activates the five subtle elements or *tanmatras* – sight, sound, smell, taste and touch.

The sage Kapila, who was active around 500 BCE, is credited as one of the founders of the system of Samkhya, one of the six schools of Vedic philosophy.

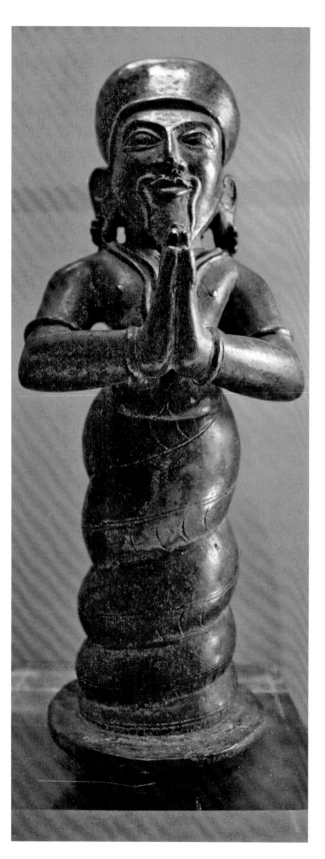

Patanjali's *Yoga Sutras*

Much of our modern yoga practice owes its survival to Patanjali's *Yoga Sutras*, but it must be made clear that there were earlier traditions in India which had adopted various yoga practices as a means of attaining liberation. What Patanjali did was to repackage these practices into a more systematic and coherent order. Today he is widely regarded as the founder of modern yoga.

The *Yoga Sutras* are the earliest extant documents outlining the philosophy, goals and techniques of yoga. Most experts date the *Sutras* to shortly after the turn of the common era – the first to second century. Some place them earlier, but all agree that they are no later than the fifth century CE. Little is known about Patanjali, not even whether he was an individual or several people compiling the *Sutras* under a pseudonym. In fact, tradition attributes the origins of yoga to a legendary figure, Hiranyagarbha, but because Patanjali collated these existing practices, his *Sutras* have become the canon for the myriad forms of meditation and yoga that exist today.

In a collection of 196 aphorisms – terse statements or 'threads', which are then expanded upon by a teacher to his students – Patanjali describes how, through yoga practice, the aspirant can gain mastery over his mind and emotions, overcome obstacles to spiritual growth and attain the goal of yoga, *kaivalya*, liberation from the bondage of worldly desires and, ultimately, union with the divine.

The first chapter (*Samadhi Pada*) provides a definition of yoga and describes the various states of the mind, its distractions and the effects that result from them. The second chapter (*Sadhana Pada*) is a more practical guide; it outlines eight limbs of yoga by which the yogi can attain liberation. The third chapter (*Vibhuti Pada*) is about accomplishments; it discusses the final steps of the spiritual practice and describes the powers and accomplishments which the serious practitioner may attain. The final section (*Kaivalya Pada*) deals with absolution and discusses yoga from a more metaphysical point of view.

The core of the *Yoga Sutras* is the eight-limbed path outlined in the second chapter, which forms the basis for modern yoga practice. These eight limbs are *yama*, abstentions and moral restraints; *nyama*, ethical observances; *asana*, posture; *pranayama*, breath control; *pratyahara*, withdrawal of the senses; *dharana*, concentration; *dhyana*, meditation; and *samadhi*, full meditative absorption.

Patanjali systematized existing yoga practices in the *Yoga Sutras*, and is considered the founder of modern yoga.

Yama – the Five Moral Commandments

The first of the eight limbs is *yama* – the ethical rules or moral commandments. These are *ahimsa*, non-violence; *satya*, truth; *asteya*, non-stealing; *brahmacharya*, continence; and *aparigraha*, non-coveting.

Ahimsa

Non-violence. The most fundamental of all moral commandments is non-harming. *Ahimsa* is usually translated as non-killing, but this doesn't convey the term's full meaning. It is non-violence in thought and action and underpins all other moral norms.

Satya

Truthfulness. To practise *satya* you must speak the truth as best you can and live truthfully through your thoughts, actions and words. However, certain truths could harm someone unnecessarily, so you have to consider how you speak the truth. If it has negative consequences for someone else, then it is better to say nothing. *Satya* should never conflict with your efforts to abide by *ahimsa*.

Asteya

Non-stealing. The practice of *asteya* implies not taking anything that has not been freely given. As long as a yogi lives in the world, he must take nothing that belongs to another without permission. *Asteya* can be compared to *ahimsa*, since the misappropriation of another's possessions leaves them feeling violated.

Brahmacharya

Continence or abstinence. In Patanjali's *Sutras* this is defined as abstaining from sexual activity through actions, thoughts or words. Sexual stimulation is thought to interrupt the path towards enlightenment by feeding the desire for sensory experience, so the energy derived from these restraints could lead to a clearer state of mind and increased vitality for the yogi to commit to his practice.

Aparigraha

Non-coveting. Renunciation is an integral aspect of yoga; by reducing his wants and needs, the yogi is encouraged to cultivate simplicity, as having or hoarding too many possessions leads to attachment and fear of loss, and is thought to distract the mind.

Nyama – the Five Observances

Once the destructive impulses are curtailed by following the *yamas*, the next stage is to cultivate *nyama* – positive actions and attitudes towards personal refinement. These rules of conduct apply to individual lifestyle, whereas the five *yamas* are universally applied.

Saucha

Purity. More than just the physical cleansing of the body, a yogi's thoughts, words and deeds must be clean and pure. Practising *asanas* or *pranayama*, eating sattvic food, being pure of thought and acting out of compassion instead of selfishness are essential for maintaining inner *saucha*.

Santosha

Contentment. A yogi must develop contentment within himself in the face of all he experiences, and cultivate the ability to experience pain or pleasure with equanimity. *Santosha* allows the yogi to feel the joys of happiness or the pain of sorrow, but not to become attached to either.

Tapas

Austerity. This *nyama* involves self-discipline in order to build a strong body and mind and a steadfast character. The Sanskrit word means 'heat', and by the practice of *tapas* one can experience liberation and mastery of the mind through imposed austerities such as thirst, heat, cold and hunger to remove impurities of the body and mind.

Svadhyaya

Study of the self. *Svadhyaya* is the study of the scriptures and any study related to one's own spiritual practice. It is believed that studying sacred texts enables the practitioner to concentrate upon and solve any of life's problems when they arise, by replacing ignorance with knowledge.

Ishvara Pranidhana

Dedication to the Lord. Devotion or surrender to the Lord is the final *nyama* and has been an integral part of yoga from its beginnings. It is said that a man's actions reflect his personality better than his words. When a yogi has surrendered all his actions to the Lord, divinity is reflected within him.

Asana

The third limb of Patanjali's yogic path is *asana* practice. By the time a yogi reaches this limb, he or she is acquainted with the causes of mental disturbances and knows how to control and reduce any unwholesome actions through regulation and mastery of *yama* and *nyama*. Accordingly, *asana* takes the practitioner to the next level, which is, by mastery and control of the physical body, to unite the body with the mind and, ultimately, the mind with the soul. To experience this awakening of consciousness it is necessary to create the right conditions on a physical as well as a subtle level. Through *asana* practice the body is maintained in a healthy, clean and pure state.

Patanjali gives no instruction about specific poses other than stating that the posture should be steady and comfortable. Most of the poses commonly practised today evolved much later. Patanjali was concerned only with enabling the yogi to sit comfortably and meditate. Certain postures bring about immediate mood-enhancing effects, facilitating the inner quiet required to concentrate and meditate. Beginners may not recognize these effects, as their awareness is directed towards the physical aspect of the pose, such as muscular tension or balancing, but with continued practice the *asana* requires less effort, so the yogi's attention can move away from the body to focus on the mind and the senses.

Pranayama

From *asana*, Patanjali states that there must be a progression to *pranayama*, breath control. The word *pranayama* combines the root *prana*, meaning life force or the vital energy that permeates and sustains all life, with *ayama*, meaning ascension, extension or expansion. *Pranayama* is the expansion of the life force through control of the breath.

Through observance of the ethical rules and moral commandments of *yama* and *nyama*, the yogi becomes more attuned to the workings of his inner environment, and through mastery of *asana*, strengthening and purifying the physical body, he is no longer distracted by muscular or physical discomfort. And so the yogi gradually becomes more aware of the subtle pranic force as it moves through the body.

Pranayama techniques enable the yogi to regulate the breath, so that the life force can be harnessed and directed to specific parts of the body. Ultimately, the goal of *pranayama* practice is to direct *prana* to the *sahasrara chakra* at the crown of the head, yielding the state of absorption or *samadhi*.

Pratyahara

Through the practices of *yama*, *nyama*, *asana* and *pranayama*, physical and mental distractions are brought into submission, leading to the fifth stage, *pratyahara* or sense withdrawal. The yogi withdraws his senses so that external stimuli can no longer govern his thoughts or actions and he is able to remain unaffected by the objects of desire. Patanjali believed that, by inhibiting his consciousness in this way, the yogi could extricate himself from his immediate surroundings. He would then be able to move on to more subtle practices to stimulate deeper levels of consciousness, remaining present in the world without attachment to it.

Dharana

After sublimation of the senses through *pratyahara*, the sixth stage of Patanjali's eight-fold path is *dharana* – intense concentration. This is no easy task. The yogi must hold his attention on a fixed internalized object through the practice of *ekagrata* – a term that can be translated as one-pointedness, or concentration. Focusing attention on a single point, perhaps a deity or a *chakra*, keeps the mind from wandering and controls the senses of cognition and volition.

Dhyana

Meaning meditative absorption, *dhyana* is reached when concentration is sustained and uninterrupted or when the object of one's concentration permeates the consciousness; the yogi then experiences supreme bliss through the integration of the body, breath, mind, senses and ego with the universal consciousness.

Samadhi

The final limb of Patanajali's eight-fold path is *samadhi*, true liberation, when the meditative state of absorption is transcended. Here we have the fusion or union of subject and object where, in the case of the yogi, his consciousness assumes the nature of the object that he is contemplating.

In the state of *samadhi* the body and senses are at rest, as if asleep, yet the mind and reason are alert and, depending on the level of absorption, a state of bliss is experienced with a sense of pure existence and wakefulness.

This icon represents the philosopher Adi Shankara of Kalady, who consolidated the doctrine of Advaita Vedanta. His teachings advocate the unity of *atman* and *brahman*.

Yoga and the Post-classical Period

The boundaries separating schools of yogic thought are not clearly defined and are impossible to date precisely, but Post-classical yoga could be regarded as a reaction to the dualism expounded in Patanjali's *Yoga Sutras* and his eight-limbed path.

Patanjali's *Yoga Sutras* were rooted in the *samkhya* belief that the transcendental self, *purusha*, was separate from the manifest world, *prakriti*. This school of thought existed alongside the non-dualistic Vedic traditions, but the succeeding Post-classical traditions believed *purusha* was inseparable from *prakriti*. This shift towards a non-dualistic world view signalled the end of the classical era.

Many parallels existed between the schools of dualism and non-dualism. Both believed in a universal consciousness that was omnipresent, immortal and could not be understood by the senses. For Patanjali this was *purusha*; the non-dualistic Advaita Vedanta called it the *atman* or self. Both believed that suffering arose out of a lack of connection with this higher self and that liberation occurred when humans realized their true nature.

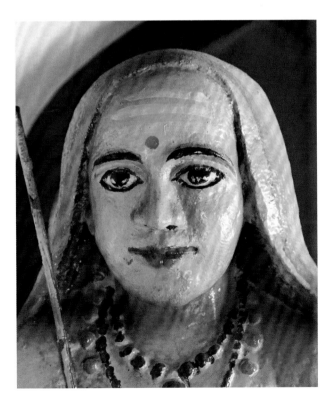

For the dualist in Pre-classical and classical yoga, this suffering occurred when someone held onto and became subsumed by everything that was not the self – when he came to believe that all he did made up his true self. A person would free himself from suffering only when he let go of his attachments to such things and realized, not with the intellect but with the heart, that the transcendental self resided within and was the ultimate reality.

For the non-dualist, suffering began when an individual tried to make a distinction between self and non-self, when he failed to understand that he was a small part of something much larger, when he forgot that everything he did and sensed was a manifestation of the transcendental *atman* or *purusha*. He released himself from suffering when he came to understand that his self was not separate, but an integral part of *atman*.

It is easier to see the divine in the mundane when you take the non-dualist view of reality, because the divine is everywhere. When *atman* or *purusha* is separate, how can anyone glimpse its luminous nature? Patanjali never answered that question, but later commentators explained that by practising the eight-limbed path, the yogi attains the highest level of existence. At this point *prakriti* becomes so transparent that *purusha* shines through. The path towards true liberation lies in experiencing, not just believing the universe as one. This combination of *Jnana* yoga and *Karma* yoga is similar to the ideas expounded in the *Bhaghavad Gita*.

Vedanta and Its Influence on Yoga

Vedanta was one of the main schools of the Post-classical Period. One of its most influential sub-schools was Advaita Vedanta. Advaita, meaning non-dualism, owes its emergence to the philosopher Shankara (c.700–750 CE) who theorized that *brahman* is real and that the world as it appears is an illusion or *maya*. As the sole reality, *brahman* cannot be said to possess any attributes and is outside time, space and causality. Vedantins believed that the dualist concept of *prakriti* represented no meaningful truth about ultimate reality. They argued that ignorance of this reality was the cause of all suffering in the world, and that only upon true knowledge of *brahman* could liberation be attained. Due to the confusing influence of *maya*, when a person tries to know *brahman* through his mind, *brahman* appears as God or Ishvara, which is separate from the world and from the individual, in the same way as the dualistic concept of *purusha* is separate from *prakriti*. In Vedanta, there is no difference between the individual soul, *atman* and *brahman*.

Tantra Yoga

More than any other school of yoga philosophy, Tantra's emergence early in the Post-classical Period, around the fourth century CE, signalled a radical departure from the classical tradition. Tantra rejected the *Vedas* and the belief that liberation could only be achieved by ascetic practices such as meditation and renunciation. Instead, it turned to the path of devotion and *Bhakti* yoga, in this case, the worship of the Goddess.

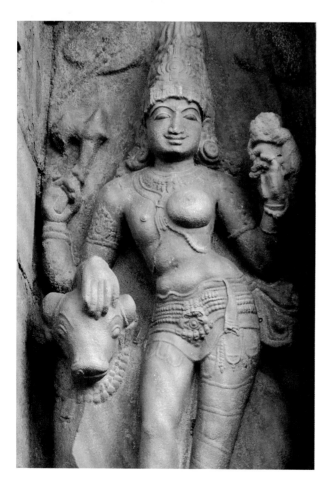

Whereas the non-dualistic traditions such as Vedanta believed that the manifest world was an illusion, Tantra believed that it was a manifestation of the divine and that all experience brought the aspirant closer to his or her own reality. Believing that all dualities existed within the universal consciousness, the only way a *tantrika* could liberate himself from suffering was to unite all these dualities in his own body.

The name Tantra comes from *tanoti*, meaning expansion, and *trayati*, liberation. Liberation occurred through the expansion of the consciousness. In Tantra, the universal consciousness referred to in classical terms as *purusha* was redefined as *shiva* and resided within the physical body. *Prakriti* became *shakti* and resided at the base of the spine. The interplay between the male energy of *shiva* and its female counterpart *shakti* took place internally, leading to final liberation, *samadhi*.

Most Westerners associate Tantra with sexual or orgiastic practices. This may have been the case with the left-handed path of Tantra, which took the concept of uniting the male and female principles literally, but the right-handed path preferred more symbolic means, through practising *asana*, *pranayama*, *mudhras* (symbolic gestures) and *bandhas* (body locks) to awaken the female *shakti* at the base of the spine and draw it up through the body, and unite it with *shiva* at the crown of the head.

However, Tantra did adhere to some of the practices outlined in the *Yoga Sutras*. In order to embark on the Tantric path, an aspirant was required to follow the ethical rules of *yama* and *nyama* and master sense withdrawal, *pratyahara*. Tantra also practised *mantra* – a sacred sound or syllable, with each letter of the *mantra* corresponding to a specific place in the body, and each place representing a force in the universe. Through *mantra*, the aspirant could awaken the body and its corresponding universal force.

As a response to dualism, Tantra recognized that our experiential nature need not be antagonistic to our spiritual evolution, and that the outer manifest world is not intrinsically different from our inner world. As in Vedanta, there is only one reality, yet in Tantra, this manifestation is more than the illusory *maya* expounded by the Vedantins.

The division between the physical experiences of body and breath and the spiritual experience of the transcendent self began to fuse as the Tantric tradition recognized a connection between the two. And so the physical practices

In Tantra yoga meditational deities such as Shakti, who personifies divine female creative power, represent archetypes of our own deepest level of consciousness.

acquired a greater prominence, and *prana* and *pranayama* in particular came to be viewed as an effective means of transforming our awareness. One of the systems that emerged out of this fusion was Hatha yoga.

Hatha Yoga

The physical postures practised in today's Western culture arose out of Hatha yoga. The term *hatha* is the combination of two *bija* (seed) *mantras: ha*, symbolizing the sun or *prana*, the vital force; and *tha*, the moon or the mind and mental energy. This system of yoga signifies the union of pranic and mental forces to awaken the higher consciousness. As a science of purification, distinct from its Tantric forebears, Hatha yoga gave more emphasis to the significance of the physical experience. Moreover, rather than trying to suppress the body, Hatha yoga attempted to overcome the dualism within ourselves by transforming the human into the divine and saw the body as an intrinsic vehicle to this transformation.

The first and primary texts on Hatha yoga are attributed to Goraksha and his guru Matsyendra around the ninth or tenth century. Often referred to as the father

Kundalini is depicted as a snake coiled at the base of the spine. The objective is to achieve liberation by raising *kundalini* up through the body, piercing the *chakras*, through yoga practices.

of Hatha yoga, Goraksha founded the Nath sect of yogis, which was a strand of Tantra. In his earliest text on Hatha yoga, *Siddah Siddhanta Paddhati*, he espoused the view that the physical body was only one level of embodiment and that there were five others, which emerged from gross to subtle, as well as nine energy centres or *chakras*, three signs or *lakshyas* and 16 props or *adhana*, which were points of focus – toes, hands and so on.

In the 15th century Swatmarama wrote the *Hatha Yoga Pradipika*, the oldest surviving manuscript devoted to the exposition of Hatha yoga. *Pradipika* is Sanskrit for 'to shed light on' and this work gives precise instruction on the path to divine union through mastery of the physical body. It names *asana* as the first accessory of Hatha yoga and lists its benefits as the attainment of steadiness (*sthira*), freedom from disease and lightness of body.

Swatwarama advocated a six-limbed, non-dualistic path, describing 15 *asanas*, positions for meditation and spinal flexibility or deep relaxation, which were mainly variations of the lotus pose; purification rituals; eight *pranayamas* or breathing exercises; and ten *mudhras* with *bandhas* or locks to constrict the flow of the vital force, *prana*.

Another important text, the *Gheranda Samhita*, dating from the late 17th century, listed seven *nyamas* necessary for yoga practice – cleanliness, firmness, stability, constancy, lightness, perception and non-defilement.

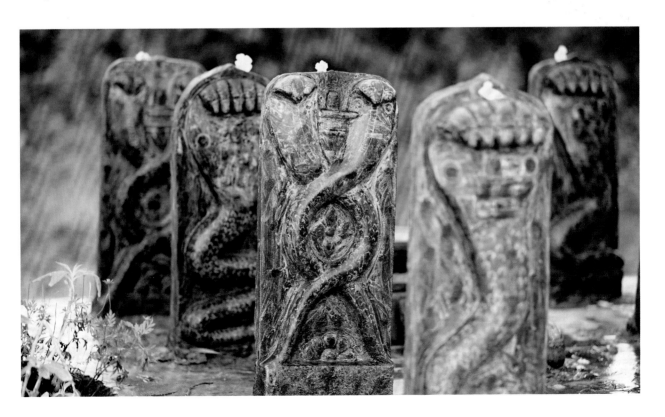

It included 32 *asanas* and 25 *mudra*s. Enlightenment was bestowed by the guru. The most comprehensive treatise on Hatha yoga appeared towards the end of the Post-classical Period in the early 18th century. Called the *Shiva Samhita*, it maintained that yoga was for the benefit of everyone, not just ascetics. It named 84 *asanas*, but describes only four seated poses, so we can see the development and the importance of *asanas*.

Purification techniques of Hatha yoga

The Hatha yogi believed that in order to purify the mind and realize one's true spiritual potential, the body must undergo a process to remove any defects or impurities that could lead to disease and decay. The first stage of this purification process was to recognize the limitations as well as the capabilities of the mind and body, and the second stage was to apply methods that would ultimately lead to expanding the consciousness.

This was achieved through six purification techniques, known as the *shat karma*s: *dhauti*, the cleansing of the stomach by swallowing a long narrow strip of cloth; *basti* or yogic enema, sucking water into the colon by means of an abdominal vacuum technique; *neti*, the cleaning of the nasal passages with salt water or a catheter; *trataka*, staring at a candle until the eyes water; *nauli*, abdominal massage effected by moving the rectus abdominis muscles in a wave-like circular motion; and *kapalabhati*, forcibly exhaling and passively inhaling through the nose by rapid contraction of the abdominal muscles. These techniques were said to prevent disease and old age by equalizing the activities and processes of the physical body. Once this equilibrium is attained, impulses are generated which awaken the central force responsible for the evolution of human consciousness.

Pranayama

Intrinsic to Hatha yoga practice is *pranayama*, which is the most effective way of controlling the life force. *Pranayama* cleanses and balances the subtle channels or *nadi*s in the body. According to Hatha yoga texts, the human body is made up of networks of these *nadi*s:

some say there are as many as 300,000 of them, but the commonly held view is that there are 72,000. There are three principal *nadi*s: a central channel, *sushumna*, with *ida* on the left side of the body, identified with the moon and carrier of the lunar force, and *pingala* on the right, identified with the sun and bearer of the solar force. The processes of *shatkarma*, *asana* and *pranayama* were devised to purify and balance these *nadi*s. Also of importance here are *chakras*, wheels or energy centres positioned at junctions along the spine and intersected by *ida* and *pingala nadi*s.

All three principal *nadi*s converge at the base of the spine, where *kundalini*, also referred to as the goddess Shakti, lies dormant and coiled, like a serpent. The objective is to gather the left and right currents of *ida* and *pingala* and draw them into the central channel, *sushumna*. Through persistent effort, *kundalini* is awakened and then drawn up along the *sushumna nadi*, piercing the *chakras* as it ascends. The result is that the life force is utilized for the transcendence of the self and the practitioner attains *samadhi*, which in turn leads to *moksha*, full liberation.

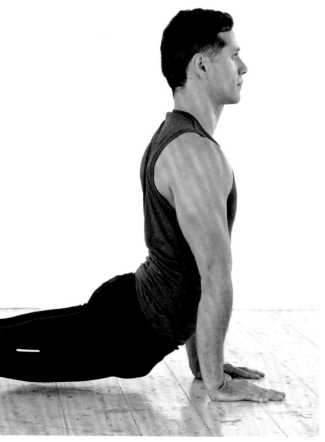

Yoga Today

There is an ever-expanding range of yoga practices to choose from. Whether your interests lead you to the more subtle psycho-spiritual nature of yoga or to the dynamic physical practices, there's likely to be something out there to suit you.

Today, we have many systems of yoga, most of which no longer reflect the practices outlined in the original Hatha scriptures. This departure from and neglect of practices such as the *shatkarmas*, *mudhras* and to some extent *pranayama* illustrate how in some schools these elements have become subordinate to the practice of *asana*.

The larger metaphysical theories and related practices are usually kept to a minimum and expressed only occasionally in yoga teaching and practice. Most teacher-training establishments require their students to have only general (if not scant) understanding of the science of yoga and its importance in raising the *kundalini*. Indeed, the average yoga class today is more likely to focus solely on the practice of *asana* and ignore the more subtle practices of Hatha yoga and the Tantric ideologies that underpin this tradition. Student yoga teachers usually learn something about *nadis* and *chakras* and many will read a modern commentary and translation of one of the seminal texts such as the *Hatha Yoga Pradipika*, but it is rare for this theoretical knowledge to be applied as part of a Hatha yoga practice as outlined in the traditional texts.

The posture-based yoga we know and practise today has emerged only over the past 120 years or so. There is little to suggest that many of the *asanas* in this book were the primary concern of any of the traditional yoga practices in India. They more likely owe their existence as much – if not more – to Western physical culture such as gymnastics and martial arts as to the Indian Hatha yoga system. In fact, most of the poses featured in this book are not referred to in any ancient texts, nor are they deemed necessary for the goal of self-realization.

Whether many of these poses existed from the outset is of little importance to the practitioners of today. Yoga is a process of transformation, and what really matters is the intention behind our practice. In our quest for liberation, our intention should be to transcend the

physical aspect and renounce the fruits of our actions. The purpose of mastery and perfection of each pose should be to awaken a different level of consciousness. Maintaining many of the poses requires not only strength and poise, but also a calm mind and for concentration to be steady and one-pointed. When we combine ancient and modern practices, the intention remains the same – integration of the mind, body and breath, leading the practitioner to a state of final liberation and union with his or her own divine nature.

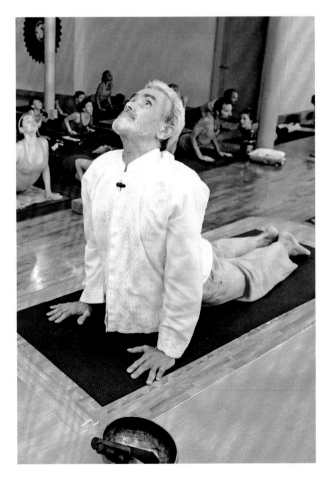

Renowned yoga teacher Sri Dharma Mittra demonstrates Upward-facing Dog Pose (see page 178) to his students in his master class at the Dharma Yoga Center, New York.

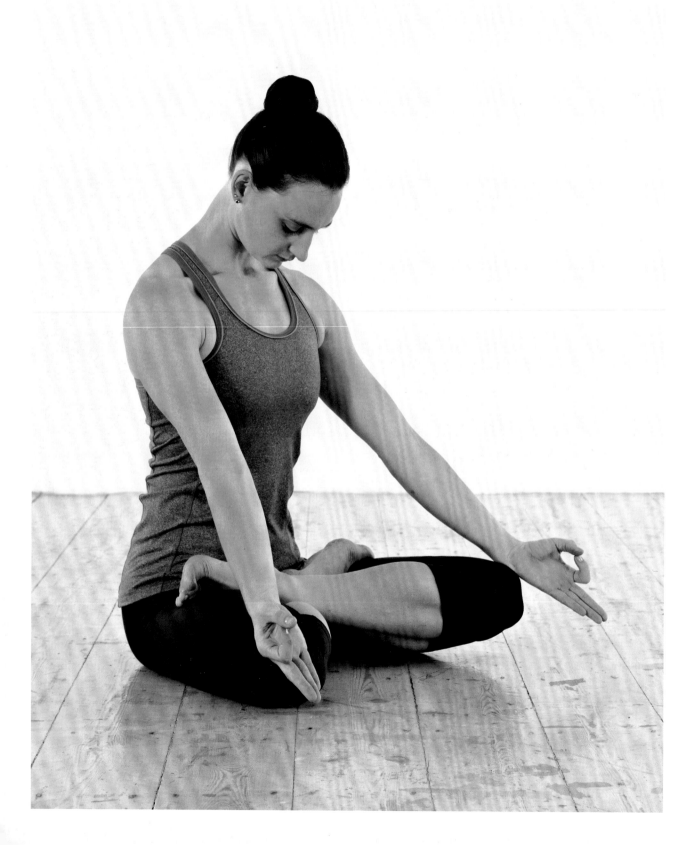

Yoga Anatomy

The body, mind and breath are an integrated system. The Hatha yoga tradition is concerned with optimizing the physical function of the body because it believes the body is the temple of the human soul and the gateway to understanding our true nature. As the sum of every part affects the whole, so our thoughts, emotions, what we eat, our professions and other lifestyle habits directly or indirectly define the body's mechanics.

Yoga and Anatomy	28
Breathing and the Respiratory System	30
The Cardiovascular System	32
The Lymphatic System	34
The Endocrine System	35
The Digestive System	36
The Nervous System	38
Cells and Tissues	40
The Muskuloskeletal System	42
The Muscular System	46
The Joints	48
Joint Movement	50

Yoga and Anatomy

To keep the body in good health is a duty … otherwise we shall not be able to keep our mind strong and clear.

Buddha

The body, mind and breath are an integrated system. Every movement and every breath requires the cooperation of all of the systems in the body, and every part of the body is connected to more than one system.

The respiratory, endocrine and digestive systems rely on the circulatory system to distribute oxygen, hormones and nutrients to the cells of the body. Without the nervous system, we couldn't coordinate the muscles of the limbs or modulate the dilation of the blood vessels to supply our vital organs with enough blood to function. Even our bones, classified as part of the skeletal system, have roles in other systems: because red and white blood cells are created in the bone marrow, they are also part of the circulatory and immune systems, for example.

It is important for a yoga teacher to have some knowledge of anatomy: the musculoskeletal system and location of the vital organs, and an understanding of the function and interplay of the body's various systems. While we are not qualified to diagnose or treat any ailments, understanding the mechanics of the body can help us determine the cause of common problems that students experience and give advice on restorative practices to resolve or prevent further occurrences.

By no means an authoritative guide to the human anatomy, this section is concerned with providing information relevant to understanding the body in relation to Hatha yoga. The *asanas* of classic Hatha yoga are simply movements and positions that the body is capable of assuming. But with some basic understanding of anatomy and physiology you can become more attuned to your own body and, as a consequence, can relate to the individual aspects shared by all bodies in order to help increase awareness in others.

The benefits of practising *asanas* include increased strength, enhanced flexibility and the abilities to relax through conscious engagement of the parasympathetic nervous system and to improve the circulation of information, energy and matter throughout the body. *Asanas* stimulate circulation by creating regions of different pressure throughout the body, taking advantage of the fact that there is a physiological tendency for energy (heat), matter (blood and intracellular fluid) and information (via the nervous system) to move from a region of higher pressure towards a region of lower pressure. An increase in pressure in one part of the body pushes energy and matter away from that region in much the same way as water is squeezed out of a sponge. In other parts of the body, reduced pressure pulls energy and matter towards that region – just as a dry sponge placed in water will expand, stretch and draw in moisture.

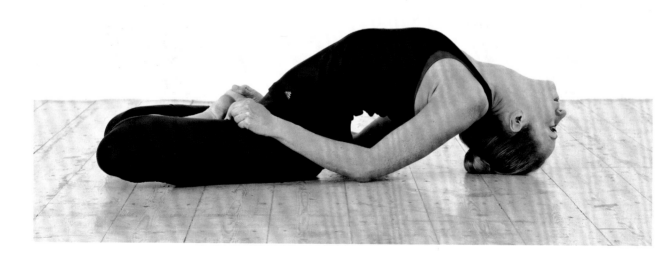

How Yoga Practices Affect Pressure in the Body

Asanas compress certain parts of the body and stretch others. In some static postures, muscle contraction increases local pressure and muscle relaxation decreases it. This is especially noticeable in inversions, semi-inversions and *Vinyasa*, which triggers the musculoskeletal pump. *Pranayama* techniques change pressure in the thorax and abdomen and normalize the action of the respiratory pump, where a reduction in abdominal and thoracic pressure causes inhalation and an increase in pressure causes exhalation. *Bandhas* stimulate the activation of opposing muscles across joints that either increase or decrease pressure.

Movement of the body and its parts, which initiates centripetal, centrifugal and inertial forces throughout the body, can affect circulation. This is especially noticeable when the movements are fast. The circulation of body substances through blood vessels and intracellular spaces increases proportionally with the difference in pressure between body parts.

To achieve maximum stimulation of circulation with minimum effort, it is important that one part of the body is kept at a very low pressure. This is one reason why the face and neck are usually kept completely relaxed while performing *asanas*. If they are not, blood pressure and stress levels can increase significantly.

The Integrated Systems of the Body

The human body is an integration of the following 12 systems, which interact to produce activity:

- reproductive
- respiratory
- cardiovascular
- circulatory
- lymphatic
- gastrointestinal
- integumentary or protective
- endocrine or hormonal
- nervous
- muscular
- skeletal
- urinary

For example, arm movement involves five different systems: the respiratory and gastrointestinal systems provide energy to the body in the form of oxygen and nutrients. Oxygen and nutrients are transported through the vessels of the cardiovascular system. The nervous system stimulates the heart to contract efficiently. This results in energy-rich blood being moved to the arm muscles. Finally, the nervous system stimulates the arm muscles to contract, causing a pulling effect on bone with consequent arm movement – an action of the musculoskeletal system.

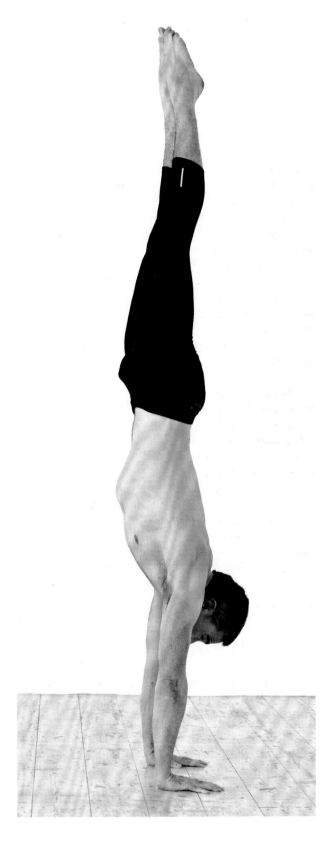

Breathing and the Respiratory System

From a yogic perspective, the breath is the gateway to purifying the mind, body and intellect. If we can control our respiration, we can control every aspect of our being and lead a better and healthier life.

Unlike our other bodily systems, breathing can be controlled voluntarily and is the key to regulating the unconscious mind. Through training, we can change the rate, depth and quality of our breathing, making it more efficient. Yoga offers us techniques to consciously regulate the breath, to pump the breath for specific purposes and also to retain it at will, but these techniques must be approached with caution and under the guidance of a teacher. To understand the benefits of these controlled methods, we must first examine the overall design of the respiratory system.

The process of taking air into and expelling it from the lungs is usually controlled by the autonomic nervous system (see page 38), which works closely with the cardiovascular system (see page 32) to deliver oxygen to the tissues and remove carbon dioxide from them. Air is inhaled through the nose, which acts as a filter to remove any impurities. It then travels down the trachea or windpipe, which branches into two main airways, the right and left bronchi, each of which connects to a lung. Many small tubes called bronchioles bring air deep into the lungs, which are moist and elastic. At the end of each bronchiole are the alveoli where gases are exchanged between blood and air.

The Thoracic and Abdominal Cavities

Breathing involves movement of the thoracic and abdominal cavities. The thoracic cavity houses the heart and lungs; the abdominal cavity houses the stomach, liver, spleen, kidneys, bladder and other organs. Each has an opening – the thoracic cavity at the top, the abdominal at the bottom. A large, dome-shaped muscle, the respiratory diaphragm, separates the two. It attaches to the inner surface of the lower ribs and the lower thoracic spine, forming the roof of the abdominal cavity and the floor of the thoracic cavity.

The diaphragm and the intercostal and abdominal muscles are the three main muscles required for breathing. The abdominal and thoracic cavities are able to change shape; without this movement, we could not breathe. They change shape in different ways, though. The abdominal cavity is like a balloon filled with water. Because water cannot be compressed, when you squeeze one end of the balloon, the water is forced to the other end. The same principle applies when the abdominal cavity is compressed by the action of breathing; a squeeze in one area produces expansion in another, so that the overall volume doesn't change. This process applies only to breathing, not to other processes within the abdominal cavity. For example, eating will cause the volume of the abdominal cavity to increase as the stomach, intestines and bladder expand and produce a corresponding decrease in the volume of the thoracic cavity. That is why it is often difficult to breathe after a big meal.

Unlike the abdominal cavity, the thoracic cavity can change in volume as well as shape, behaving rather like a pair of bellows. When you squeeze the bellows, you reduce their volume and force air out. When you pull the bellows open, the volume increases and air is sucked in again. If we imagine the thoracic and abdominal cavities as a pair of bellows on top of a water balloon, we get a sense of how the two operate when we breathe. Movement in one will necessitate movement in the other.

Yoga and the Respiratory System

Asanas and *pranayama* improve the efficiency of the respiratory system by increasing air intake and breath control through breathing exercises such as *Kapalabhati*, which exercises the diaphragm. As well as developing strong muscles and elastic tissues, *Salabhasana* and *Mayurasana* also deepen the inhalations and improve breath retention, while *Nauli* and *Uddiyana Bandha* encourage deeper exhalation.

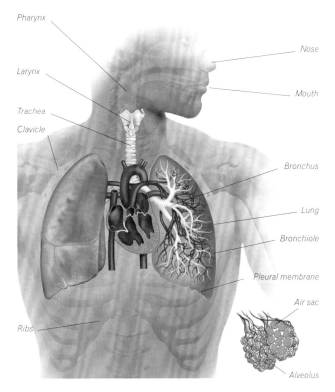

Pharynx

Nose

Larynx

Mouth

Trachea

Clavicle

Bronchus

Lung

Bronchiole

Pleural membrane

Air sac

Ribs

Alveolus

Oxygen is inhaled as air, taken to the lungs and diffused through the alveoli walls into the blood cells. Carbon dioxide is absorbed from the blood into the alveoli and expelled through exhalation.

Inhalation and Exhalation

So we can see how volume and pressure are intrinsically related. When volume increases, pressure decreases, and vice versa. During an inhalation, air isn't drawn into the body, in spite of how it might feel; it is in fact *pushed* into the body by the surrounding atmospheric pressure, because air always flows towards an area of low pressure. So when the volume inside the thoracic cavity increases, there is a decrease in pressure, causing air to flow into it.

As the thoracic cavity expands, it pushes down on the abdominal cavity, which changes shape as a result. A passive exhalation is a reversal of this process. The thoracic cavity and the lung tissues which were stretched open during the inhalation return to their initial volume, pushing the air out and returning the thoracic cavity to its previous shape. This process is known as passive recoil. Exhalation is usually a relaxation of the diaphragm. Because the lungs are naturally elastic, they are able to recoil and expel air without the help of muscular contractions.

When more oxygen is needed, such as during exercise, forced exhalation occurs. The abdominal muscles and pelvic-floor muscles may be contracted to expel more air

faster. The intercostal muscles can also aid in depressing the ribcage.

Breathing patterns such as speaking, singing or blowing up a balloon, which require active or conscious exhalation, cause the muscles surrounding the cavities to contract in such a way that the abdominal cavity is pushed up towards the thoracic cavity, or the thoracic is pushed down towards the abdominal, or a combination of the two.

Any reduction in the elasticity of these tissues will result in a reduction of the body's ability to exhale passively, leading to a host of respiratory problems. The surfaces of air tubes are covered in tiny hair-like projections called cilia that sweep dust and microorganisms up to the pharynx where they are coughed out. Repeated damage to these structures can lead to scarring and infection.

Function of the Respiratory System

The primary function of the respiratory system is to exchange oxygen and carbon dioxide between the external atmosphere and the bloodstream. This process is known as ventilation.

Oxygen is the primary source of energy for all cells. It is inhaled through the nose, makes its way through the respiratory system, is absorbed into the circulatory system and transported to the cells. When the cells use oxygen for energy, the resultant waste product is carbon dioxide, which travels from the cells and is exhaled out of the body via the respiratory system, being pushed out of the lungs through the nose or mouth as the diaphragm relaxes.

The major functions of the breathing and respiratory systems are to:

- Transport nutrients from the digestive tract to all parts of the body.
- Transport oxygen from the lungs to all parts of the body.
- Transport carbon dioxide and other wastes from cells to excretory organs such as the lungs, the sweat glands of the skin and the urinary system.
- Transport hormones from the endocrine glands to various parts of the body.
- Help to maintain body temperature.
- Help to maintain fluid balance.
- Protect the body against disease.

The Cardiovascular System

Some 80 per cent of the human body is made up of fluid, which needs to be moved and maintained by the two systems that form the circulatory system – the cardiovascular and lymphatic systems.

The cardiovascular system is responsible for the movement of nutrients, gases, waste products and hormones. Its function is to pump and carry blood around the body, which results in nutrients being sent to the cells and wastes being removed from them. It is regulated by the endocrine and nervous systems; many other systems depend on it for their primary function. Regular practice of *asana* and *pranayama* increase the efficiency of the cardiovascular system.

The Heart

The most important component of the cardiovascular system is the heart, which pumps blood around the body, supplying cells with oxygen and nutrients. To achieve its pumping effect, the heart contracts and relaxes. It is a double pump with four chambers: the right side pumps blood to the lungs; the left pumps it around the body. A muscular wall called a septum separates the two sides.

Each side of the heart has an upper chamber (atrium) and a lower chamber (ventricle). Blood enters the heart through the right atrium from the superior vena cava, and is pumped through the tricuspid valve into the right ventricle. When the right ventricle contracts, the blood is pushed into the pulmonary arteries, which carry it to the lungs, where it is oxygenated. The re-oxygenated blood enters the left atrium and passes through the mitral valve into the left ventricle, from where it is pumped via the body's main artery, the aorta, to the circulatory system.

Blood flow passes from the right to the left side of the heart via the lungs, hence the right side is low in oxygen and the left rich in oxygen. The right-side flow is called pulmonary circulation and the left systemic circulation.

During the relaxation or diastole period, the heart chamber fills with blood; during contraction – the systole period – it expels it. The terms diastolic and systolic are used in the measurement of the blood pressure against the arterial wall: a normal resting blood pressure measurement is 120 systolic over 80 diastolic. A resting or calm healthy heart beats 70 times a minute, but during stress, exercise or excitement this could rise as high as 200 beats a minute. The heart rate can be measured by the pulse of an artery expanding and contracting.

The nervous system has a profound influence over the heart rate, altering it to meet the demands of the body, for example during exercise or when experiencing excitement or fear.

The Blood Vessels

The heart regulates the flow of blood via an intricate network of blood vessels. Most arteries carry rich, oxygenated blood to the cells of the body; the exceptions are the pulmonary arteries, which carry de-oxygenated blood to the lungs for oxygenation. Arteries have thick walls that can expand to absorb the surge of blood

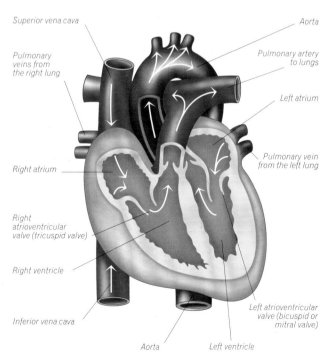

Superior vena cava

Pulmonary veins from the right lung

Right atrium

Right atrioventricular valve (tricuspid valve)

Right ventricle

Inferior vena cava

Aorta

Aorta

Pulmonary artery to lungs

Left atrium

Pulmonary vein from the left lung

Left atrioventricular valve (bicuspid or mitral valve)

Left ventricle

Oxygenated blood from the lungs arrives in the left atrium of the heart and then moves on to rest of the body. De-oxygenated blood is deposited in the right atrium and pumped to the lungs.

resulting from each beat of the heart. The smaller arteries, known as arterioles, branch into tiny vessels, the capillaries. Their thin single-cell walls allow nutrients and oxygen to pass through into the surrounding tissues.

Veins carry blood that is low in oxygen – again with the exception of the pulmonary veins, which return oxygenated blood from the lungs to the heart. Veins are thinner-walled than arteries and have valves to prevent any back-flow of blood. The smallest veins are called venules.

Blood

The average body has 5–6 litres of blood, which circulate every 60 seconds. The blood has four main functions:
- Transports oxygen, nutrients and hormones to the cells.
- Carries waste products from the cells.
- Protects against disease-producing organisms.
- Produces clots to prevent haemorrhaging.

Blood is composed of plasma, a straw-coloured liquid that is 90 per cent water and 10 per cent protein and other solutes, and which has millions of cells suspended in it. The principal ones are:
- **Red blood cells** (erythrocytes), the most numerous of the blood cells. Their functions include transporting oxygen to cells and carbon dioxide from the cells to the lungs. They contain haemoglobin, an iron protein complex that carries oxygen. These cells live only nine days and are recycled by the spleen and liver (the iron is then excreted in the faeces).
- **White blood cells** (leukocytes), which act as part of the immune system – they can identify foreign cells, viruses and cancer cells. They form antibodies against disease, protect the body from infection, aid in the body's healing process and remove debris from injured tissue.
- **Cell fragments** (platelets), activated whenever blood clotting or repairs to blood vessels are necessary.

Yoga and the Cardiovascular System
An efficient circulatory system requires a healthy heart, and arteries and veins to be clear and unobstructed. All *asanas* improve circulation – especially *Sirsasana* and *Sarvangasana*. These inverted poses reverse the effect of gravity, resting the valves and vein walls. The increase and decrease in pressure on the heart strengthens the heart muscle, while the practices of *Nauli* and *Kapalabhati* massage the heart.

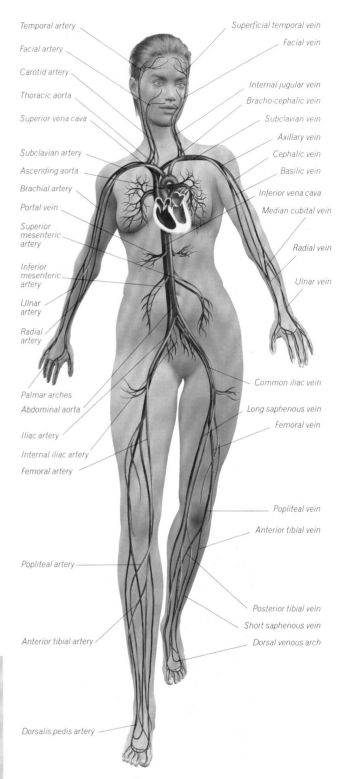

Temporal artery
Facial artery
Carotid artery
Thoracic aorta
Superior vena cava
Subclavian artery
Ascending aorta
Brachial artery
Portal vein
Superior mesenteric artery
Inferior mesenteric artery
Ulnar artery
Radial artery
Palmar arches
Abdominal aorta
Iliac artery
Internal iliac artery
Femoral artery
Popliteal artery
Anterior tibial artery
Dorsalis pedis artery

Superficial temporal vein
Facial vein
Internal jugular vein
Bracho-cephalic vein
Subclavian vein
Axillary vein
Cephalic vein
Basilic vein
Inferior vena cava
Median cubital vein
Radial vein
Ulnar vein
Common iliac vein
Long saphenous vein
Femoral vein
Popliteal vein
Anterior tibial vein
Posterior tibial vein
Short saphenous vein
Dorsal venous arch

A system of veins, arteries and capillaries allows blood to circulate all around the body, enabling the transportation of nutrients and oxygen and the removal of waste products.

The Lymphatic System

This secondary circulatory system is the body's waste-disposal unit. It is composed of lymph vessels, nodes and ducts, as well as lymphoid organs and tissues, including the thymus, spleen and tonsils.

The lymphatic system functions in a similar way to the cardiovascular system, with vessels that branch through the body. A clear watery fluid, lymph, removes pathogens, excess fluids, waste products, dead blood cells and toxins that are present in the interstitial fluid between the cells within the tissues.

Lymph originates as plasma, the fluid portion of the blood. Arterial blood, flowing away from the heart, slows as it moves through a network of capillaries to an organ. Due to this slow movement, some plasma is able to flow into the tissues, where it becomes known as tissue fluid or extracellular fluid. It then flows between the cells and

delivers nutrients, oxygen and hormones to them. As it leaves the cells, it takes with it waste products and protein cells. Approximately 90 per cent of this tissue fluid now enters the venous circulation as plasma. The remaining 10 per cent is known as lymph.

The Movement of Lymph

A series of one-way valves move most of the lymph forward to the biggest lymph vessel, the thoracic duct or left lymphatic duct. This runs up the front of the spine and empties into the left subclavian vein, re-entering the blood circulatory system. Lymph from the upper right area of the torso, however, passes into the smaller right lymphatic duct and enters the bloodstream via the right subclavian vein. The process is aided by the activity of the skeletal muscles, pulsation of the neighbouring arteries and 'suction' from the respiratory system.

At various points the lymph passes through small, bean-shaped structures called lymph nodes where debris is removed and cleansed by white blood cells. The purified lymph is then returned into the blood. Clusters of lymph nodes are found in the armpits, groin, chest and abdomen. During an infection the immune system is activated and these lymph nodes can swell to the size of marbles or larger, until the infection is reduced.

The two main organs of the lymphatic system are the thymus and the spleen. The thymus is located in the upper chest, behind the sternum, and plays a key role in the body's immune system by secreting the hormone thymosin. This stimulates the development of lymphocytes, a type of white blood cell that plays a vital role in the body's immune system (see page 40). The spleen is located in the upper left area of the abdomen. With its many blood vessels, it serves as a reservoir for blood cells, destroys old red blood cells and platelets and also plays a part in the body's immune system.

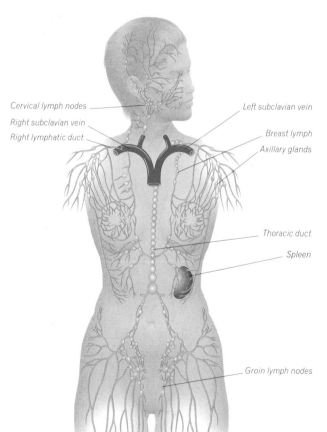

Cervical lymph nodes

Right subclavian vein

Right lymphatic duct

Left subclavian vein

Breast lymph

Axillary glands

Thoracic duct

Spleen

Groin lymph nodes

The lymphatic system has no pump, relying on the movements of the skeletal muscles to move lymph around the body. Practising *asanas* helps ensure proper lymph circulation.

The Endocrine System

The endocrine system is a collection of glands that produce chemical messengers called hormones that regulate mood, metabolism, sleep, growth and other vital functions.

Compared to the nervous system, the endocrine system works slowly, because hormones must travel through the circulatory system to reach their target. It works on a principle of equilibrium: one hormone stimulates responses and another inhibits them. Together with the sympathetic nervous system, the endocrine system is the mediator of an often complex relationship of body and mind. Emotions such as fear or love reflect hormonal activity and influence the function of the endocrine system. The major endocrine glands are as follows:

The Hypothalamus
Hormones are produced in response to signals from the hypothalamus, an area of the brain that acts in conjunction with the pituitary gland. This gland links the nervous and endocrine systems, and regulates body temperature, hunger, thirst and certain emotional states. It synthesizes and releases neurohormones, which act on the pituitary, causing it to secrete further hormones.

The Pituitary Gland
This pea-sized master gland regulates the activity of most endocrine glands in the body. Controlled by the brain, it produces three key trophic hormones – thyroid-stimulating hormone (TSH), adrenocorticotrophic hormone (ACTH) and gonadotrophic hormone – that act to increase production of other hormones. It also produces growth hormone and prolactin.

The Pineal Gland
The pineal gland secretes melatonin, which regulates our waking and sleeping cycles.

Thyroid and Parathyroid Glands
These are situated in the neck. The thyroid regulates the metabolism, growth and normal nervous activity and causes bones to retain calcium. The parathyroid regulates calcium levels in the bloodstream.

Pancreatic and Adrenal Glands
Located beside the stomach, the pancreas produces insulin, which regulates blood sugar. It is also part of the digestive system (see page 36). The adrenal glands sit on top of the kidneys and regulate stress response.

Ovaries and Testes
These produce sex hormones and regulate reproduction.

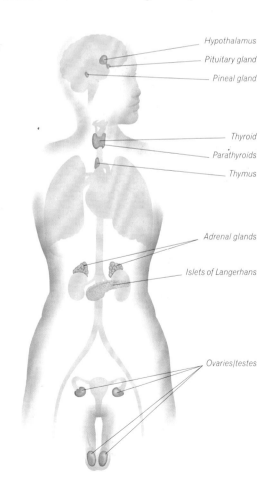

Hypothalamus
Pituitary gland
Pineal gland
Thyroid
Parathyroids
Thymus
Adrenal glands
Islets of Langerhans
Ovaries/testes

Regular yoga practice can have a positive influence on the endocrine system: inversions such *Sirshasana* increase blood flow to the thyroid, and *Yoga Mudra* stimulates the pineal gland.

The Digestive System

Food and drink in their gross state are not in a form that the body can use. They must be broken down into smaller molecules that can be absorbed into the blood, carried throughout the body and used to nourish cells and provide energy. This process is called digestion.

Also known as the alimentary or gastrointestinal tract or canal, the digestive tract consists of the mouth, oesophagus, stomach, small intestine, large intestine or colon, rectum and anus. The lining of these 'hollow' organs is called the mucosa. In the mouth, stomach and small intestine, the mucosa contains tiny glands that produce juices to help digest food. The liver and the pancreas are also part of the digestive system, producing digestive juices. The gallbladder stores the liver's digestive juices until they are needed in the intestine. Parts of the nervous and circulatory systems also play major roles in the digestive system.

How Food Is Digested

Digestion involves mixing food with digestive juices, moving it through the digestive tract and breaking down large molecules of food into smaller ones. The process begins in the mouth, when you chew and swallow, and is completed in the small intestine. All the main organs of the digestive system have a specific role in ingesting and extracting components from food and drink as they pass through the digestive tract. There are five stages to the digestive process:

- **Ingestion** or the taking of food into the body. In the mouth, the salivary glands secrete saliva, which contains enzymes to begin the digestive process.
- **Movement of food** along the digestive tract. The hollow organs contain a layer of muscle that enables their walls to propel food and liquid along. This process is called peristalsis and it looks like an ocean wave travelling through the muscle. The first major muscle movement occurs when food or liquid is swallowed. Although you are able to start swallowing by choice, once swallowing has begun, it becomes involuntary and proceeds under the control of the nerves.
- **Digestion** or the mechanical and chemical breakdown of food into simple molecules that can be absorbed and used by all the cells in the body. Mechanical digestion

is the process of chewing and churning food. Chemical digestion occurs when enzymes aid in turning food into solutions and simple compounds that can be easily absorbed.
- **Absorption**, the chemical process of breaking down food matter and utilizing the nutrients extracted, involves the accessory glands of the digestive system – the salivary glands, pancreas, gallbladder and liver. Solutions and simple compounds in the gastrointestinal tract pass into the cardiovascular and lymphatic systems for distribution to the cells.
- **Defecation** or the elimination of substances that cannot be absorbed by the body. Any waste products from the digestive process, including undigested parts of the food, known as fibre, and older cells that have been shed from the mucosa, are pushed into the colon, where they remain until the faeces are expelled by a bowel movement.

The Organs of the Digestive Process
- **Mouth**: it is here that the teeth mechanically break down food into small particles (mastication).
- The **salivary glands** begin the chemical breakdown of starches by secreting saliva, which moistens food, making it easier to chew and swallow.
- The **tongue** assists in mastication and swallowing.
- The **pharynx** is the passageway between the mouth and oesophagus which also serves as the respiratory tract. A cartilaginous flap called the epiglottis covers the opening to the larynx and trachea, preventing food and fluids from entering the lungs. When this malfunctions, it is commonly known as 'going down the wrong way'.
- The **oesophagus** is a muscular tube approximately 25 cm (10 in) long that connects the pharynx and the stomach. Food is pushed through this tube by muscle contractions called peristalsis. Reverse peristalsis or emesis is vomiting.

- The **stomach** is located at the end of the oesophagus, in the upper left quadrant of the abdominal cavity, under the diaphragm. The abdominal cavity is lined with a membrane called the peritoneum. The stomach stores swallowed material and secretes hydrochloric acid and enzymes to aid in chemical digestion. It churns food with gastric juices into a mixture called chyme. Very little absorption occurs in the stomach.
- The **small intestine**, about 6.4 m (21 ft) long, is where most absorption of food occurs. It is connected to the stomach by the pyloric sphincter, a one-way passage that prevents the back-flow of partially digested food. The small intestine is lined with fibre-like projections called villi, which aid absorption. After eating, it takes from 20 minutes to two hours for the first portion of food to pass through the small intestine.
- Larger in diameter than the small intestine, but much shorter (only 1.5 m/5 ft long), the **large intestine** is divided into four major regions: the caecum, colon, rectum and anal canal. It receives watery residue from the small intestine and stores flatus (gas) and faeces.
- The **colon** is divided into four portions: ascending, transverse, descending and sigmoid. The rectum curves into the short anal canal. The anus is the external opening of the rectum. It is kept closed through the action of a strong, muscular ring called the anal sphincter, which opens for defecation.

Accessory Organs of Digestion

The **liver**, the largest gland in the body, is located in the right upper quadrant of the abdominal cavity. It secretes bile, which breaks down fats and allows them to be absorbed. The liver has many functions outside digestion. It removes excess sugar from the blood and stores it for future use; it also removes and neutralizes toxins from the blood. Additionally, some vitamins are stored in the liver.

The **gallbladder** is a pear-shaped sac behind the liver. It receives bile from the liver – hence its dark-green appearance – and stores it until the small intestine is stimulated by fat. The gallbladder then releases bile in order to emulsify fats.

A large gland lying behind the stomach, the **pancreas** secretes pancreatic juices, which contain many enzymes important for the digestion of proteins and other food molecules. The pancreas also contains endocrine cells called the islets of Langerhans which secrete the hormone insulin, needed for the utilization of sugar.

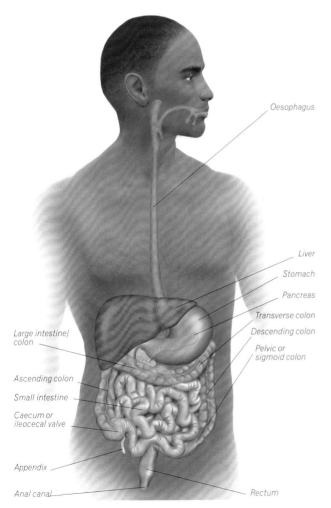

Oesophagus

Liver

Stomach

Pancreas

Transverse colon

Descending colon

Pelvic or sigmoid colon

Large intestine/ colon

Ascending colon

Small intestine

Caecum or ileocecal valve

Appendix

Anal canal

Rectum

The food we ingest is broken down in the alimentary tract to a form that can be assimilated by the body.

Yoga and the Digestive System

A regular yoga practice can help maintain a healthy digestive system and aid in alleviating many common digestive ailments, from indigestion to constipation. *Asana* practice improves blood circulation in the digestive tract, thereby improving the digestive capacity of the stomach. Forward-bending postures such as *Paschimottanasana* and the purifying practice *Nauli*, one of the *Shatkarmas*, have a massaging effect on the abdominal organs and will speed up a sluggish digestion and help to eliminate gases. Strengthening and toning the muscles surrounding these organs also helps improve the digestion process.

The Nervous System

This is the body's information highway. Monitoring and controlling almost every organ system, it is made up of billions of nerve cells that transmit, process and store information throughout the body.

Specialized cells called sensory receptors are sensitive to temperature, pain and touch. Often located in the sense organs, they detect changes in the environment or stimuli and turn them into electrical impulses, sending a signal along the nerve cells or neurons to the brain. The brain then coordinates the response. When there's nerve damage, pain is the last sensation to be lost.

The **central nervous system** (CNS), containing the brain and spinal cord, processes and stores information. The **peripheral nervous system** (PNS) transmits sensory information to the CNS, which in turn processes it and delivers instructions back to the PNS in the form of motor responses to the muscles, glands and organs. The PNS is made up of 12 pairs of cranial nerves linking the brain with sensory receptors and muscles, and 31 pairs of spinal nerves linking the spinal cord with various structures.

There are two types of nerve fibres: dendrites, which receive neural messages, and axons, which transmit neural messages from cell bodies to other neurons, muscles or glands. A nerve is a bundle of axons wrapped in connective tissue and each nerve cell has only one axon.

The Peripheral Nervous System

The PNS includes the autonomic (involuntary) nervous system (ANS) and the somatic nervous system (SoNS). The SoNS is associated with the voluntary or conscious control of body movements via the musculoskeletal system. It consists of nerves that stimulate muscle contraction.

The ANS is responsible for unconscious sensations and responses, changes in blood pressure, heart rate, respiration and digestive functions. It is in the ANS that the hypothalamus (see page 39) plays its part as a control centre that responds to emotions and sensory information such as smell, taste and temperature.

The ANS has two specialized branches: the parasympathetic nervous system (PSNS) and the sympathetic nervous system (SNS). One or other of these two branches is dominant in the body at all times.

The PSNS is usually dominant during day-to-day functioning. Its parasympathetic nerves cause the body and mind to relax and conserve energy. By contrast, the sympathetic nerves of the SNS usually act as an accelerator, an example being the 'fight or flight syndrome'. The SNS is often activated by physical or emotional stress such as an accident, embarrassment, excitement or exercise. The effects of the SNS, once triggered, can be long-lasting.

The Brain

One of the body's largest organs, the brain contains billions of neurons or nerve cells, the basic building blocks of the nervous system. Neurons transmit information throughout the body in both chemical and electrical forms. They use glucose as their energy source, and as glucose cannot be stored, a continuous supply of oxygen is needed to break it down, which is why oxygen deprivation kills brain cells in minutes. Sensory neurons carry information from the sensory receptor cells throughout the body to the brain, while motor neurons transmit information from the brain to the muscles.

The **cerebrum** is the largest and most highly developed part of the brain. It is divided into right and left hemispheres and each hemisphere is divided into four lobes. The frontal lobe is responsible for higher intellectual processes such as judging and decision-making, personality, voluntary skeletal muscle movement and speech. The parietal lobe is

The Function of the Nervous System

The nervous system transmits nerve impulses to:

- Detect internal and external changes.
- Stimulate activities such as muscular contraction and glandular secretion.
- Coordinate body activities.
- Stimulate brain activity such as interpretation, reasoning and memory.

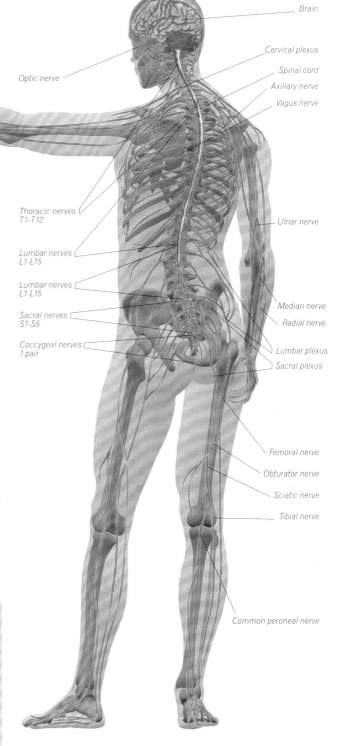

responsible for sensations such as pain, heat and cold, speech comprehension and taste. The temporal lobe is responsible for hearing, smell and taste. The occipital lobe is responsible for vision.

The **cerebellum** is the second largest portion of the brain. It governs balance and fine-tunes motor impulses sent to the skeletal muscles. The **medulla oblongata** governs the heart rate, breathing and blood pressure. The **thalamus** relays nerve impulses throughout the brain. The **hypothalamus** regulates the Autonomic Nervous System, pituitary gland, body temperature and appetite. The **meninges** are three protective layers of tissue that cover the brain and spinal cord.

Cerebrospinal fluid is made up of water, mineral salts, glucose and proteins; it cushions the CNS and acts as a shock absorber, protecting the brain from injury. It circulates through the **ventricles** (cavities) and spaces of the brain and spinal cord, carrying nutrients and removing waste from the nerves.

The **spinal cord** is a freeway enabling nerve impulses to travel to and from the brain. It runs in the vertebral canal of the spine, extending from the brain to the lumbar region. Its function is to control reflexes and transmit information back and forth from the PNS to the brain through ascending and descending pathways.

Labels on figure:
- Brain
- Cervical plexus
- Spinal cord
- Axillary nerve
- Vagus nerve
- Optic nerve
- Thoracic nerves T1-T12
- Lumbar nerves L1-L15
- Lumbar nerves L1-L15
- Sacral nerves S1-S5
- Coccygeal nerves 1 pair
- Ulnar nerve
- Median nerve
- Radial nerve
- Lumbar plexus
- Sacral plexus
- Femoral nerve
- Obturator nerve
- Sciatic nerve
- Tibial nerve
- Common peroneal nerve

Yoga and the Nervous System

Yoga can influence the response of the nervous system to stressful situations. *Asanas*, *pranayama* and meditation increase activity of the parasympathetic nervous system, clearing toxins. This inhibits muscular tension produced by alerts from the central nervous system and controls symptoms such as fear, aroused by the sympathetic nervous system. The raising of *kundalini* energy is thought to support the sympathetic nervous system.

The Central Nervous System includes the brain and spinal cord, and integrates all nervous activities, while the sensory and motor nerves pass infomation to and from the CNS.

Cells and Tissues

A cell is the smallest unit of life. The human body is made up of approximately 100 trillion cells, which, through their individual functions, form the basic characteristics of all living matter.

Each cell consists of three parts: the membrane, the nucleus and the cytoplasm. The size and shape of each cell depends on its specific function.

The **membrane** is a thin layer that separates the cell's external environment, which it relies on for nutrients, from its internal environment, which contains the nucleus and cytoplasm. It is permeable enough to allow nutrients to penetrate. The cell turns these nutrients into the energy that fuels its life. This metabolic activity generates waste, which must then be allowed to exit through the membrane. If this process becomes impaired, with nutrients unable to enter and waste to exit, the cell will die of starvation or toxicity. The membrane plays an important role in helping the cells to regulate body temperature, blood-sugar levels, metabolism, water and mineral levels.

The **nucleus** contains genetic material and regulates activities of the cell. It determines how the cell will function, as well as its basic structure.

The **cytoplasm** consists of everything that is outside the nucleus but still enclosed within the cell membrane. All the functions for cell expansion, growth and replication are carried out in the cytoplasm. Small organs called organelles are scattered throughout the cytoplasm and perform specific functions: they store and transport food and manufacture substances in the cell. Cells depend on them to survive, and organelles cannot live outside a cell.

There are over 200 types of cell in the human body, each with a specific function. Some cells are designed for secretion or storage, some trigger movement, some are responsible for our immune system and others transmit messages throughout the body. The size and shape of a cell will differ according to its function. In some parts of the body, such as the lining of the respiratory tract, cells have tiny hair-like processes called cilia on their surfaces. These help move materials that are outside the cell.

In addition to the nerve cells or neurons (see page 38), some of the more important types of cell are:

Epithelial cells: found throughout the body. They join to make up the tissues that cover the body surfaces and line body cavities. Epithelial cells resemble building blocks and can be flat, cuboid or column-shaped, depending on where they are situated.

Lymphocytes: small white blood cells that are responsible for immune responses and therefore play a vital role in defending the body against disease. There are two main types: B cells and T cells. The B cells make antibodies that attack bacteria and toxins, while the T cells attack body cells themselves when they have been taken over by viruses.

Muscle cells are classified as skeletal, cardiac or smooth, but the function of all three is to produce force and cause motion. Voluntary contraction of the skeletal muscles is used to move the body and can be finely controlled. Examples are movements of the eye, or gross movements like the quadriceps muscle of the thigh, used in walking. With cardiac and smooth muscles, contraction occurs involuntarily and is necessary for survival. Cardiac muscle is concerned with the contraction of the heart, while an example of smooth-muscle action is the peristalsis that pushes food through the digestive system.

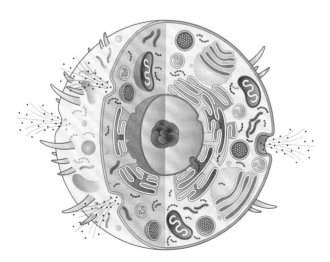

The basic unit of all living organisms, a cell is bounded by a membrane of lipids and proteins that controls the passage of substances in and out of the cell.

Body Tissues

Similar cells will group together to form tissue. There are four primary tissue types in the body:

Epithelial tissue covers all body surfaces, lines body cavities and hollow organs, and is the major tissue in glands. Examples of epithelial tissue are the outer layer of the skin and the inside of the mouth and stomach.

Connective tissue binds structures together and forms a framework for organs and the body as a whole. It stores fat, transports substances and helps repair tissue damage. Most types contain fibrous strands of the protein collagen, which gives it strength. Examples include the inner layers of the skin, tendons, ligaments, cartilage, bone and fat tissue. Blood is also considered a form of connective tissue.

Muscle tissue is composed of cells that are able to contract in order to produce movement of body parts. It has elasticity and can respond to nerve impulses. Examples are the smooth muscle of the digestive tract, the cardiac muscle of the heart and the skeletal muscles.

Nerve tissue is found in the brain, spinal cord and nerves. It is made up of neurons (see page 38) and glial cells that can receive and transmit messages through nerve impulses. Nerve tissue is responsible for coordinating and controlling many body activities.

Body Membranes

The two main categories of these thin sheets of tissue are epithelial and connective-tissue membranes. There is also the cutaneous membrane, better known as the skin.

Epithelial membranes consist of epithelial tissue and the connective tissue to which it is attached. Mucous membranes line the body cavities that open directly to the outside, including the respiratory and digestive tracts. Serous membranes line body cavities that do not open to the outside, and cover the organs within them. Serous fluid lubricates the membrane and reduces friction when organs move against each other or the cavity wall.

The main types of **connective-tissue membrane** are synovial membranes and the meninges. Synovial membranes line the cavities of movable joints such as the shoulder, elbow and knee. They secrete synovial fluid into the joint cavity, which lubricates the cartilage on the ends of the bones so that they can move freely. The connective-tissue covering on the brain and spinal cord, within the dorsal cavity, is called the meninges. This provides protection for these vital structures.

As our bodies age, our tissues become less supple. *Asana* practice, particularly prolonged stretches, keeps tissues lubricated and increases the elasticity of connective tissues.

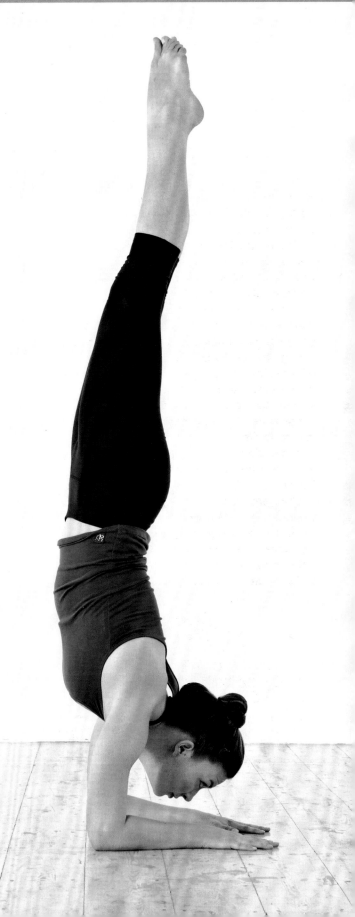

The Musculoskeletal System

Our muscles and bones work together to negotiate our relationships to gravity and space and enable us to move. If we consider how movement is generated, it seems logical to treat the skeletal and muscular systems as one combined system.

One function of the bones it to bear weight and transmit force, while the ligaments direct that force along specific pathways. This weight and force might be generated by gravity or by the muscles that propel the leg through space to take a step. The role of the muscular system is to move the bones into positions where they can function as effectively as possible. This part of the system is made up of the muscles and tendons that attach to the bones, as well as the nerve endings that organize the timing of our muscles' actions. All of these tissues are either composed of or wrapped in layers of connective tissue (see page 41).

The Human Skeleton

The skeletal system comprises the bones and the cartilage, ligaments and other connective tissues that stabilize or connect them. In addition to supporting the weight of the body, bones work with muscles to provide form, support, stability and movement. Muscles need the structure and support of the skeleton, without which our muscles would be a pile of contractile tissue with nothing to move. Without muscles to enable movement, our bones would be unable to move through space. And without connective tissue such as ligaments and tendons, bones and muscles would have no way to relate to each other.

There are approximately 206 bones in the human body, making up about 13 per cent of a person's body weight. Together, they form the skeleton, which serves as a scaffold to anchor the muscles, protect and support the body's vital organs and also function as part of the endocrine system, producing osteocalcin, the hormone which regulates blood sugar and bone density.

Bones change over time and benefit from weight-bearing activities. When ideally aligned, the skeleton creates support and structure to the body, enabling the muscles and joints to move freely. For most of us, this is not the case. Due to poor diet and bad postural habits, lack of exercise and other factors, the muscles have to work harder and do most of the work the bones should be doing, which leads to tension, fatigue and discomfort.

The **axial skeleton** consists of the 80 bones along the central axis of the human body: the skull, ribcage, sternum and vertebral column, which guards the spinal cord. The **appendicular skeleton** contains the other 126 bones: the hip and pectoral girdles and the limbs responsible for locomotion – the arms and legs.

The Functions of Bones

The bones of the body perform five main functions. They:

- **Support:** the skeletal system provides structural support for the entire body. Individual bones or groups of bones provide a framework for the attachment of soft tissues and organs.
- **Store minerals and lipids:** calcium is the most abundant mineral in the body and 99 per cent of it is found in the skeleton. The bones also store energy reserves as lipids in areas filled with yellow marrow.
- **Produce blood cells:** red and white blood cells and other blood elements are produced in the red marrow, which fills the internal cavities of many bones.
- **Protect body organs:** many soft tissues and organs are surrounded by skeletal elements. For example, the ribcage protects the heart and lungs, the skull protects the brain and the vertebrae protect the spinal cord,
- **Provide leverage and movement:** many bones function as levers that can change the magnitude and direction of the forces generated by muscles.

Yoga and the Musculoskeletal System

The physical practice of yoga stretches and strengthens the joints, which reduces pressure on the protective cartilage and helps restore correct alignment to the bones. Keeping muscles and ligaments healthy through *asana* practice improves posture and inhibits joint damage. Weight-bearing *asanas* may also help prevent osteoporosis.

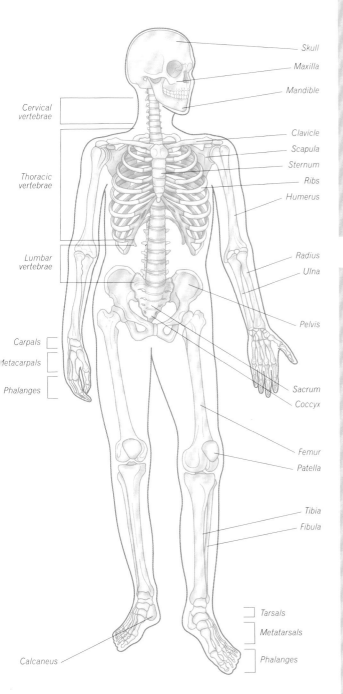

Cervical
vertebrae

Thoracic
vertebrae

Lumbar
vertebrae

Carpals

Metacarpals

Phalanges

Calcaneus

Skull

Maxilla

Mandible

Clavicle

Scapula

Sternum

Ribs

Humerus

Radius

Ulna

Pelvis

Sacrum

Coccyx

Femur

Patella

Tibia

Fibula

Tarsals

Metatarsals

Phalanges

Types of Bone

There are five general classifications of bone, based on their shape:

- **Long** – the length is greater than the width (e.g. humerus).
- **Short** – length, width and depth are similar (e.g. tarsal).
- **Flat** – broad and flat, for attachment and protective purposes (e.g. scapula).
- **Sesamoid** – small and round, developed in tendons (e.g. patella).
- **Irregular** – any bone that does not fit another classification (e.g. vertebra).

Bones of the Axial Skeleton

Skull or cranium
29 bones consisting of: 8 Cranial (frontal, nasal, orbit, maxilla, mandible, zygomatic, parietal, occipital) (F), 14 Facial (I), 6 Ear ossicles (I), 1 Hyoid (Se)

Vertebral column
26 bones consisting of: 24 Articulating Vertebrae (I), 1 Sacrum (I), 1 Coccyx (I)

Thoracic cage
25 bones consisting of: 24 Ribs (F), 1 Sternum (F)

Bones of the Appendicular Skeleton

Pectoral or shoulder girdle
4 bones consisting of: 2 Clavicles (L), 2 Scapula (F)

Upper limbs
60 bones consisting of: 2 Humerus (L), 2 Radius (L), 2 Ulna (L), 16 Carpals (S), 10 Metacarpals (L), 28 Phalanges (L)

Pelvic girdle
2 bones consisting of: 2 Coxa or hip bones (ischium, ilium, pubis fused together) (F)

Lower limbs
60 bones consisting of: 2 Femur (L), 2 Patella (Se), 2 Tibia (L), 2 Fibula (L), 14 Tarsals (S), 10 Metatarsals (L), 28 Phalanges (L)

L – Long; **S** – Short; **F** – Flat; **I** – Irregular; **Se** – Sesamoid

The axial skeleton consists of the basic structure of skull, vertebral column, ribcage and sternum, while the appendicular skeleton comprises the bones of the limbs.

The Spine

Nature's ingenuity is fully evident in the formation of the human spine, more than in any other vertebrate structure. If you were to remove all the muscles that attach to it, the spine would not collapse, because it is a self-supporting structure bound together under mechanical tension.

The human spine is distinct among mammals in that it is characterized by a primary and secondary curve, which give the natural S shape. This provides support, balance and, most important, shock absorption. The normal curvature of the lower spine is called lordosis; in the thoracic spine it is kyphosis. The primary curve comprises the kyphotic, thoracic and sacral curves; the secondary, lordotic curves are present in the cervical and lumbar regions.

The spinal column is specifically designed to neutralize the effects of stretching and compression to which it is subjected by the forces of gravity and movement. Its 24 articulating vertebrae are bound together by cartilaginous discs, capsular joints and spinal ligaments. These pads of cartilage have a soft gelatinous centre and act as buffers to absorb shock and allow movement. In repose, each disc has a rounded shape and, in a normal standing position, the centre of the disc is compressed due to the body's weight.

Viewed from the side, the spine can be divided into two columns (diagram): on one side, the anterior column of vertebral bodies and discs, which deals with weight-bearing and compressive forces, and on the other, the posterior column of arches and processes, which deals with tensile forces resulting from movement. In the anterior column, the vertebral bodies transmit compressive force to the discs, which resist compression by pushing back. In the posterior column, the arches transmit tension to all the attached ligaments, which resist stretching by pulling back. All this protects the central nervous system by neutralizing the forces of tension and compression: every movement that produces disc compression in the anterior column necessarily results in a tensile response to the corresponding ligaments in the posterior column.

From the top of the cervical spine to the base of the lumbar spine, the shape of each vertebra differs according to the functional demands of that area, but each also has common elements.

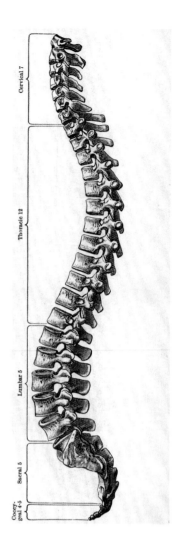

Structure of the Spine

The 33 vertebrae of the spine can be subdivided into:
Seven cervical: found at the top of the spine and involved in motion. The seventh cervical vertebra is the most prominent.
Twelve thoracic: in the mid-spine, where each vertebra is connected to a rib.
Five lumbar: at the base of the spine, in the lower back, and also involved in motion.
Five fused sacral: the number of fused/vestigial vertebrae in the sacrum varies from person to person.
Four fused coccyx or tailbone: the number of vertebrae in the tailbone below the sacrum varies.

Types of Spinal Movement

The human body has evolved to allow a remarkable range of movements of the limbs and spine, but most of us never fully explore this, partly due to a lack of awareness of the body's potential and partly because we allow the ligaments of the joints, spine and muscles to tighten through lack of use. There are four types of spinal movement: flexion (forward bending), extension (backward bending), axial rotation (twisting) and lateral rotation (side bending). The limit of movement is determined by three factors – the knobbed construction of the vertebrae, the length of the spinal ligaments and the condition of the antagonistic muscles. The flexibility of the spine varies between individuals and with use. The most basic movement of the spine is the one that emphasizes its primary curve – flexion.

Back problems are a common side-effect of today's sedentary lifestyles. Long-term benefits of *asana* practice include improved posture and reduced back pain.

The Muscular System

Muscles move the bones and internal organs. Any function of the body that involves movement, from standing to breathing to pumping blood, requires muscle power.

The muscular system consists of two categories of muscle. Involuntary muscles such as the heart (see page 32) work without conscious effort and cannot be controlled at will – they move automatically in response to messages from the brain. Voluntary muscles are controlled at will and can be made to contract whenever we want to move. They are arranged in layers, symmetrically on each side of the body, and tend to work in groups.

Muscles can only contract. For example, they can pull, but cannot push. Muscles engage in two ways: isotonically and isometrically. Isotonic engagement produces movement. Isometric engagement produces no movement. This is an important distinction to make with regard to *asana* practice. To move into a posture, we use isotonic muscle contraction and to hold the posture we use isometric muscle contraction. The science behind the practice of *asana* becomes evident as it lengthens and strengthens every muscle group in the body, creating ease and symmetry.

Muscles are infused with blood and, when irritated or injured, become hypertonic (a state of contracture or shortening), draining our energy and pulling our bodies out of alignment. When the injury is close to a tendon attachment, it takes longer to heal than if it were located in the belly of the muscle, but in general muscles heal fast and perform much better when they are warm, which makes them more elastic, contractile, pliable and flexible.

in pairs and lie on opposite sides of a joint, the two halves of each pair will work in an opposing manner, so that as one muscle contracts to produce movement, another relaxes and stretches to allow it – for example, when you bend your knee, the flexor muscle contracts in order to pull (this is the prime mover or agonist) and the extensor muscle (the antagonist) relaxes and extends in order to allow the bend. When you straighten it, the reverse happens. Muscles that help the agonist are called synergists and those that help the antagonist to stabilize the joint are called fixators. Similarly, we have elevator and depressor muscles to raise and lower parts of the body, and adductor and abductor muscles to move the part towards or away from the centre line. There are also rotator muscles to help pivot a joint and tensors that make the joint rigid.

Muscles are made up of elongated cells called fibres that have a rich supply of blood vessels, lymph vessels and nerves and are covered by the connective tissue, fascia. There are two different types of muscle fibre: slow fibres, which contract slowly, but keep going for a long time, and fast fibres, which contract quickly, but get tired rapidly. When a signal is received from the brain, the muscle cells become shorter and fatter as filaments within the cell slide against each other until they completely overlap. This causes the muscle as a whole to contract.

How Muscles Work

Muscle is attached by tendons to a bone at each end. The origin is at the fixed end of the muscle, the insertion is the moving end of the muscle. The action is the change that occurs to a joint when the muscle contracts. This action or movement and its direction can be identified by the origin and insertion of the muscle.

Skeletal muscles are ranged symmetrically left to right and front to back. Each muscle has an insertion at the pulling point and an origin at an anchoring point. Muscles function in a variety of ways depending on the role played in a specific action. As they often work

Yoga and the Muscular System

Muscles in the body are arranged symmetrically, left to right and front to back and usually work in pairs. Bending the knee requires both a flexor muscle to contract and pull it and an extensor muscle to allow it to bend. Stretching the muscles through *asana* practice systematically works each opposing set of muscles, and stretches tendons and connective tissues to their full capacity. This prevents muscles from shortening over time, maintaining elasticity.

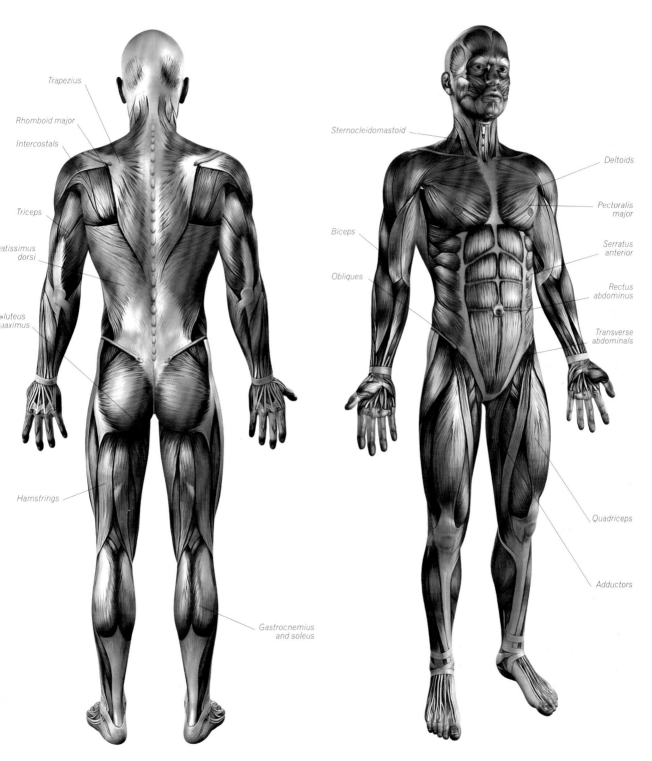

Trapezius

Rhomboid major

Intercostals

Triceps

atissimus dorsi

luteus aximus

Hamstrings

Gastrocnemius and soleus

Sternocleidomastoid

Deltoids

Pectoralis major

Biceps

Serratus anterior

Obliques

Rectus abdominus

Transverse abdominals

Quadriceps

Adductors

Movement occurs due to the combined efforts of muscle groups that surround the joints.
When one muscle group contracts to produce movement, the other relaxes and lengthens.

The Joints

Joints exist wherever two bones attach to each other. Whereas bones provide a solid framework to which muscles attach, joints enable movement and are classified depending on their range of motion.

- **Fibrous joints** are immobile and held together by cartilage or fibrous tissue: examples are the skull sutures and the joint between the radius and ulna in the arm.

- **Cartilaginous joints** are slightly movable. They fall into two categories: primary joints, where the two bones are held together by cartilage (for example, the tibia and fibula joint just below the knee); and secondary joints, where the bone ends are covered by cartilage and there is a disc of fibrocartilage between the ends.

- **Synovial joints** are freely movable. They differ from other types in that the space between the bones, known as the joint cavity, is filled with a lubricant called synovial fluid. This allows the bones to move smoothly past each other, rather like oil in an engine. A layer of hyaline cartilage covers each bone at the joint, acting as a shock absorber. This whole construction is held together by a fibrous capsule of connective tissue lined with a synovial membrane. Most of the body's joints are synovial, such as the knees, hips, shoulders and wrists.

Problems with Joints

Joint flexibility refers to the range of motion of a joint. Yoga *asana* deals primarily with the cartilaginous and synovial joints (spine, shoulders, elbows, wrists, fingers, hips, knees, ankles and toes). Overstretching the ligaments and joint capsules can lead to instability of the joint complex. With age or an excessively acidic diet, insoluble mineral salts in cartilage can lead to stiffness or brittleness.

Problems with joints occur when they are used in a way they were not designed for. For example, the wrist joint is not load-bearing and too much weight on a flexed wrist can lead to injury. There is a relationship between the stability of a joint and its articulation – the more secure and solid the joint, the less mobile it is. The shoulder joint has the most flexibility. To enable this it sits in a shallow socket, which makes it more vulnerable to injury than the hip joint, which sits in a deeper socket and has a more limited type and range of movement.

Connective Tissues

The connective tissue that helps form joints takes various forms:

- **Cartilage** is a Teflon-like coating that mostly covers the bones where they articulate or join with each other and thus reduces friction. Unlike other connective tissues, it does not contain blood vessels. Because of this, if damaged it heals very slowly.

- **Ligaments** are bands of tough fibrous tissue that connect the ends of bones. Most ligaments limit dislocation, or prevent certain movements that may cause breaks. Their elasticity means they can increasingly lengthen when under pressure. Ligaments may also restrict some actions, such as hyperextension and hyperflexion.

- **Tendons** are similar to ligaments in their composition, the difference being that they connect muscle to bone, rather than bone to bone. As muscle contracts, the tendon transmits force to the bone, which pulls on it, causing movement. Tendons can stretch substantially, allowing them to function like a spring during locomotion.

- **Fascia** is similar to ligamental tissue and is stronger than steel, pound for pound. It covers every tissue in the body, often forming web-like strands. It separates muscles into groups and binds or connects muscle to another structure. Scar tissue is clumped fascia.

Yoga and the Joints

A balanced *asana* practice ensures that all joints are regularly moved through their full range of motion, increasing flexibilty. Maintaining healthy muscles and ligaments and correct posture can prevent damage to the joints.

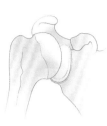

Ball and socket
A round ball fits into a concave, cup-shaped socket, allowing it to move around many axes

Examples
Hip and shoulder joints

Type of movement
Flexion, extension, abduction, adduction, rotation, circumduction

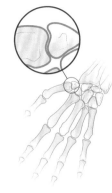

Saddle
Both joint surfaces are concave and convex and fit onto each other, allowing movement around two axes

Example
Carpometacarpal joint of the thumb

Type of movement
Flexion, extension, abduction, adduction, rotation, circumduction

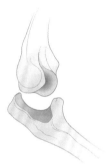

Hinge
The convex surface of one bone fits into the concave surface of another, allowing movement in one axis in a hinge action

Examples
Elbow and ankle

Type of movement
Flexion and extension

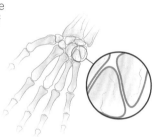

Gliding
The articular surfaces glide over each other, allowing movement around many axes

Examples
Carpal and tarsal joints

Type of movement
Flat gliding

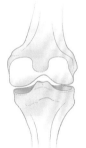

Ellipsoid or condyloid
Two convex surfaces fit into two concave surfaces, allowing movements around two axes

Example
Wrist

Type of movement
Flexion, extension, abduction, adduction

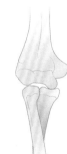

Pivot
A small projection of one bone pivots in a ring-shaped socket of another bone, allowing movement in one axis

Example
Joint between the first (atlas) and second vertebrae (axis)

Type of movement
Pivoting

The Types of Synovial Joint of the Appendicular Skeleton
There are six types of synovial joint, which are named according to their shape or movement:

The shoulder girdle

Acromioclavicular	Gliding
Sternoclavicular	Ball and socket

The upper limb

Shoulder	Ball and socket
Elbow	Hinge
Radio-ulnar, proximal and distal	Pivot
Wrist	Ellipsoid or condyloid
Intercarpal	Gliding
Carpometacarpal	Gliding
Metacarpophalangeal	Ellipsoid or condyloid
Interphalangeal	Hinge

The lower limb

Hip	Ball and socket
Knee	Ellipsoid or condyloid
Tibiofibular, proximal and distal	Pivot
Ankle	Hinge
Tarsals and metatarsals	Gliding
Metatarsophalangeal	Ellipsoid or condyloid
Interphalangeal	Hinge

There are five basic movements of the body that take place in three planes, which intersect at right angles to each other. This system helps us understand the form and function of the *asanas*.

Coronal plane

This divides the body into **front** and **back.** Movements along this plane are called **abduction** and **adduction**.

Abduction is the movement of a body part away from the midline.

- **Shoulder abduction – moving the arm from the midline** – occurs as a result of the contraction of the deltoid and the supraspinatus muscles. The arm moves away from the midline. *Virabhadrasana* II (Warrior II Pose, see page 88) is an example of shoulder abduction.

- **Hip abduction – drawing the thigh away from the midline** – occurs as a result of the contraction of the gluteus medius muscle. This results in the leg moving away from the midline. *Natyasana* (Ballet Pose) is an example of hip abduction.

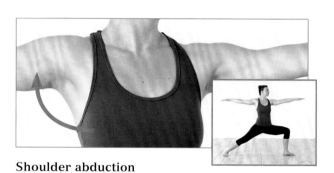

Shoulder abduction

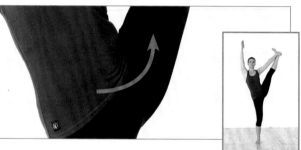

Hip abduction

Adduction is the movement of a body part towards the midline.

- **Shoulder adduction – moving the arms towards the midline** – occurs as a result of the contraction of the pectoralis major and the infraspinatus muscles. This results in the arm moving towards the midline. *Garudasana* (Eagle Pose, see page 98) is an example of shoulder adduction.

- **Hip adduction – drawing the thigh towards the midline** – occurs as a result of the contraction of the adductor brevis, adductor longus and adductor magnus muscles. This results in the leg moving towards the midline. *Garudasana* (Eagle Pose, see page 98) is an example of hip adduction.

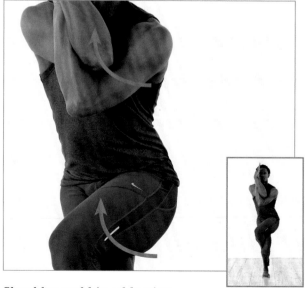

Shoulder and hip adduction

Transverse or horizontal plane

This divides the body into **upper** and **lower** halves. **Rotation** is a turning and twisting movement. It is further classified as medial rotation (towards the midline) or lateral rotation (away from the midline), also referred to as internal and external rotation.

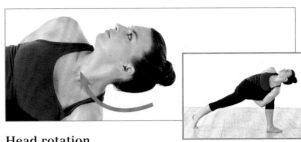

Head rotation

- **Head rotation** occurs as a result of contraction of the sternocleidomastoid muscle. *Parivrita Parsvakonasana* (Extended Side Angle Twist, see page 92) is an example of head rotation.

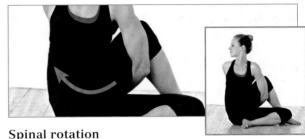

Spinal rotation

- **Spinal rotation** occurs as a result of the contraction of the erector spinae and oblique muscles. *Ardha Matsyendrahsana* (Half Spinal Twist, see page 122) is an example of spinal rotation.

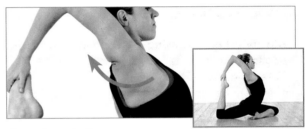

Scapula rotation

- **Scapula rotation** occurs as a result of contraction of the rhomboid muscles. *Eka Pada Raja Kapotasana* (King Pigeon Pose I, see page 198) is an example of scapula rotation

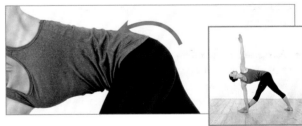

Leg rotation

- **Leg rotation** occurs as a result of contraction of the sartorius and hamstring muscles. *Parivritta Trikonasana* (Revolving Triangle Pose, see page 91) is an example of leg rotation.

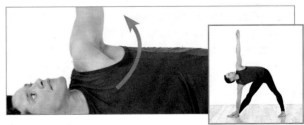

Arm rotation

- **Arm rotation** occurs as a result of contraction of the rotator cuff muscles. *Uttitha Trikonasana* (Extended Triangle Pose, see page 90) is an example of arm rotation.

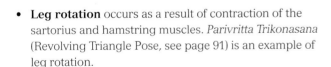
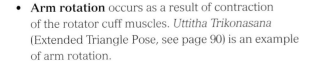

Saggital plane

This divides the body into **right** and **left**. Movements along this plane are called **flexion** and **extension**.

A **bending** movement, **flexion** usually moves the extremity **forward**, except at the knee, where it moves it backwards.

- **Elbow flexion** occurs when the biceps brachii muscles contract. This results in the bending of the arm at the elbow joint. *Gomukhasana* (Cow Face Pose, see page 139) is an example of elbow flexion.

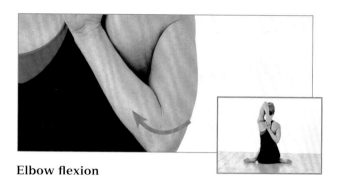

Elbow flexion

- **Knee flexion** occurs when the hamstrings contract. This results in the bending of the leg at the knee joint. *Eka Pada Rajakapotasana* (King Pigeon Pose I, see page 198) is an example of knee flexion.

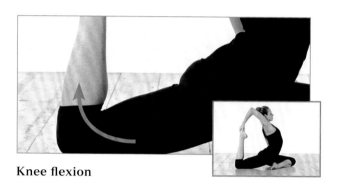

Knee flexion

- **Spinal flexion** occurs when the rectus abdominus, oblique and psoas major muscles contract. This results in the bending of the spine. *Balasana* (Child's Pose, see page 115) is an example of spinal flexion.

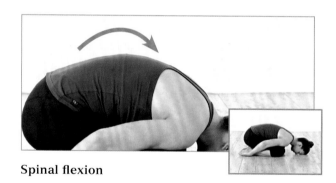

Spinal flexion

- **Hip flexion** occurs when the iliopsoas, rectus femorius, sartorius, tensor fasciae latae and pectineus muscles contract. This results in bending at the hip joint. *Uttanasa* (Forward Bend, see page 94) is an example of hip flexion.

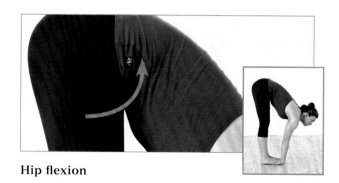

Hip flexion

Extension is a **straightening** movement, which moves the extremity **backwards**.

- **Elbow extension** occurs when the triceps brachii muscle contracts. This results in the straightening of the arm at the elbow joint. *Utthita Parsvakonasana* (Extended Side Angle Pose) is an example of elbow extension.

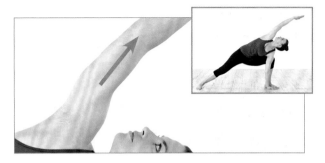

Elbow extension

- **Knee extension** occurs when the quadriceps contract. This results in the straightening of the leg at the knee joint. *Paripurana Navasana* (Boat Pose, see page 140) is an example of knee extension.

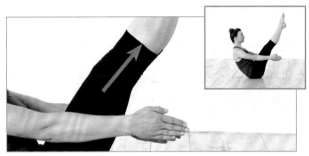

Knee extension

- **Spinal extension** occurs when the erector spinae muscles contract. This action brings the torso away from the front of the legs. *Bhujangasana* (Cobra Pose, see page 208) is an example of spinal extension.

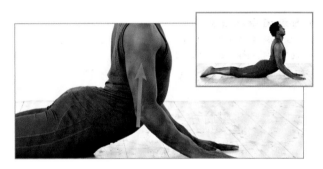

Spinal extension

- **Hip extension** occurs when the gluteus maximus and hamstrings contract. This results in straightening at the hip joint. *Salabhasana* (Locust Pose, see page 206) is an example of hip extension.

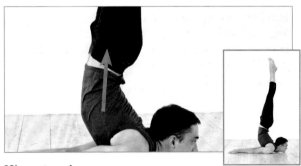

Hip extension

Movement and Actions of Specific Limbs

Some joint actions have terms that are used for specific parts of the body.

Hand

Rotation – Rotation around the long axis of the hand is called **eversion (1)** when it lifts the outer edge of the hand, and **inversion** when it lifts the inner edge of the hand.

Wrist

Dorsiflexion (2) – Movement when the angle between the back of the hand (dorsal surface) and the forearm decreases.

Palmar flexion (3) – Movement when the angle between the palm and the forearm decreases

Forearm

Rotation – Rotation of the radius and ulna so that they cross each other is **pronation (4)** – sometimes described as 'palm down'. Rotation of the radius and ulna so that they are uncrossed is called **supination (5)** – or 'palm up'.

Foot

Rotation – Tilting the foot inwards is called **inversion (6)** and tilting the foot outwards is called **eversion (7)**.

Ankle

Dorsiflexion (8) – Movement when the angle between the foot and the shin decreases.

Plantarflexion (9) – Movement where the sole of the foot presses down is plantarflexion, increasing the distance between the foot and the shin.

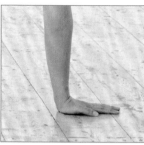

1

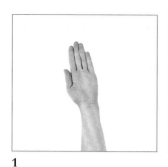

2

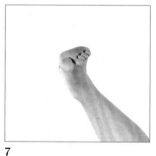

3

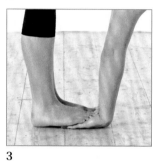

4

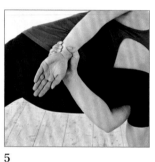

5

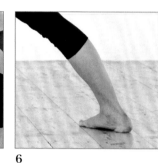

6

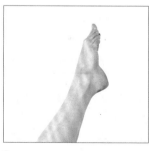

7

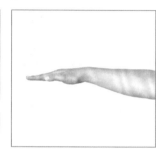

8

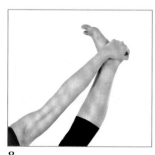

9

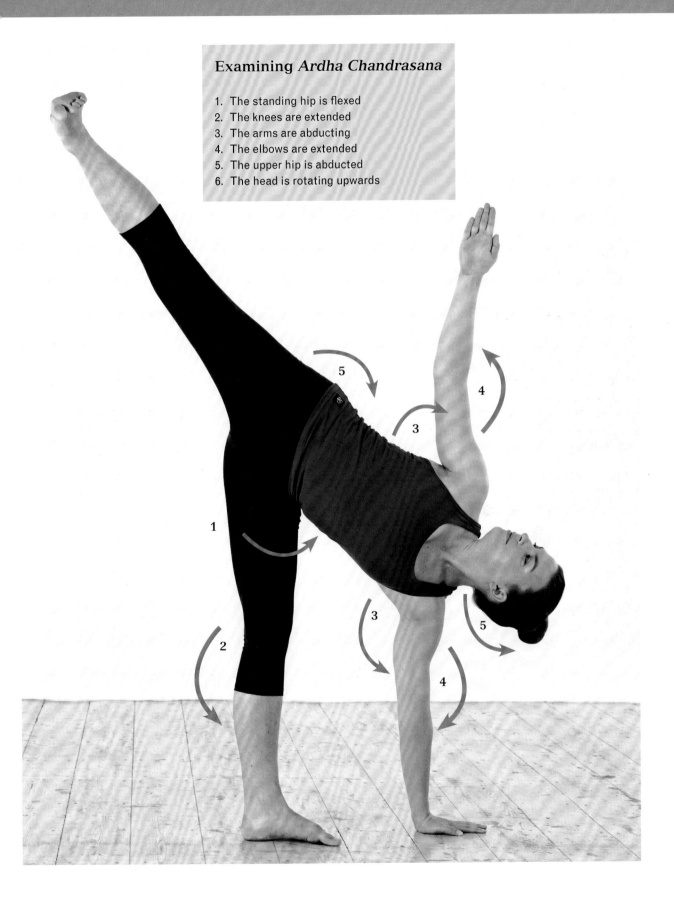

Examining *Ardha Chandrasana*

1. The standing hip is flexed
2. The knees are extended
3. The arms are abducting
4. The elbows are extended
5. The upper hip is abducted
6. The head is rotating upwards

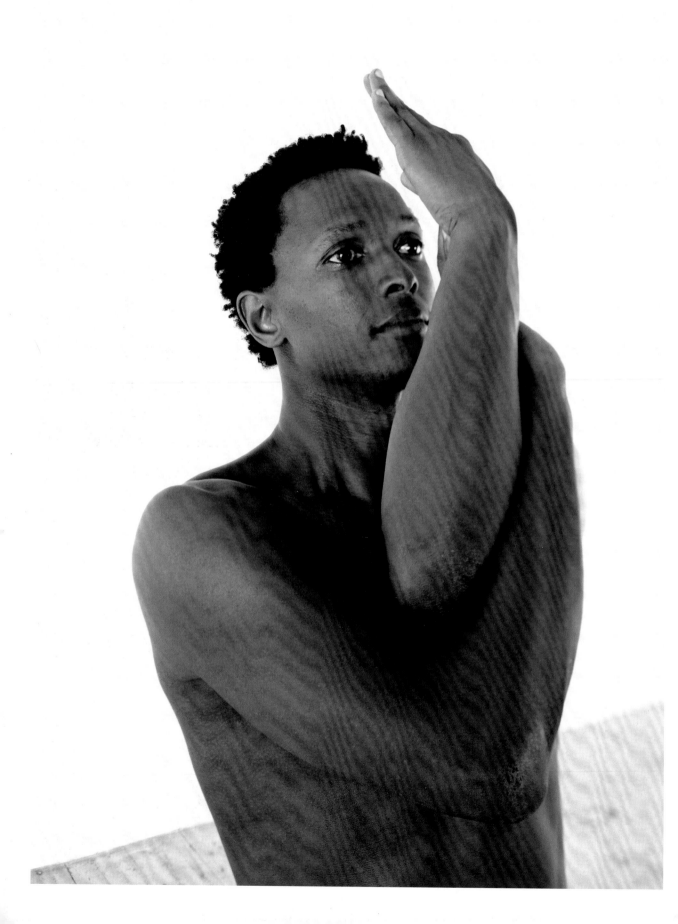

The Science of Yoga

The goal of yoga is to lead us to a true understanding of what is; the exploration of our consciousness leading us to a direct understanding of the nature of all things – this is self-realization. Yoga is a science, a quest to know the truth. Just like a scientist, a yogi applies a logical approach to his search for the truth. This chapter examines the science that underpins our yoga practice; the ethereal or subtle body; *prana*, the vital life force; the *nadis* and the *chakra* system; the five sheaths we must penetrate to arrive at the core of our being and the purification practices we can employ to lead us there.

The Astral Body   58
The Pranic Body and the Five *Pranas*   60
The *Nadis*   62
The *Chakra* System   64
The Five Sheaths or *Koshas*   66
The *Shatkarmas* and *Kriyas*   68
Karma   72
Yoga and Diet   74

The Astral Body

It is a fundamental premise of all esoteric schools of thought that the world we perceive through our ordinary senses is only a minute slice of a much larger reality and that there are many more subtle planes of existence.

Georg Feuerstein, *The Yoga Tradition*

The first texts on Hatha yoga expounded by Goraksha around the ninth century speculated on a subtle physiology, made of a finer substance or energy than the physical body, which yogis believe man possesses. This subtle counterpart is usually referred to as the astral or causal body or *sukshma sharira*. Although modern science dismisses these claims due to the lack of any empirical proof, the organs of this astral body are thought by yogis to be as real as those of its physical equivalent and even visible to clairvoyant sight.

The anatomy and physiology of this subtle body became the subject of intense investigation by the ancient yogis, who refined and expanded Goraksha's earlier anatomical model in an effort to understand how yoga can transform the physical body. They believed that, through knowledge of this subtle physiology, the yogi could transcend his material existence. Diligently they mapped out its basic structures, detailing the currents and pathways through which the vital force, *prana*, circulates; the psycho-energetic centres, which we call *chakras*; and the five elements of nature inherent in the body itself.

The astral body and the activity of its subtle organs can vary according to the physical and mental wellbeing of each individual, so the *chakras* and *nadis* or subtle channels may be more or less active and more or less defined depending upon your psycho-spiritual disposition. This could explain why descriptions of the *chakras* as given in various texts are inconsistent.

Another reason is that the descriptions serve only as idealized models, which are meant to guide the yogi's visualization and contemplation. Thus the depiction of the *chakras* as lotuses whose petals are inscribed with Sanskrit letters is clearly an idealization, not an empirical observation. But it is an idealization based on actual perception. The activated *chakras* are, as the literal meaning of the Sanskrit word suggests, wheels of energy with radiant spokes that lend themselves to representation as lotus petals.

While Western science is still struggling to find explanations for such phenomena as acupuncture meridians, *kundalini* awakenings and Kirlian photography (techniques used to capture electrical coronal discharges on film), yogis continue to explore and enjoy the pyrotechnics of the subtle body as they have done for hundreds of generations.

Kundalini Shakti

The most significant aspect of the subtle body is the psycho-spiritual force known as the *kundalini shakti*.

Metaphysically speaking, *kundalini* is a microcosmic manifestation of the primordial energy or *shakti*. It is the universal power as it is connected with the finite body and mind. This is sometimes misinterpreted as meaning mere force, but most authorities refer to it as divine intelligence.

Kundalini means 'she who is coiled' and the term refers to the fact that the energy is envisioned as a sleeping serpent, coiled three and a half times around a phallus (*linga*) in the lowest bio-energetic centre of the human body. That serpent blocks the central pathway with its mouth at the place of the first knot. This symbolism suggests that *kundalini* is in a state of dormancy. Through controlled breathing in which the life-energy *prana* is withdrawn from the left and right *nadis* and forced into the central pathway, the dormant *kundalini* is awakened and the *shakti* ascends to the crown centre where the blissful union between *shakti* and *shiva* occurs.

Depicted as a sleeping serpent coiled up at the base of the spine, *kundalini* is the latent female energy that can be awakened and released through *pranayama* pracice.

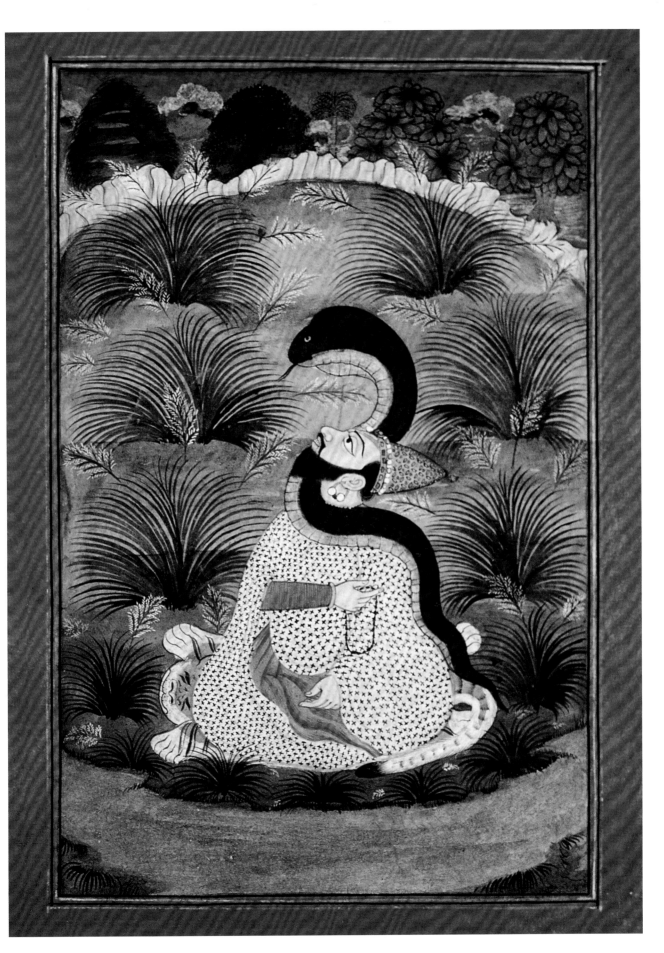

The Pranic Body and the Five *Pranas*

Prana is central to all yoga practice. More than just the air we breathe, it is the energy that keeps us alive and through which everything is able to exist and move and permeates the universe on all levels – physical, mental, intellectual, sexual, spiritual and cosmic.

Hatha yoga uses *prana* – the vital life force – as the vehicle through which we can expand our consciousness and achieve self-realization. Within the individual subtle body, *prana* separates out into five primary and five secondary energy flows, each of which has its own specific function.

The five primary flows are known as *prana, apana, samana, udana* and *vyana*. The two most important are *prana* and *apana*, which underlie the breathing process. Their incessant activity is seen as the principal cause for the restlessness of the mind, and their suspension is the main purpose of breath control. This individualized *prana* is different from the life force described above.

Prana

In this context, *prana* is the ascending life energy seated in the thoracic region between the larynx and the top of the diaphragm. It is associated with *ida nadi* and is also referred to as the *in breath*. It draws the life force into the body and governs inhalation and the organs of respiration as well as their corresponding muscles and nerves; it also stimulates cardiovascular health.

Apana

Apana is the descending life energy seated in the lower half of the body below the navel region. It is associated with *pingala nadi* and is also referred to as the *out breath*. It provides energy for the intestines, kidneys, anus and genitals and governs exhalation, elimination and the reproductive organs.

Samana

Samana is the middle-life energy located between the heart and the navel. It controls the digestive system, stimulates the heart and circulation and is responsible for assimilation and distribution of nutrients. According to the *Hatha Yoga Pradipika*, this is the most important *prana*, as it is related to the central or *sushumna nadi* and is also referred to as the *middle breath:* the time between inhalation and exhalation. In the *samana* region, assimilation through the suspension of *prana* and *apana* takes place to awaken *kundalini* power (see page 58).

Udana

Udana is the upward-rising energy seated in the throat region and controls everything above the neck. Movement in the throat, such as speech and swallowing, and the sensory receptors – eyes, nose and ears and facial expression – are stimulated by *udana*, making thought and awareness of the external world impossible without this energy.

Vyana

Vyana pervades the entire body, regulating and controlling all movement. It governs the circulatory system and the distribution of *prana* throughout the body.

As well as the five main *pranas*, there are the five minor ones, also known as *upa-pranas* or *sub-pranas*: these are *naga, kurma, krikara, deva-datta* and *dhanam-jaya*. The precise functions of these subsidiary energies are unclear, but they are said to control various responses in the body.
- **Naga** means serpent and controls belching, vomiting and hiccups.
- **Kurma** means tortoise and controls the opening and closing of the eyes and blinking.
- **Krikara** governs hunger and thirst, sneezing and coughing.
- **Deva-datta** governs yawning and sleepiness.
- **Dhanam-jaya** governs the decomposition of the body.

Pranic Energy

There are many ways of redirecting the vital life force from the lower to the higher centres and Hatha yoga uses practical methods to achieve this – through the physical body. *Prana* underpins all life and can be harnessed through the breath. Its impulse is to move upwards (making it afferent by nature), but it also manifests as negative energy through *apana*, whose efferent nature is to move downwards. That energy which enters the body is called *prana* and that which leaves is called *apana*.

Through the breath, *prana* and consciousness are essentially linked and can be separated by a scientific means which starts with the yogic technique of retaining the breath. *Prana* is the energy that keeps us alive and is regarded as the tangible manifestation of the higher self.

Pranic energy is affected by our lifestyles. Activites such as sleep, work, exercise, diet and sexual activity all influence the flow of *prana* in the body. Emotions and thoughts also have an impact on the pranic body. Lifestyle habits such as poor diet and stress deplete and block the pranic flow and can leave us feeling drained of energy. This eventually leads to disease and dysfunction in the particular areas of the body where the pranic flow is most obstructed. Techniques that help us redirect our *prana* such as *pranayama* (breathing exercises) help to reverse this process by energizing and balancing the *pranas*.

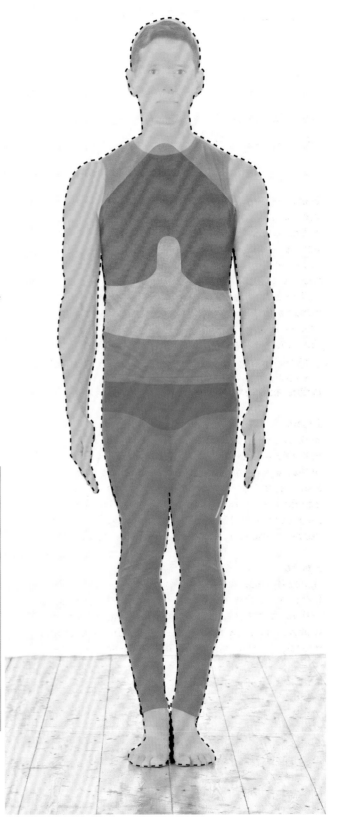

The pranic body

The five primary energies that flow in and around the subtle body have different functions. The two main *pranas*, **prana** and **apana**, are associated with the breathing and elimination processes.

udana – upward-rising energy, seated in the throat

prana – ascending life energy, seated in the thoracic region

samana– middle-life energy, seated between heart and navel

apana – descending energy, located below the navel

vyana – pervades the whole body, controlling the circulation of *prana*

The illustration shows the five primary *pranas* throughout the body, with *vyana* pervading the whole body. *Prana*, *samana* and *apana* are concentrated in the torso, while *udana* is in the throat.

The *Nadis*

The *nadis* are a series of pathways or psychic channels that carry the life force, *prana*, throughout the subtle body. Invisible to the naked eye, some are a thousand times thinner than a hair.

The word *nadi* means duct or conduit, but *nadis* should not be mistaken for veins or arteries, or for the nerves that correspond with the physical body, even though some traditional yoga texts might describe them as such. *Nadis* are more like electric currents or flow patterns within the energy field comprising the subtle body.

The idea of the existence of *nadis* in the subtle body first appears in the earliest *Upanishads* – the heart was said to be the centre of 72,000 *nadis*. The concept was developed in the later *Upanishads* and the nascent Yoga and Tantric schools.The classical drawings of the networks of the *nadis* fail to convey the living, vibrant radiance of the supra-physical vehicle that, to the trained eye, looks like a shimmering, shifting mass of light with foci of different colours and sometimes dark areas suggesting physical weaknesses, perhaps even disease.

The Principal *Nadis*

Although the *nadis* are vast in number, three principal *nadis* are universally recognized in the yogic literature. All originate at the *kanda kanda*, an egg-shaped bulb which, according to some claims, lies between the anus and the penis or clitoris; others locate it in the region of the navel.

Sushumna *Nadi*

Sushumna, the central pathway, runs along the spine. Referred to as the royal pathway to God, it is also called *brahma nadi* because it is through *sushumna* that *kundalini shakti* ascends and leads to liberation. On a physical level it corresponds with the central nervous system.

Ida *Nadi*

Ida lies to the left of *sushumna*. It corresponds with the left nostril and the right-brain hemisphere, and is called *ida* because it is pale in colour. It is symbolized by the moon and is known as the channel of comfort, possessing cool and negative attributes. Physiologically it is associated with the parasympathetic nervous system and relaxes and restores the body's equilibrium. On a pranic level it governs functions on the left side of the body.

Pingala Nadi

Pingala lies to the right of *sushumna*. It corresponds with the right nostril and the left-brain hemisphere and gets its name because it is reddish in colour. It is symbolized by the sun, heat and positive attributes; physiologically it is associated with the sympathetic nervous system. It is said to energize the body and invigorate the whole system, regulating respiratory and cardiovascular function.

The seven lesser *nadis* are: *ghandari* (which ends at the left eye), *hastijihva* (ends at the right eye), *pusha* (ends at the right ear), *yashasvini* (ends at the left ear), *alambusha* (ends in the mouth), *kuhu* (situated above the sexual organ) and *shamkini* (in the *muladhara* or anus region).

Both *ida* and *pingala* wind around *sushumna* to form a helix. They converge at each of the first six *chakras* (see page 64), and terminate at the penultimate, *ajna chakra*, behind and between the eyebrows. Only *sushumna nadi* extends all the way from the base *chakra* to *sahasrara chakra*, the seventh or crown *chakra*.

Harnessing the Flow of the Life Force

One of the key intersections for *ida* and *pingala nadi* is at the base of the spine, where a gate blocks the entrance to *sushumna*, preventing *kundalini shakti* (see page 58) from ascending. The yogi's principal objective is to harness the flow of energy in this central pathway.

As long as the life force oscillates up and down *ida* and *pingala nadis*, the yogi's attention will remain externalized and his or her consciousness will be dominated by the lunar and solar forces or negative and positive aspects. Engaging *bandhas* (locks) during retention of the breath in *pranayama* forces *prana* and *apana* to fuse at the navel region and beat against the gate. Performing this action regularly with great

Sushumna is the central *nadi*, which runs along the spinal axis, towards the crown of the head. It is flanked on either side by the two other principal pathways, *ida nadi* and *pingala nadi*.

determination will eventually force the gate to open; the dormant *kundalini* energy will be awakened and forced up *sushumna nadi*. As the energy rises up, the major *chakras* along the spine open up, like the blooming petals of a flower, and begin spinning. Thus *hatha,* the union of sun and moon, is the convergence of the life force that ordinarily travels along the *ida* and *pingala* pathways.

Knowledge of the function and characteristics of *ida* and *pingala nadis* is central to Hatha yoga. On a physical level, their activity governs the responses of the sympathetic and parasympathetic nervous systems. There is evidence that, through the designated breathing practices, both heart rate and metabolism can be accelerated when the *prana* is directed along *pingala nadi*, or decelerated when it is conducted along *ida nadi*. Clinical studies have shown that, as a result, some yogis are able to survive underground in a sealed container for hours, and even days.

But the rationale of breath control – *pranayama* – is different. Yogis do not seek merely to stop their breath to bring about a hibernating condition, but to transcend the human condition and awaken faculties dormant in the ordinary human being, and to break through the domain of the transcendental: a higher state of consciousness, an enhanced state in which attention is improved and refined, where thought and perception are transcended and a greater awareness of reality is experienced. To do this, they need to channel the life force along the spinal axis towards the crown of the head, which is the location of the major etheric centre.

More will be said about *kundalini* shortly, but here it is important to point out that the life force, which is responsible for the functioning of the body and mind, and *kundalini* are both an aspect of the divine power or *shakti*. If we compare the life force to electricity, *kundalini* can be likened to a high-voltage electric charge. Or if we regard the life force as a pleasant breeze, *kundalini* is comparable to a hurricane. Once its power is unleashed in the body, it produces far-reaching changes in our physical and mental being. If properly managed, this incredible power can, as the adepts of Tantra and Hatha yoga promise us, refashion the body and mind into a divine vehicle capable of incredible feats.

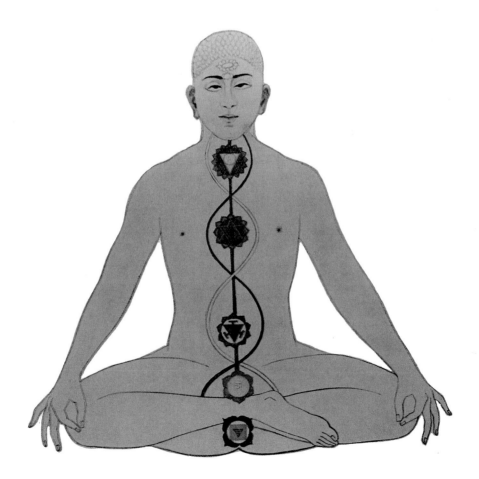

The *Chakra* System

Chakras are centres of energy in the astral body that vibrate at different speeds. The seven major *chakra*s are arranged vertically along *sushumna*, the principal channel through the body.

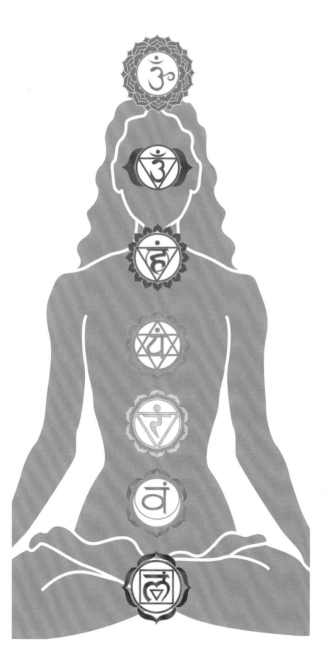

Each *chakra* is associated with specific functions and corresponds with the nerve plexuses of the physical body, and each exists at a point where at least two *nadis* intersect. Each *chakra* is traditionally depicted as a lotus flower with a certain number of petals, corresponding to the number of *nadis* emanating from it, and each petal represents a sound vibration produced when *kundalini shakti* passes through the *chakra*. Additionally, all except the crown *chakra* have their own colour and *bija* or seed mantra; the first five are also associated with one of the five elements of nature.

Each *chakra* has influence over the function and health of the glands and organs near which it is located in the physical body. As *kundalini shakti* rises, the major *chakras* are activated. Most of the time, energy is expended at the level of the first three *chakras*, as we are consumed with matters of food, survival, sex, fame and the acquisition of power. Occasionally, awareness rises to the level of the fourth or heart *chakra*, but it can always sink back down.

When awareness reaches the fifth *chakra*, at the base of the throat (*vishuddha chakra*), the aspirant becomes deadly serious about spiritual matters. Even this stage is not permanent, as energy keeps moving from one place to another according to previous and present actions, thoughts and deeds. Through the practices of meditation, *pranayama*, surrendering to the Lord (*isvara pranidhana*) and steady purification of the heart (*tapasya*), consciousness can eventually reach the sixth *chakra* (*ajna*). Only then will it remain permanently raised. At this stage the mind gains divine perception which, once acquired, is never relinquished. The final stage is the abode of the seventh and final chakra, *sahasrara*, the centre of consciousness, where integration of all polarities is experienced, and the act of transcendence is accomplished.

The Sanskrit word *chakra* means 'wheel' or 'disk'. The seven major *chakras* positioned along the spinal column, or *sushumna nadi*, correspond with the organs where each *chakra* is located.

Muladhara Chakra

root support (mula – root; adhara – support)

Situated at the perineum, the root *chakra* – also known as *adhara* – influences the excretory and reproductive organs. It is connected with the sense of smell and associated with the earth element *prithvi*, the *mantra lam* and the elephant, symbol of strength. The presiding deities are Brahma, the creator, and the goddess Dakini. *Muladhara* is usually depicted as a red, four-petalled lotus and marks the point of origin of *sushumna nadi*, from which the *kundalini shakti* emerges.

Swadisthana Chakra

own base (sva – own; adhisthana – base)

Located at the genitals, just above *muladhara*, *swadisthana chakra* is connected to the sacral plexus and the urinary and reproductive organs. It is associated with *tattvas*, the water element, the sense of taste, the hands, the *mantra vam* and an aquatic monster resembling a crocodile – a symbol of fertility. The presiding deities are Vishnu and the goddess Rakini. This centre is depicted as an orange six-petalled lotus.

Manipura Chakra

jewel city (mani – jewel, pura – city or fortress)

Situated behind the navel and also called *nabhi chakra* – navel wheel – *manipura* is connected with the solar plexus and influences the assimilation of food and *prana*. It is associated with the fire element *agni*, the visual sense, the anus, the *mantra ram* and with the ram, symbol of fiery energy. The presiding deities are Rudra and the goddess Lakini. *Manipura* is portrayed as a bright yellow lotus of ten petals. When *kundalini* energy reaches this level the consciousness is still bound by the grosser levels of existence and sensualities.

Anahata Chakra

unstruck

Connected to the heart and respiration, *anahata* is located at the heart and is also widely known as the *hrid padma* – heart lotus. It is at the heart that the transcendental sound – *nada* – can be heard. Responsible for the emotions of love, hate, compassion and cruelty, *anahata* is associated with the air element *apa*, the sense of touch, the penis, the *mantra yam* and a black antelope – symbol of swiftness. It is depicted as a green lotus of 12 petals. The presiding deities are Isha and Kakini.

Vishuddha Chakra

pure

Situated at the throat, this *chakra*, which is depicted as a smoky, turquoise, 16-petalled lotus, is connected with the laryngeal plexus and is believed to maintain purity in the body and mind. It is associated with *akasha*, the ether element, the ears, the throat, speech, the *mantra ham* and a snow-white elephant – symbol of pure strength. The presiding deities are the androgynous Ardhanarishvara (a composite of Shiva and Parvati) and the goddess Shakini. It is at this centre that the yogi tastes the secret *soma* secretion which drips from the *lalana chakra*, a minor structure located behind *vishuddha*.

Ajna Chakra

command

Located in the brain, midway between the eyes at the medulla oblongata, this is one of the most important *chakras*, also known as the third eye. It is sometimes referred to as the guru *chakra*, as it is through this *chakra* that a disciple can communicate telepathically with his teacher. *Ajna* is depicted as a violet or blue two-petalled lotus, which contains a symbolic representation of the phallus placed within a downward-pointing triangle. This centre corresponds with the cavernous plexus and is associated with the *manas* or the aspect of the mind concerned with higher intelligence, known as the gateway to liberation. *Ajna* is also connected with the sense of individuality and with the *mantra om*. The presiding deities are Parama Shiva and the goddess Hakini.

Sahasrara Chakra

thousand-petalled (sahasra – thousand; ara – petal)

The seventh and last *chakra*, *sahasrara*, has no associated element, colour or sound. Situated at the crown of the head, this is the thousand-petalled lotus. This *chakra* marks the final destination of *kundalini shakti* and represents pure consciousness, the union of the male principle, *shiva*, with the female principle, *shakti*. It corresponds with the pituitary gland. As we have seen, as *kundalini* ascends and passes through each *chakra*, different states of consciousness are experienced. When *sahasrara* is activated, it is the highest experience of human evolution, the centre of quintessential consciousness and where the state of *samadhi* is attained.

The Five Sheaths or *Koshas*

From the physical body we move inwards to the vital body, which supports our breathing and emotions; to the mental body, where thoughts and obsessions can be controlled; to the intellectual body, where we find intelligence and wisdom; and finally to the divine body, the domain of the universal soul.

Each one of us is searching for our true nature – the *atman* or small portion of God that lies deep within the heart of every being, but for most, it remains hidden. We needn't look beyond ourselves to experience the higher self; instead we need to move within, to the very core of our being, and allow our inherent nature to reveal itself.

Yoga releases the higher potential for life by showing how we can progress in our quest to experience our divine origin. Through the practice and techniques that have evolved in the classical yoga system, the yogi is able to achieve his or her primary goal – self-realization.

According to yogic physiology, the human framework comprises five sheaths or layers (*koshas*), which form the different dimensions of human existence. Through the study and understanding of this five-fold sheath, we can move closer to revealing our innermost being. The ancient yogis viewed the physical body as only one layer of an individual, a layer through which the transcendental self could emerge. Starting with the outermost layer, the physical body, and progressing through the layers of the mind and intelligence, they came ultimately to the centre of their being, the layer of the soul.

When these bodies or sheaths are misaligned, we encounter the alienation and fragmentation that so trouble our world. When we are able to bring the various sheaths into harmony, integration is achieved and unity is established. The physical body must connect with and thereby imprint on the energetic and organic body, which must in turn accord with the mental body, the mental body with the intellectual body and the intellectual body with the blissful body.

The Hatha yoga concept of the five sheaths divides the individual into five selves. The five *koshas* are said to obscure the true self, like a set of Russian dolls – as you remove the top from one, another is revealed. Starting from the periphery of the body and moving steadily inwards to the core of the self, these sheaths become successively finer, with each layer being interdependent and unable to exist without the others.

The anatomical layer, the *annamaya kosha*, comprises the physical body, which includes skin, muscle and bone and the five gross elements (*bhutas*) – earth, water, fire, air and ether. When a yogi practices *asanas*, he is working with the *annamaya kosha*. The next layer, the *pranamaya kosha* – the sheath composed of life force – exists on a slightly deeper level and represents the physiological body, including the circulatory, respiratory, excretory, digestive, nervous, glandular and reproductive systems. *Pranayama* practice touches this *kosha*.

On a deeper level still is the *manomaya kosha*, the sheath composed of the mind. It is the mental or psychological body and includes the emotions as well as the mind. Meditation reaches this layer. The *vijnanamaya kosha* – the sheath composed of awareness – represents the intellectual body. The serious study of scripture – *jnana marga* – awakens this sheath. And at the very deepest level, the *anandamaya kosha*, the bliss sheath, represents the spiritual body that encompasses the transcendental self.

When a yogi performs *asanas*, *pranayama* or any meditation, all the *koshas* reap the benefits – what he does for or to his body ultimately affects his mind or spirit. For example, meditation relieves the stress that muscles and joints feel in the *annamaya kosha*, which in turns quiets the sympathetic nervous system, *pranayama kosha*, which calms the emotions, *manomaya kosha*. This then quiets the mind, allowing the yogi to see more clearly, *vijnanamaya kosha*, which puts him in closer touch with his divine self, *anandamaya kosha*.

Annamaya Kosha

This is the first of the five *koshas* and consists of the physical body and its component parts: blood, flesh, bones, skin and hair – the parts that depend upon food and oxygen for survival. Anyone who identifies predominantly with the *annamaya kosha* believes that he or she is only the physical body, and is attached to and involved solely with the state of the physical form.

Pranamaya Kosha

This second layer or sheath consists of the vital life force *prana* and animates the *annamaya kosha*. It contains all the five *pranas*, including *prana* and *udana*, as well as the organs of action – the *karmaindriyas*: hands, feet, voice, genitals and anus. The *pranamaya kosha* is associated with feelings of hunger and thirst and the processes of elimination and procreation. It is more important and subtler than *annamaya kosha*, since without *prana* the body would cease to function.

Manomaya Kosha

The third *kosha* is defined as the mental sheath, but it represents the lower aspect of the mind, *manas*: the volitional and emotional aspect, which is governed by the five sense organs or *jnanaindriyas* – touch, taste, smell, hearing and sight. The yogi residing in this layer has thoughts and desires that identify with name and form. He experiences pain, pleasure, longing, doubt and fear – the tides of human emotion. But the lower mind lacks the cognitive ability to reason and is unable to discriminate objectively. Because it is governed by emotions and desires, this sheath is in a constant state of flux.

Vijnanamaya Kosha

This fourth sheath is the intellectual one (*vijnana* means knowing). It represents the wisdom that lies beneath the processing, thinking aspect of the mind. This aspect of the mind decides, judges and discriminates according to the information being processed. *Vijnanamaya kosha* is the realm of higher wisdom, wherein one seeks the truth by diving within towards the eternal consciousness.

Anandamaya Kosha

The innermost and finest of all the *koshas*, and the one closest to the pure consciousness of *atman*, *anandamaya kosha* is also known as the bliss sheath, which permeates and influences all the other *koshas*. The yogi who resides here experiences absolute peace, joy and love. *Anandamaya kosha* is a perfect reflection of *atman*, suffused with a spontaneous and effortless joy that is independent of any reason or stimulus that could provoke a mental reaction.

The goal of yoga, the science of self-realization, is to directly experience and realize the *atman* or soul. In doing so, the yogi merges completely with the divine. *Atman* is omnipresent, omniscient and omnipotent, beyond consciousness, form, name and time: to attempt to describe its true nature is impossible. Through constant study of the Five-fold Sheath, the yogi can make rapid progress in the quest to realizing the truth within his or her own heart.

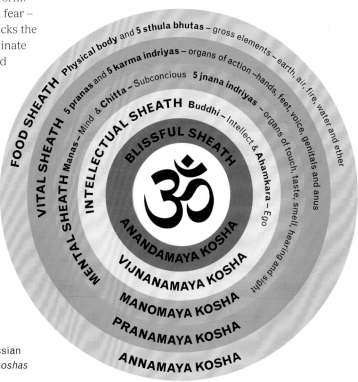

The five sheaths or *koshas* are nested like a set of Russian dolls, with each layer containing the next. Aligning the *koshas* helps facilitate the mind–body connection.

The *Shatkarmas* and *Kriyas*

In Hatha yoga, internal purification occurs when the psychic channels are cleared of any blockages. The ancient yogis devised six ways to purify the physical and subtle bodies before embarking on the higher stages of practice.

Described in the *Hatha Yoga Pradipika* and the *Gheranda Samhita*, the cleansing methods are referred to as either the *shatkriyas* (six cleansing duties) or the *shatkarmas* (six cleansing actions). These techniques were devised to remove phlegm, wind, bile and excess fat or other impurities from the physical body. Practice of these cleansing techniques also improves concentration and willpower. The yogis believed that using them together with *pranayama* and meditation practice would stimulate the life force, leading to the awakening of *kundalini*.

Most yogis practise only a few *kriyas* daily. As with most yoga practices, these techniques should initially be attempted under the guidance of a qualified teacher, who should demonstrate them first. As well as the main six methods, I have chosen to describe extra *kriya* techniques for the benefit of the practitioner.

Dhauti

Dhauti (literally 'to wash') is the internal cleansing of the body. The most common of the *dhauti* practices is *vastra dhauti* or cloth cleansing, in which a swallowed cloth absorbs phlegm, bile and other impurities in the stomach.

Soak a long strip of cloth or gauze no wider than the tongue in warm water or milk. In a squatting position, slowly and carefully swallow the cloth while holding onto one end. Initially it may catch in the back of the throat, causing a retching reflex, but don't panic: keep swallowing slowly or sip some water to help the cloth move down the throat. Let it remain in the stomach for 10–15 minutes before slowly pulling it back out. (If it remains there longer, it will begin to pass through the digestive system.) The body's gagging reflex may occur during the first attempts, but this will be overcome with practice. In the beginning, swallow only 60–90 cm (2–3 ft) of cloth, then gradually increase to 4.5 m (15 ft) or more as the body becomes accustomed to it. This *kriya* has many therapeutic benefits and is prescribed to cure diseases caused by an imbalance of phlegm in the body.

Danta Dhauti

Danta-mula-dhauti is the practice of brushing or rubbing the teeth and gums. Traditionally, this is done using betel-nut plant powder, *neem* or pure earth. Tongue-cleansing or *jihva-shodhana* may be done with a metal tongue-scraper, a spoon or the fingers.

Kama Dhauti

This is literally the cleaning of the ears. The *Gheranda Samhita* concisely states: 'Clean the two holes of the ears with the index or ring fingers. By engaging in this practice daily, the mystical sounds (*nada*) will be heard.' It is of course important to be careful when cleaning the ears, as the ear canal is delicate and easily damaged.

Vamana Dhauti

Swallow two to four glasses of warm water with a small amount of salt dissolved in it, then insert three fingers into the throat and vomit the water out. With regular practice, you should be able to vomit the water back out without using the fingers at all.

Jala Dhauti

This practice cleanses the stomach and assists in bowel movements on waking. Drink a glass of warm water with lemon and, if needed, a little honey. Vegans may substitute agave nectar or maple syrup for the honey, but use just a little. The lemon juice should be fresh: a half-lemon for a small glass and a whole one for a larger glass.

Basti or Vasti

The *Gheranda Samhita* describes two kinds of *vasti*: *jala vasti* (water *vasti*) and *suska vasti* (dry *vasti*). The first was originally performed by rolling a large banana leaf into a straw, inserting it into the anus, squatting in water up to the navel and contracting and dilating the sphincter of the anus. This action draws water into the colon, where you hold it for a short time and churn it about. The water is then released by relaxing and physically opening the anal sphincter. Performing *uddiyana bandha*, the lock focusing on the area between the diaphragm and the pelvic floor (see page 70), while squatting creates a vacuum in the colon and the water is then churned around by means of *nauli* (see page 70). Today you can use an anal douche, but be careful: the water must not be allowed to rise too high in the colon. *Suska vasti* involves assuming *Paschimottanasana* or Seated Forward Bend (see page 116), moving the intestinal tract slowly downwards while in this posture, and performing *asvini mudra* (contraction of the anal sphincter). Dry *vasti* is said to increase the gastric fire *agni*, and be a cure for constipation.

Neti

Used for cleansing the nostrils and nasal sinuses, this practice has two forms: *sutra neti*, using a rubber catheter, linen or gauze cord, and *jala neti*, using warm, salty water.

Sutra Neti

Pass a thin rubber catheter or linen or gauze cord up one nostril until the end appears at the back of the throat. This can be difficult at first: turning the catheter is usually an effective way to direct it. Once it appears in the back of the throat, grasp it between the index and middle finger of the right hand and draw it out through the mouth.

Jala Neti

Makes sure to clear the nasal passages gently prior to performing this *kriya*.

1. Dissolve a quarter of a teaspoonful of salt in warm water in a *neti* pot (a small pot with a narrow spout). Be careful not to add too much salt or you will experience a burning sensation. Too little salt will also cause pain.

2. Tilt the head 90 degrees to the side with the mouth open so that you can breathe. Insert the spout of the pot into the left nostril. Pour the water in slowly; it should pass out through the right nostril.

2. After all the water has passed through the right nostril, hang the head and torso down in *Uttanasana* or Standing Forward Bend (see page 94) and perform four gentle expulsions of all the air in the lungs. This will remove any excess water from the back of the nose. After exhaling, allow the lungs to refill automatically, as in *kapalabhati* (see page 71). Be careful not to exhale too forcefully or water may end up in your inner ear or sinuses, causing discomfort and/or pain.

3. Repeat the process, pouring the salt water through the right nostril.

Jala neti is the *kriya* with the most benefit for the least amount of discomfort. Aspiring yogis should make it a part of their morning routine on arising for meditation.

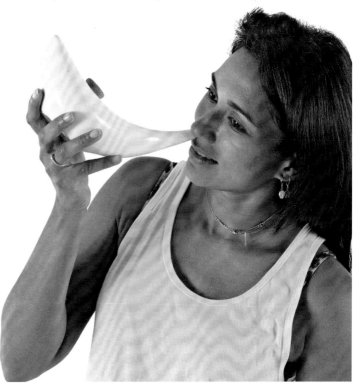

The practice of *jala neti* – flushing waste matter from the nasal passages and sinuses – is advised as part of the yogi's daily *pranayama* practice.

Nauli

Abdominal churning is the most effective and important of all the cleansing techniques and signifies ultimate control over the abdominal region. Regular practice stimulates digestion and tones the abdominal muscles, the intestines and the reproductive, excretory and urinary organs. It improves the elasticity of the lungs and the strength and mobility of the diaphragm, and massages and stimulates the liver, pancreas, kidneys and adrenal glands. There is a direct link between *nauli* and sexual vigour, and with overcoming sexual disabilities. Regular practice can alleviate constipation and control appetite, indigestion, acidity, flatulence and even hormonal imbalances and emotional disturbances.

In this practice, the rectus abdominis muscles are repeatedly contracted and isolated from right to left and left to right in a continuous wave-like motion. This takes place during breath retention, and the number of repetitions depends on how long you can retain the breath without struggling.

1. Stand with the feet a little wider than hip width apart with the knees slightly bent and the palms resting just above the knees. Breathe in through the nose and exhale forcefully through the mouth. At the end of the exhalation, suck the abdomen in towards the spine. This is *uddiyana bandha*.
2. Without leaning to the right, lift the right hand off the knee while maintaining pressure on the left knee with the left hand. This isolates the rectus abdominis muscles on the left. This is *vama nauli*.
3. Exhale and release *uddiyana bandha*.
4. Now do the same with the right side, lifting the left hand off the knee and isolating the rectus abdominis muscles on the right. This is *daskina nauli*.
5. Practise both sides until you are able to isolate both left and right sides at the same time, which will cause the rectus abdominis muscles to protrude from the centre. This will require you to have both hands above the knees at the same time. This is *madhyama nauli*.
6. Once you are able to isolate the muscles in the centre, you can begin to practise churning: isolating one side and then the other, moving first clockwise and then anti-clockwise. The number of repetitions depends on how long you can retain the breath without struggling. Check your progress in a mirror so you can see how to control the muscles in order to create this movement.

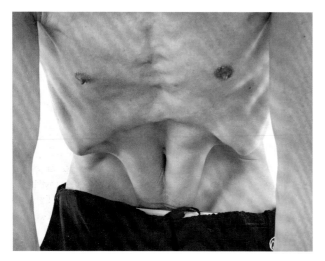

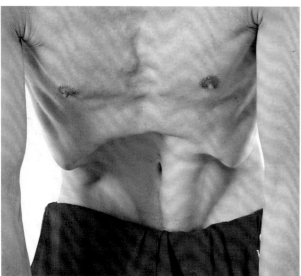

The rectus abdominis muscle is isolated and churned from side to side in a wave-like motion. An advanced technique, *nauli* should be practised under the guidance of an experienced teacher.

Trataka

This is concentrated gazing. It has two forms: external, *bahiranga*, and internal, *antaranga*. The more common is external gazing. Position a candle flame at eye level, about an arm's length away. The flame must be still and the room darkened. Fix your gaze on the flame without blinking. This will cause the eyes to water, washing away any impurities. This *kriya* can be a little uncomfortbale at first, but there is nothing dangerous about it. *Trataka* can be followed by the Clock Exercise – rolling the eyes like the hands of a clock. Make several rotations in a clockwise direction, then do the same number of rotations in the opposite direction. Conclude the practice by closing the eyes for a few minutes of quiet rest. .

Kapalabhati

This breathing exercise invigorates the brain, strengthens the lungs, oxygenates the blood and eliminates toxins from the body. Normally when we breathe, our inhalation is active and exhalation is passive, but this exercise reverses the process. This is often compared to a pair of bellows: when you close the bellows, air is forced out and when you release them, a vacuum is created and air is sucked back in. Likewise, in *kapalabhati* the inhalation is an involuntary reaction to a forceful exhalation.

The forced exhalation is said to have a massaging effect on the brain. Most people take an average of 15 breaths per minute, which means the brain is compressed upon inhalation and decompressed on exhalation that many times. In a *kapalabhati* cycle, the breath is accelerated to the rate of 50–100 per minute, so the brain is stimulated much more frequently. The exercise also removes more carbon dioxide and other waste gases from the cells and lungs than when we breathe normally.

1. Sit comfortably with the legs crossed or in Lotus position and straighten the spine.
2. Close the eyes. Place the palms face upwards on top of the knees with the index finger and thumb of each hand touching. Alternatively the index finger can touch the base of the thumb.
3. Begin with an inhalation and then exhale forcefully by pumping the breath out through the nose. The force of the exhalation should pull the abdomen in towards the spine and the inhalation should become involuntary. Continue for 20–30 seconds. You may choose to count the number of breaths, beginning with 20 pumpings per round and gradually increasing by 10 breaths per round each week until you reach 100. Or you can time yourself. Increase the duration of the exercise to as much as two minutes per round as your stamina improves. Exhalations should be two or three times faster than the passive inhalations that follow, and performed at the rate of one or two per second.
4. At the end of each round, inhale a full breath and hold it. This retention is called *kumbhaka*. Advanced practitioners may apply the root lock, *mula bandha*, and chin lock, *uddiyana bandha* (see page 70), during breath retention and hold for a comfortable length of time without strain, as any sense of suffocation not only disturbs the mind but can harm the nervous system.

Breathing exercises such as *kapalabhati* and *nadi sodhana pranayama* (alternate nostril-breathing) should be performed as part of your regular yoga practice.

Vahnisara

Also known as fire purification, this is performed in a similar way to *kapalabhati*. Standing with knees bent and hands on the thighs, exhale forcefully, with the navel contracting towards the spine, but in this case release the stomach before inhalation. This *kriya* massages the internal organs and stimulates the internal gastric fire *agni*, which is said to reside behind the navel; it is believed to cure diseases of the stomach and aid digestion. Begin by performing five contractions of the navel towards the spine, one per exhalation. Over time, increase the number of contraction-exhalations to ten.

Nadi Sodhana Pranayama

Also known as *Anuloma Vilmoma*, alternate nostril-breathing is the most efficient nerve purifier. It is also recommended for high blood pressure or any sort of physical imbalance. It is practised by inhaling and exhaling gently through alternating nostrils without holding or suspending breathing. Use the right hand in *vishnu mudra* and the left hand in *jnana mudra* (see *Mudhras* on page 222) and inhale slowly through the left nostril according to your capacity. Close the left nostril with the ring finger and immediately open the right nostril by letting go with the thumb. Exhale and inhale, close the right nostril, then exhale through the left. This is one complete cycle. Start with 12 cycles, and gradually increase the cycles according to your capacity. The longer you can practise this exercise, the greater the benefits.

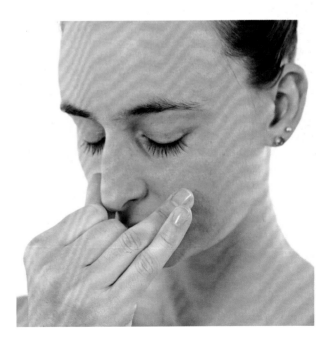

Karma

Karma is the universal principle of cause and effect, which governs all consciousness. All deeds, thoughts, vibrations of any sort, are ruled by a law that demands perfect rebound.

The concept of *karma* lies at the very heart of Hindu and Buddhist philosophy. The word comes from Sanskrit *kri*, meaning 'to do'. *Karma* is not fate, for we have free will to create our own destinies; but the result of action. The consequence or fruit of an action is part of the action, and cannot be separated: sooner or later it returns upon the doer, either in this life or in a future one. According to the *Vedas*, a person consists of desires and, as is his desire, so is his will. As is his will, so is his deed. It is complex to predict which *karma* will yield exactly which result, but generally 'as you sow, so shall you reap'.

All living creatures are bound by the laws of *karma*. We humans are said to produce it through thoughts, words, actions that we perform ourselves or through actions others perform under our instructions. Everything we have ever thought, spoken, done or caused is *karma*, as is everything we are thinking, speaking or doing this very moment. The innumerable karmic seeds we create will produce a positive or negative result, sooner or later in this life, or some future one. Hindu scriptures divide *karma* into three kinds: *sanchita*, *prarabdha* and *agami karma*.

Sanchita Karma

Acquired Karma
This is the accumulated *karma* from all previous births yet to be resolved – the sum of yet unrealized *karma*s committed during previous existences. This is your total cosmic debt. At every moment an individual is either adding to or reducing his or her cosmic debt. It would be impossible to experience and endure all *karma*s in one lifetime, so it needs to be fulfilled in your future births until the balance is exhausted. The imprints we inherit from past lives create our personality, inclinations and talents. Our likings, abilities, attitudes and inclinations are based on the thoughts and actions of past lives.

Prarabdha Karma

Present Karma
From the stock of *sanchita karma* a handful is taken to serve one lifetime: *prarabdha karma*, which is Sanskrit for 'action that has been unleashed or aroused'. It also refers to the action that manifests now. It is the portion of *sanchita karma* that was earned in the past and is already occurring. The *karma*s of destiny are like arrows already in flight; it is almost impossible to change their direction. You cannot erase this *karma*, you must go through it, because it is already in process with no way to change it.

Agami Karma

Approaching Karma
This is the *karma* of the present life over which we have control. It embraces everything that we produce in this life. Through it we create our *karma* for this life and lifetimes to come. Some *agami karma* bears fruit in the current life; the rest is stored for future births as *sanchita karma*. While we are free to choose our actions, our old tendencies and habits (from *sanchita karma* and *prarabdha karma*) influence *agami karma*. An individual fully aware of his actions can choose the good *karma* that will yield good future results.

Can we change or erase our *karma*?

Karma is infinite. Every habit is *karma*. The result can be good or bad, depending on our perception. Being aware of our tendencies may help to bring them under control. But *karma* that has already yielded a result (or is in the process) cannot be changed. So *prarabdha karma* must be endured. However, spiritual masters believe it is possible to erase *sanchita karma* through practices that help us to make right choices: prayer, meditation and selfless service. *Agami karma* can be erased through greater awareness.

To conclude, all individual souls must experience *karma* if they live in the phenomenal universe. To escape the cycle of life, death and rebirth, the individual must exhaust his *karma* and realize his true self as the highest truth of oneness that is Brahman, the supreme Godhead.

In Hindu and Buddhist philosophy, *karma* is the sum of a person's actions in this and previous lives, which will affect their fate until all of their karmas have been exhausted.

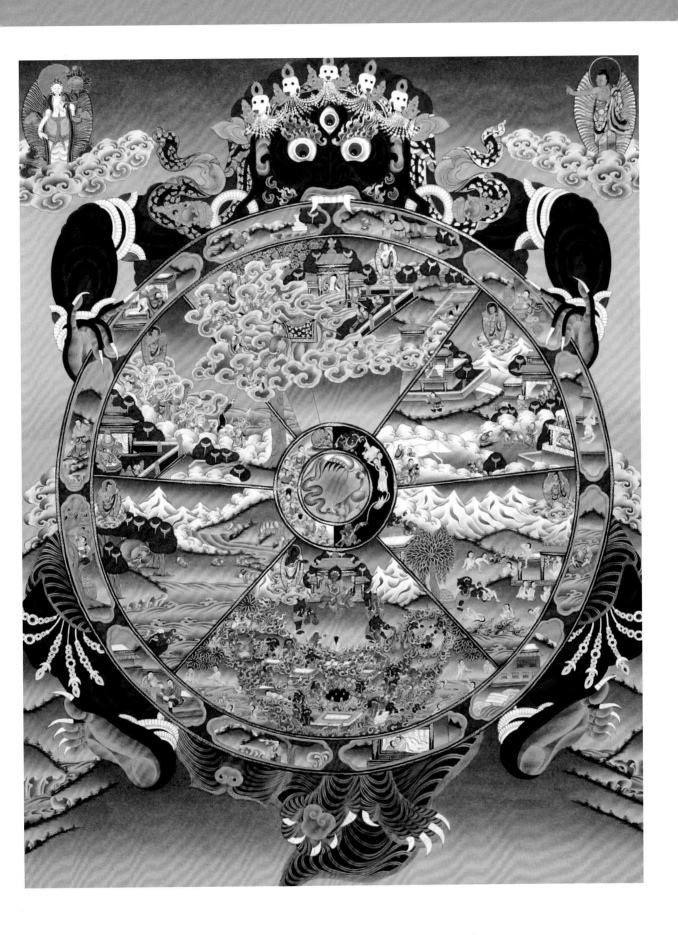

Yoga and Diet

Let thy food be thy medicine and thy medicine be thy food.
Hippocrates (460–370 BCE)

The yogic diet is a natural one. Anyone following the principles of yoga must, when choosing what to eat, take into consideration the ecological implications, conserving natural resources, as well as ethical and moral issues regarding cruelty to animals. Traditionally the yogic diet was called a diet of 'fruits and roots' (*phala mula*). It would consist largely of whole grains, beans, root vegetables, seeds and nuts, fruits and leafy vegetables, and some dairy foods in the form of milk. When a yogi eats, he or she should recognize not only that the food nourishes the body, but that its inherent qualities will also have an effect on the mind.

However, there is often confusion around the right foods to eat in order to nourish and develop body and soul. Many yogis today adopt a vegan diet because of the ethical issues regarding the farming and consumption of dairy produce, and some exist on a diet of only raw foods.

Choosing the Right Foods

Since the essence of food forms the mind, a pure and moderated diet of foods produced by the combined effects of sun, air, soil and water is the best prescription for physical and mental wellbeing. The goodness we gain from these foods comes at first hand, bringing harmony and vitality to the aspirant. Full of *prana*, it keeps the body lean and supple and the mind clear and focused.

To coin a phrase, you are what you eat. We should aim to eat food that will increase our *sattvic* qualities (see box on opposite page) and increase *prana*.

The three *gunas*, *sattva*, *rajas* and *tamas*, exist together in equilibrium (see page 17). These qualities encompass all existence and all actions. In our manifest world, any one of these qualities is always dominant, but can exist only when the other two are present. Each individual's dominant *guna* is reflected in our thoughts, actions and

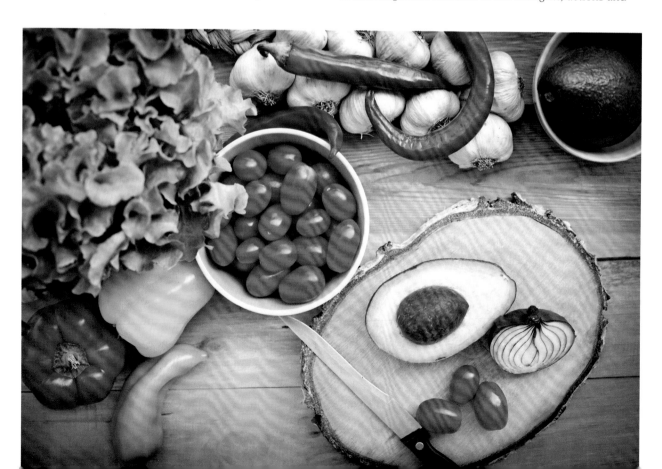

the foods we choose to eat. Purity of food is followed by purification of the inner nature. A purer, more *sattvic* diet will change our consciousness, and eventually *rajassic* and *tamasic* foods will lose their appeal, making our *asana, pranayama* and meditation practice easier.

When eating, one half of the stomach should be filled with solids (food), one quarter with liquid (water or any healthy juice) and the other quarter left empty to allow for ease of digestion. This also prevents mental stress afterwards.

The importance of raw food for the purpose of purification cannot be underestimated. Raw food is our most direct source of *prana,* and by eating raw foods we can directly increase *prana,* not only in the body, but also in the mind.It also cleanses the *nadis* or nerve channels. For optimum physical and spiritual health 50–80 per cent of a person's diet should be made up of raw food.

In contrast, meat comes from creatures that have already processed the optimal natural energy drawn from different plants. Animal flesh contains a high proportion of toxins and lacks vital vitamins and minerals. Human anatomy and physiology bear a closer resemblance to that of fruit-eating primates than to carnivorous animals, so that by eating meat we compel our bodies to adapt to a diet for which they were not designed.

Apart from questions of health and nutrition, there are other significant implications to eating meat. Ecologically it is inefficient and wasteful: 50 per cent of the world's cereal is fed to livestock, and, as protein converters, livestock are inefficient. One hectare (2.5 acres) of cereal will produce five times more protein than the same area devoted to raising animals for our meat consumption. The figure for legumes is ten times higher, and for leafy vegetables higher than that.

Protein deficiency

These days people are better informed about vegetarianism, but a vegetarian diet is still not appealing for many. One of the meat-eater's main objections to it is a concern over protein deficiency. Westerners are obsessed with protein, believing that they need far more than they actually do. On the contrary, research has shown that a balanced vegetarian diet provides all the protein the body requires. Nuts, dairy produce, spirulina and legumes all supply high-class protein. Ironically, meat-eaters obtain the worst-quality protein from their food – animal protein

Eating mostly plant-based foods is better for you and also for the planet – raising livestock for meat requires significantly more energy and natural resources than growing crops.

Yogic Diet and the Three *Gunas*

The three *gunas* of *sattva, rajas* and *tamas* can be applied to our choice of food, and, as in ourselves, these qualities also exist in the foods we eat. Again, these qualities are in a state of flux and any one can predominate. However, we should, for optimum health, focus on food that is predominantly *sattvic,* in order to increase our *sattvic* nature.

Sattva and its constituent foods

Sattva is the quality of purity and harmony, the balancing force that embodies spiritual evolution. A *sattvic* diet consists of neutral, natural, organic, simple, clean, fresh foods grown in harmony with nature, in good soils, ripened naturally and either eaten raw or cooked with an attitude of devotion. Such a diet brings optimum health, nourishing the body and purifying the mind.

Sattvic food: fruit, vegetables, cereals, grains, legumes, nuts, seeds, wholemeal bread, sprouted seeds, honey.

Rajas and its constituent foods

Rajas is the active quality, the stimulating force that initiates change and disturbs the equilibrium. It embodies emotional fluctuations of fear and desire, attraction and repulsion, agitation, speed and movement.

Rajassic foods are hot, bitter, sour, dry or salty. This affects the equilibrium between mind and body, feeding the body at the expense of the mind. Too much *rajassic* food will over-stimulate the body and excite the passions, making the mind restless and uncontrollable.

Rajassic food: hot spices or strong herbs. Coffee, tea, fish, eggs, salt and chocolate.

Tamas and its constituent foods

Tamas is the passive quality. A negative and obstructive force that resists change, it embodies darkness, non-feeling, attachment, depression, lethargy, dullness, heaviness, stagnation and ignorance.

Tamasic food benefits neither the mind nor the body. The body's resistance to disease is reduced and the powers of reasoning become affected. Emotions such as anger and greed predominate.

Tamassic food: meat, onions, garlic, fermented foods such as vinegar and stale or overripe foods. Alcohol.

contains high levels of uric acid which, can't be broken down by the liver; some is eliminated, but the rest is deposited in the joints, causing stiffness and eventually leading to problems such as arthritis.

The Benefits of a Vegetarian Diet

A vegetarian diet is rich in fibre and high in polyunsaturated fats. Lack of the dietary fibre that unrefined plant food contains can lead to a number of disorders of the intestine. The health of the entire body begins with the state of the colon, so eat to live and don't live to eat. Vegetarians consume almost twice as much fibre as meat-eaters. They also consume less fat, and the fats they do eat tend to be polyunsaturated and not the saturated animal fats that raise cholesterol.

Statistically, vegetarians have a lower incidence of heart disease, kidney disease and cancer. Their resistance to disease is generally higher than that of meat-eaters and they are less likely to suffer from obesity. Studies have shown that a vegetarian diet is a prime preventer of osteoporosis, to the extent that vegetarian women suffer from it less than meat-eating men.

Switching to a Vegetarian diet

- Make it a gradual transition: slowly begin to reduce your intake of meat or fish and replace it with fresh vegetables, fruit, nuts, grains and pulses.
- Make sure you have a regular intake of good protein foods – nuts, pulses, whole grains and cheese.
- Buy a juicer or blender. If there are some fruits and vegetables you don't enjoy eating, juicing is a great alternative and brings the same nutritional benefits.
- Eat a salad of raw vegetables each day. Include plenty of green vegetables in your diet.
- Don't overcook vegetables or they will lose their nutritional value. Steaming or stir-frying will preserve their goodness.
- Eat some fresh fruit every day.
- Avoid processed foods such as white flour, white bread, cakes and refined cereals, canned fruit, vegetables and drinks, and saturated fats.
- Avoid reheating food, as it will lose its goodness.
- Drink plenty of water and replace tea and coffee with herbal teas or fruit juices.

And there is no truth in the oft-repeated claim that a vegetarian diet is boring. The choice of vegetarian foods is abundant and they can be prepared in a multitude of ways to offer a range of tastes and textures. The less meat you eat, the more flexible you will become and the more the fluctuations of the mind will reduce.

Making the transition to a vegetarian diet

If you do decide to become vegetarian, start by integrating small changes one by one, observing moderation all along the way. Every change should come from a natural inclination and not from a feeling of guilt or obligation. Some people become disillusioned or disaffected because they can't cope with being vegetarian – some even give up yoga altogether – but if this happens to you, it is better to follow a diet that suits you and continue with yoga than to abandon your practice because you can't adjust to the dietary restrictions.

Try cutting out red meat first, then poultry and finally fish and seafood; replace them with fresh fruit and vegetables and raw nuts. There are some great vegetarian recipe books available and plenty of free recipes online. Be imaginative about your food choices – it will be easier to make the transition if you are enjoying what you eat.

The philosophy of vegetarianism

While we reflect on a vegetarian diet, we should also ask ourselves whether we can consume with a clear conscience the flesh of a living being that has been slaughtered, often under the most barbaric conditions. It's easy to ignore the horrors of the meat industry when we are faced with neatly packaged portions of meat or fish at the supermarket. We no longer make the connection between the product and the animal that has been killed for our consumption. *Ahimsa* – non-harming and non-violence – is among the highest laws in yogic philosophy and cannot be ignored if we are to grow spiritually. For a yogi all life should be sacred. Once you become conscious of where your food comes

What the Body Needs

Carbohydrates and fats provide energy; proteins, vitamins and minerals are the essential body-building materials. The exact requirements vary from person to person. Active people need more carbohydrates and fats, while children and pregnant women need more protein and calcium.

from and how it affects your body and your mind, you will gradually become more receptive and realize that all creatures are as divine as you are.

Fasting

Fasting is another way to bring the mind and the senses under control and to cleanse and rejuvenate the body. A lot of energy is spent digesting food. Resting the digestive system allows the energy to be used for spiritual development and for healing, expelling the body's toxins. On no account should fasting be confused with dieting: its purpose is solely for purification and self-healing.

Fasting need not be the restriction of all food and drink. There are different types of fasting, for example liquid or juice fasts, which involve the intake of liquids only – water, fruit or vegetable juices. Some fasts involve the intake of just one food for a period of time, such as water melon, to purify and cleanse the body. Another fast involves eating just one meal at the start of the day and nothing for the rest of the day for two days each week. This has been scientifically proven to improve health.

Fasting is best done communally and under the guidance of a teacher. In isolation, it is perhaps best to fast just one day a month. A fast should begin on a day of rest and is facilitated by quietude and meditation with some light exercise and fresh air. Do not fast for more than 36 hours at a time. As the body cleanses old impurities, you may experience aches and pains, weakness and nausea. Excessive discomfort shows that the cleansing is proceeding too rapidly, and the process should be moderated by the intake of heavier foods.

Freshly squeezed juice is a quick, easy and delicious way of adding more raw vegetables and fruits to your diet – experiment to find the healthy combinations that taste best to you.

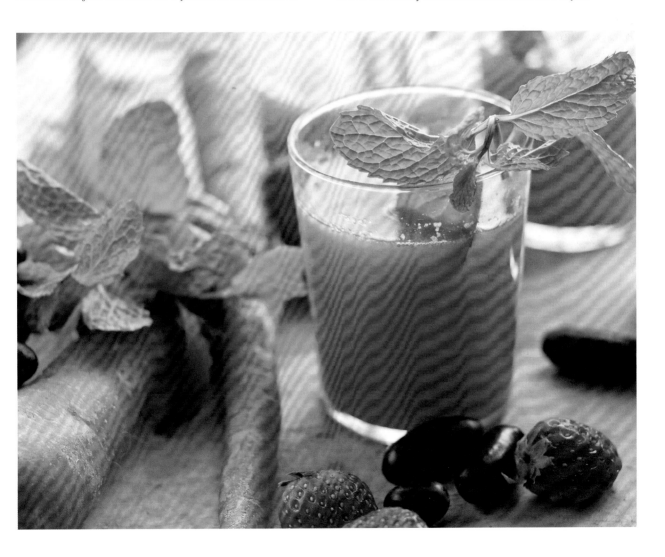

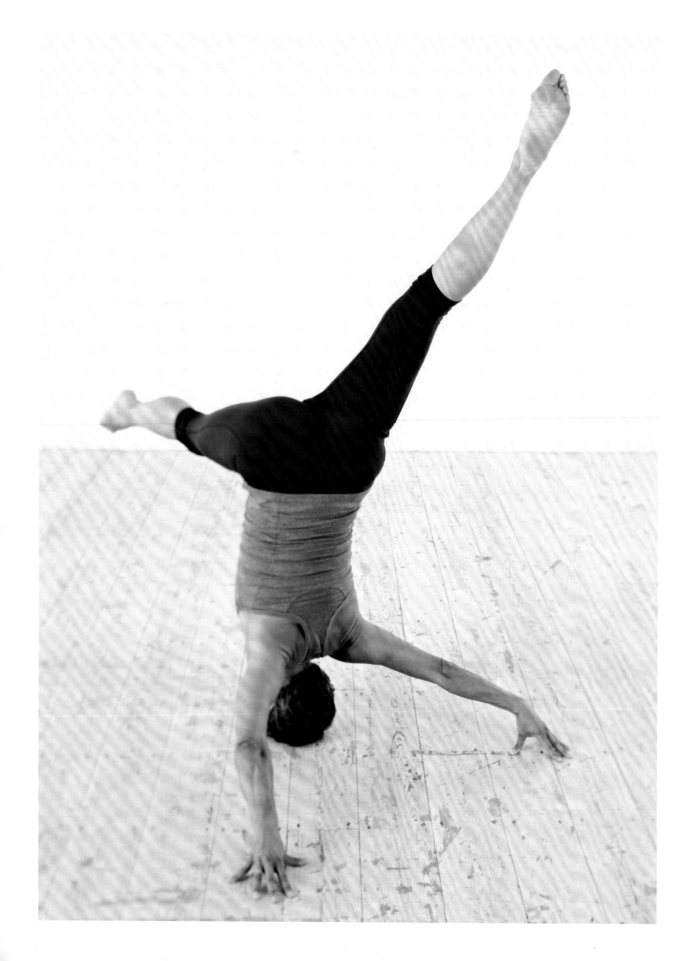

Asanas

For most of us, our experience of yoga begins on a physical level through *asana* practice, and so our initial understanding of yoga comes through the experiences of the physical body. *Asanas* are the gateway to higher states of awareness, providing us with the foundation necessary for exploring the body, breath and mind. *Asanas* originally referred to the sitting positions that ancient yogis assumed for long periods while performing spiritual practices. Today the word has a broader and more holistic approach. *Asanas* are now practised not only for meditative purposes, but also to bring radiant health and help in our quest for spiritual enlightenment.

The Benefits of *Asana* Practice	80
The Postures	82
Standing Poses	85
Seated Poses	117
Supine Poses	147
Balancing Poses	155
Inverted Poses	181
Back-bending Poses	191
Surya Namaskara (The Sun Salutation)	209
A Daily Practice Plan	212

The Benefits of Asana Practice

The body and mind are not separate from each other. The renowned yogi B.K.S. Iyengar refers to the body as the gross form of the mind and the mind as the subtle form of the body, and *asanas* as the means to integrate and harmonize the two.

In the *Yoga Sutras*, asana is the third of Patanjali's eight-limbed path, which provides the foundation for our yogic life. Patanjali's definition of *asana* is *Sthira sukham asanam*, generally translated as 'steady, comfortable postures'. However beautifully we perform an *asana*, unless we integrate the body with the breath and mind we cannot claim that what we are doing is yoga. The essence of yoga is not external display, but internal cultivation. Regular *asana* practice brings optimum health. The exercises strengthen and tone the muscles, improve balance, increase bone mass, help digestion and calm the nerves. While practising *asanas* to keep fit is a legitimate place to start, it isn't the goal. *Asana* is a preparation for *pranayama* and meditation practice. Only when the mind is calm can it find the uninterrupted flow of concentration that is meditation.

When an *asana* is performed correctly and practised with awareness, the movements are fluid and there is a lightness in the body that generates a sense of freedom in the mind. *Asana* is an exploration of one's individual consciousness. Through *asanas*, our physical body becomes a vehicle to discipline the mind and examine obstacles in our daily life to discover how we can overcome them. Practising with this awareness is integral to Hatha yoga – and more important than flexibility or achieving the advanced poses.

Asanas are the gateway to the core of our being. When we working from the periphery to the core, we can embark on an inner journey to penetrate the soul.

Asana practice

Keeping an awareness of how you move and breathe brings control and grace in the pose, even for beginners. *Asana* practice helps to train the body and mind through endurance, as both are subjected to difficulties. This is known as *tapas*, or the acceptance of pain as a means of purification. If we remind ourselves that the journey is more important than the destination, then the effort involved in trying to achieve a pose can have more value than actually achieving it.

When we practise and focus our attention within the body, this is advanced yoga, no matter how easy the pose. Practising with scattered attention is the action of a beginner. Hold your attention within the body, either on the breath or on the tissues being stretched, the joints or the fluidity of your movements.

Many *asanas* are named after animals. The ancient *rishis* observed how animals live in harmony with their environment and the *asanas* reflect the movements of these animals. Mastery of a posture allows us to experience a different state of consciousness when we achieve or inhabit the pose fully. If an *asana* feels too heavy or awkward, something is wrong.

Try to move in and out of poses gracefully, like a dancer. Sometimes, it's good to imagine yourself performing in front of an audience. It can make you practise with greater attention to detail.

Attending class

Even as a teacher, attending the occasional class can be a great help to your practice. Observing others and imitating them physically and mentally, moving in sync with one another, develops a collective consciousness and you can learn a great deal this way.

Additionally, practising with others provides mutual support and encouragement. If you practise alone, since there is no-one there to witness, it's easy to avoid certain poses or to break a pose too soon when the mind or body says it's had enough. A teacher may make an adjustment when you practise in class. Remember that he or she is only correcting you to help you progress a little faster. After all, if the posture looks odd, it's likely that it will feel odd too.

Some students feel concerned if their mat is not arranged in a certain way, or if they don't have the appropriate cushion. But remember that you don't need anything to practise yoga – the body is all that's required.

Being patient

It is important to develop patience in your practice. Progress in *asana* is achieved by advancing slowly and steadily, according to your capacity. A yoga practice should be well-structured, containing a balanced range of *asanas* – a forward bend, back-bend, twist, inversions and balancing poses; and developed daily, depending on how much time you have and what your objectives and requirements are.

It is recommended that you practise on an empty stomach, leaving at least two hours after you've eaten. If your schedule allows, try to practise at the same time and in the same place every day. This will enable you to recognize any day-to-day changes. It's great to practise *asana* after noon; after 4 p.m. is even better and after 6 p.m. is ideal. However, if you need to do all of your *sadhana* (spiritual practice) in one sitting, early morning is the ideal time.

How we accomplish the poses is a matter of divided opinion: there are disagreements about how they should be approached or taught. Remember that yoga practice is an exploration of your individual body and you have to find what works best for you. The steps to mastering the poses featured in this section are suggestions rather than instructions. It is up to you to 'find your own tricks', as my Guru says, and, if they work, to share them with others.

Avoiding injury

When we perform *asanas,* we are physically demonstrating our strength of will and tenacity through the expression of the muscles. The challenge of yoga is to go beyond our perceived limits, but within reason. *Asanas* teach us to develop greater tolerance physically and mentally. Through our bodies we discover how to tolerate the pain that can't be avoided and how to transform the pain that can. When we practise, we experience a level of pain that can even be exhilarating and constructive, leading to physical and spiritual transformation.

However, the pain that comes through practising with a lack of awareness can be destructive and often leads to suffering. Failure to listen and respond to the body's warnings can result in pulled muscles, torn ligaments, nerve damage or ruptured discs. If today's practice impacts on tomorrow's, then you are doing something wrong. Try to focus on relaxing when you're holding a pose. This relaxes the brain as well as the body.

Making progress

It's important to repeat new or difficult poses at least three times or more. With each repetition, the pose becomes easier as the mind and body begin to understand and recognize it.

The most efficient place to focus the inner gaze in most postures is the space between the eyebrows, also known as the third eye or *Trikuti*. Where the attention goes, the blood goes, and where the blood goes, *prana*, the vital life force, follows. Fixing the attention at the third eye stimulates the pituitary gland deep in the base of the brain. In yoga, the pituitary gland is seen as the true sixth sense, so stimulating this gland is of critical importance.

Anything found can easily be lost, so if you have worked hard over a period of time to achieve a pose, practise it every day. If you don't do it for three days, you may have to find it all over again.

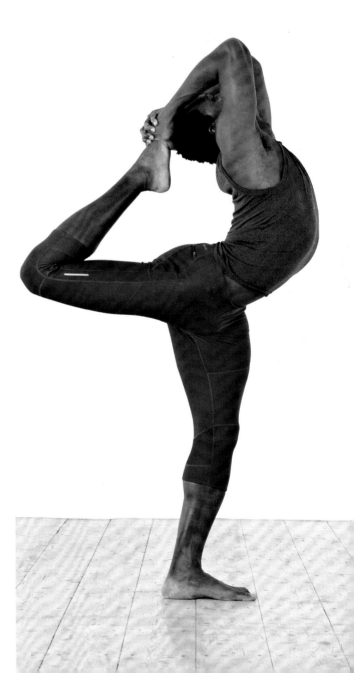

The Postures

This section contains 65 of the most commonly practised *asanas* in Hatha yoga. They enable you to explore your body and recognize any limitations and how to overcome them. There are more challenging variations for each pose, depending on the experience of the individual and are intended to expand the physical and mental capabilities of the practitioner.

To illustrate the poses, I have chosen people whom I teach and whose progress I have observed, in some cases, over several years. I have tried to achieve a balance between technical accuracy and maintaining the essence of the pose. Each pose brings a different state of awareness. If we become too obsessed with technical accuracy we risk losing this awareness. Of course I am looking for correct alignment, not for visual reasons, but for the benefit of the student. Correct execution and alignment of the pose avoids pain or injury and brings grace and poise. When the pose is held correctly, there is fusion of the body and mind.

How we transcend our physical limitations depends on our mental determination. Developing a little more tolerance to discomfort in order to master the poses is fundamental to *asana* practice. Often people come to yoga expecting some gentle stretching to prepare them for meditation, but if the body hasn't been prepared, then it can't sit for more than ten minutes without becoming uncomfortable, leading to more restlessness in the mind.

We have to be realistic about the age we live in. Our society is goal-driven and our minds are increasingly restless, always searching for another challenge – financial, romantic, career. I teach many professionals who sit in front of computer screens all day long. They come to class for the body–mind connection, but my experience tells me that they're not going to make that connection by sitting still and meditating. If I was to have them do this, I know their minds would be filled with distracting thoughts: what to have for supper, what's on TV later. The challenge lies in finding stillness in the demands that these *asanas* bring.

I prefer to keep these students focused on where they are and what they are doing, totally in the present moment. In order to achieve this, the poses are often stimulating, both physically and mentally, to take them out of the mental space they usually inhabit.

I hear excuses from students about why they can't do a pose – my arms are too short, my legs are too long. From my own experience, I believe that anything is possible,

and this attitude is the gateway to your own success, either in *asana* or in your profession. Today I practise some *asanas* that I never imagined I would be able to do – and that I had no interest in attaining when I began my practice. I always suggest to students that they try a pose, because they might just surprise themselves by what they can achieve. The human body is a fascinating machine capable of much more than what we limit it to. It is the students I teach who are my inspiration, and it is them I practise for – so that I can continue to encourage and inspire them.

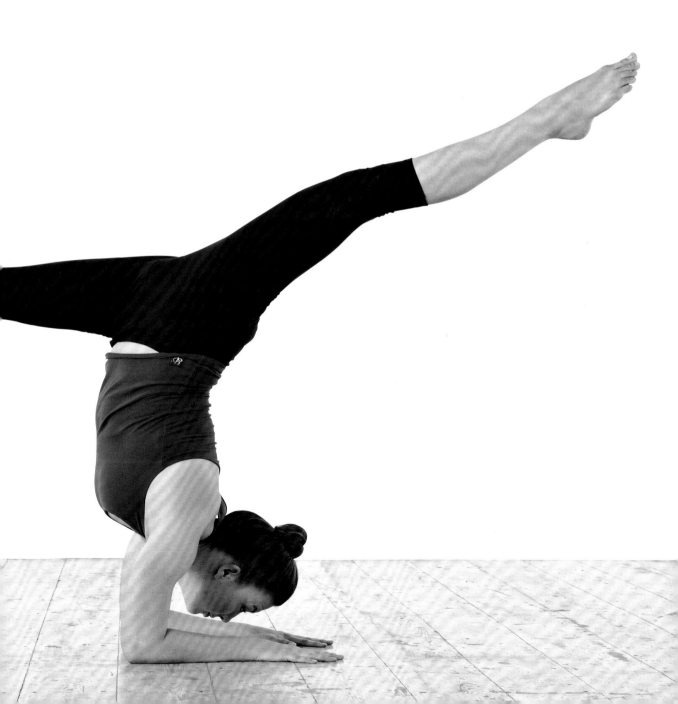

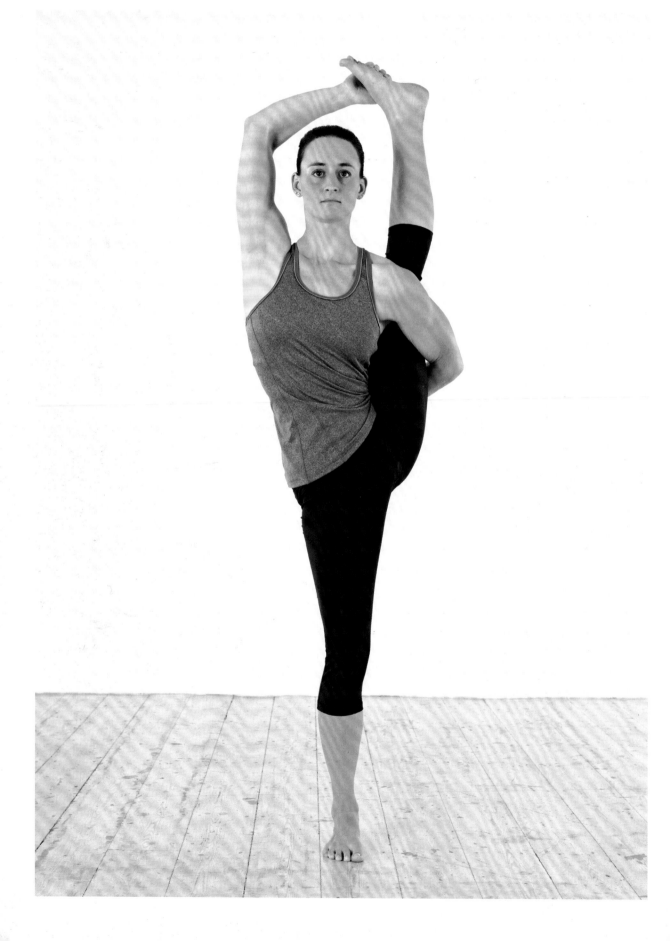

Standing Poses

Standing bears weight on the feet, the only parts of the body that have evolved to maintain our unique bipedal stance. Footwear and paved floors mean we no longer use our feet in the way they were engineered to be used. The standing poses in yoga connect our feet to the earth and give us the foundation on which to build our *asana* practice, restoring flexibility to the foot and lower leg and strengthening the leg muscles and ankle and knee joints. The poses also keep the spine flexible and long, help to maintain its upright posture and help to circulate blood to the lower extremities.

Tadasana 86

Virabhadrasana I 87

Virabhadrasana II 88

Virabhadrasana III 89

Uttitha Trikonasana 90

Parivrtta Parsvakonasana 92

Uttanasana 94

Urdhva Prasarita Eka
  Padasana 95

Utkatasana 96

Malasana 97

Garudasana 98

Vatyanasana 99

Vrikshasana 100

Ardha Baddha
  Padmottanasana 101

Prasarita Padottanasana 102

Utthita Tittibhasana 104

Uttitha Hasta
  Padangusthasana 106

Svarga Dvijasana 107

Ardha Chandrasana 108

Patan Vrikshasana 110

Parsvottanasana 111

Natarajasana 112

Uttan Pristhasana 114

Balasana 115

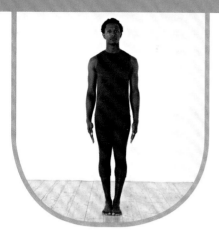

Tadasana
Mountain Pose

Also known as *Samasthiti* ('equal standing'), *Tadasana* is the basic standing pose and starting position for the standing poses, as well as for the Sun Salutation sequence. The aim of this pose is alignment, to stand as firm and erect as a mountain.

1. Stand with the feet together, heels and big toes touching, then lift and spread the toes and the balls of the feet evenly. The weight of the body should be distributed evenly across both feet, not in the heels or toes. Draw the thighs and kneecaps up and tighten the muscles on the backs of the thighs.

2. Pull the abdomen in and lift the chest, keeping the spine and neck straight. Relax the shoulders away from the ears and hang the arms beside the torso with the palms beside the thighs. Hold for 30–60 seconds.

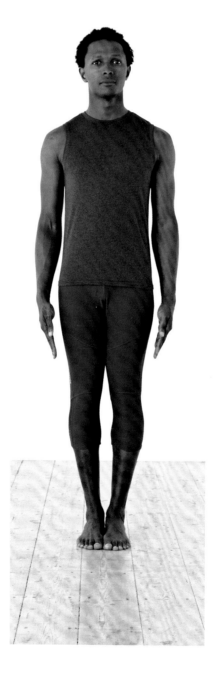

Benefits

- Improves posture.
- Strengthens the thighs, knees and ankles.
- Firms the abdomen and buttocks.

Cautions

- Not recommended for those with low blood pressure.

Anatomical Function

Upper body

- The erector spinae muscles work with the muscles in the small of the back to keep the spine upright.

- The abdominal and back muscles support and balance the torso.

- The rhomboids work with the middle part of the trapezius muscle, drawing the shoulder blades in and opening the chest.

Lower body

- The psoas and glutei muscles lengthen in order to keep the pelvis upright and balanced.

- The knees are kept straight by the shortening of the quadriceps muscles on the front of the thighs.

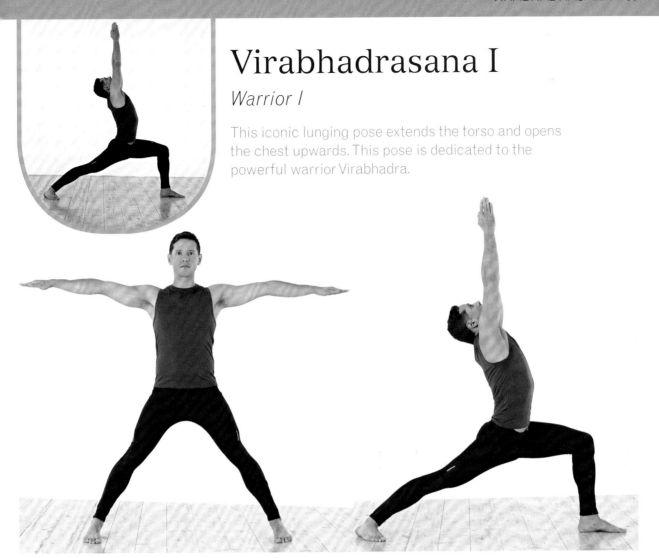

Virabhadrasana I

Warrior I

This iconic lunging pose extends the torso and opens the chest upwards. This pose is dedicated to the powerful warrior Virabhadra.

1. From *Tadasana* (see opposite), step the feet wide apart and take the arms out to the side. Turn the left foot to the left and turn the right foot in 45 degrees.

2. Bend the left knee and draw the left hip back and the right hip forward, so that the pelvis is square. Raise the arms and bring the palms together, drawing the shoulders down. Keep the head in a neutral position, or tilt it back and look up. Hold for 30–60 seconds. Exhale and release the arms down, straighten the right knee and turn the feet forward. Take a few breaths, then repeat the pose on the left side.

Benefits

- The chest is fully expanded to enable deep breathing.
- Strengthens the shoulders, arms and back; strengthens and stretches the thighs, calves and ankles.

Cautions

- Not recommended for those with high blood pressure or heart problems.
- Students with shoulder problems should keep their raised arms parallel to each other.
- Students with neck problems should keep their head in a neutral position.

Anatomical Function

- The erector spinae and quadratus lumborium muscles lift and arch the back; the abdominal muscles contract.
- Spinal rotation; scapular abduction and upwards rotation as the triceps assist in rotating the shoulder blade.
- Front leg: hip flexion; the quadriceps contract to support the body weight; also knee flexion and ankle dorsiflexion.
- Back leg: hip extension; the quadriceps straighten the knee; also ankle dorsiflexion and stretching of the calf muscles on the back of the leg.

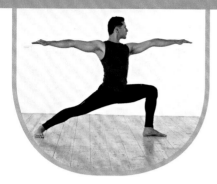

Virabhadrasana II

Warrior II

This pose develops strong muscles in the legs. The Warrior series is good preparation for the advanced standing poses and forward bending.

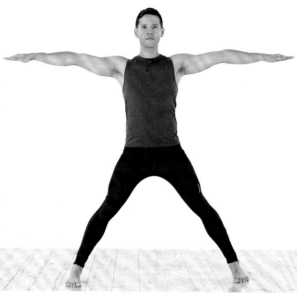

Anatomical Function

Upper body

- The erector spinae and quadratus lumborium muscles lift the back and arch it slightly, and the abdominal muscles contract to protect the lower back.

- The triceps straighten the elbows; the deltoids and rotator cuff muscles raise the arms and open the chest.

Lower body

- Front leg: hip flexion; the quadriceps contract to support the body weight; also knee flexion and ankle dorsiflexion.

- Back leg: the buttock muscle extends to enable hip extension.

- The quadriceps straighten the knee and the muscles along the front shin shorten to enable ankle dorsiflexion and to stretch the calf muscles on the back of the leg.

1. From *Tadasana* (see page 86), step the feet wide apart and take the arms out to the side. Turn the left foot to the left and turn the right foot in 45 degrees.

2. Bend the left knee and bring the thigh parallel to the floor. Extend the right hip back, keeping keep the right leg straight. Look over the left hand. Keep the shoulders level. The legs, dorsal region and hips should be in a straight line. Hold for 30–60 seconds. Exhale and release the arms down, straighten the right knee and turn the feet forward. Take a few breaths, then repeat the pose on the left side.

Benefits

- Strengthens and tones the calf and thigh muscles and relieves cramp.

- Tones the back muscles and the abdominal organs.

Cautions

- Not recommended for those with high blood pressure or heart problems.

- Students with neck problems should keep their head in a neutral position and not look over the left hand.

- Students with shoulder problems may place the hands on the hips or waist.

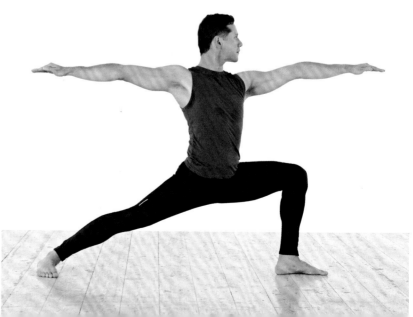

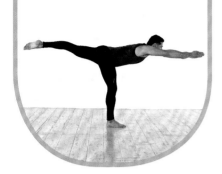

Virabhadrasana III
Warrior III

Warrior III is a more intense variation of Warrior I, bringing harmony, balance and poise. Standing firmly on the soles of the feet controls the abdominal muscles and develops agility.

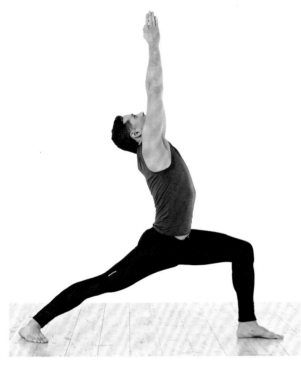

Anatomical Function

Upper body

- Scapular rotation, abduction and elevation due to the action of the upper trapezius.

- The anterior deltoids lift the arms, and the triceps straighten the elbows.

Lower body

- Standing leg: hip flexion and adduction; the gluteus medius muscle keeps the pelvis from rotating outwards.

- Knee extension is the action of the quadriceps, and ankle dorsiflexion the action of the peroneus longus and brevis muscles along the outside of the shin, which press the sole of the foot into the floor.

- The combined efforts of the gluteus maximus and gluteus medius muscles lift the raised leg; the erector spinae and quadratus lumborum in the small of the back lift the pelvis and spine; the rectus abdominus stabilizes the torso.

- The quadriceps straighten the knee.

1. From Warrior I (see page 87), bring the arms forward so they are in line with the shoulders. Inhale, lift the left heel and come onto the ball of the foot.

Benefits

- Strengthens and stretches the legs and ankles; stretches the groin, chest and lungs, and shoulders.

- Stimulates the abdominal organs.

Cautions

- Not recommended for those suffering from high blood pressure.

2. Exhale and bend the right knee as you bring more weight onto the right foot and raise the left leg. Keep the leg straight and bring it in line with the left hip. Straighten the right knee and bring the torso horizontal with the floor. Imagine someone pulling you by the hands and the foot as you lengthen the torso forward and back. Hold for 30 seconds and repeat on the left side.

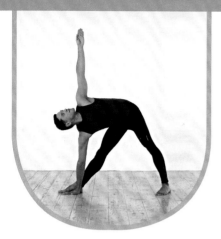

Utthita Trikonasana

Extended Triangle Pose

This pose stretches the hamstrings and calf muscles and also the abdominal and back muscles on the upper side of the body. Instead of stretching the top arm towards the ceiling, you can also stretch it over the back of the top ear, parallel to the floor.

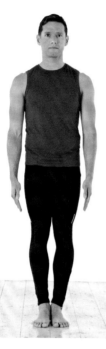

1. Starting in *Tadasana* (see page 86), step the left foot back approximately one leg length and line up the heels by turning the left heel 45 degrees in to the right.

2. Extend the right arm forward and the left arm back, keeping the arms in line with the shoulders and the palms facing down. Draw the shoulders down by pulling the shoulder blades into the middle of the back.

Benefits

- Strengthens and stretches the legs.
- Stretches the hips and spine.
- Opens the chest to improve breathing.
- Relieves mild back pain.
- Stimulates the abdominal organs.
- Improves the sense of balance.

Cautions

- Anyone suffering from back or spine injuries or low blood pressure should avoid this pose.

Anatomical Function

Upper body

- The triceps straighten the elbows; the serratus anterior muscle draws the lower arm towards the foot.
- The rhomboids and back of the deltoid draw the upper side of the trunk deeper into the twist.

Lower body

- Front Leg: the psoas works with the buttock muscles to create a wringing effect across the pelvis and stabilize the pose. The psoas works with the pectineus and adductor muscles to bend the hip over the front leg. The back-leg buttock muscle extends the leg behind the body and turns it outwards.
- Back Leg: The ankle turns slightly inwards, drawing the top of the foot towards the shin, which stretches the muscles in the back of the calf.

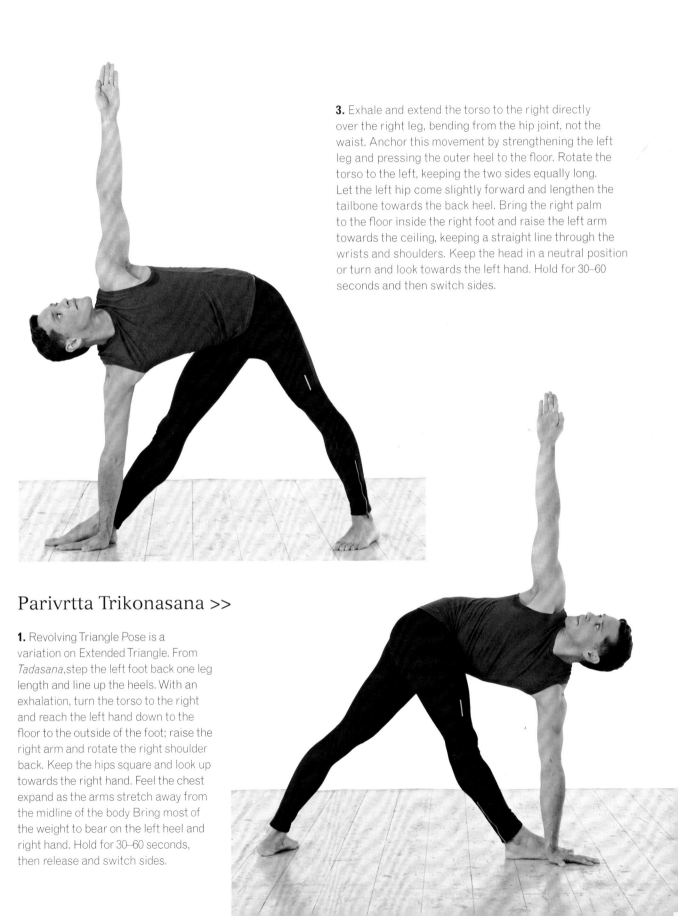

3. Exhale and extend the torso to the right directly over the right leg, bending from the hip joint, not the waist. Anchor this movement by strengthening the left leg and pressing the outer heel to the floor. Rotate the torso to the left, keeping the two sides equally long. Let the left hip come slightly forward and lengthen the tailbone towards the back heel. Bring the right palm to the floor inside the right foot and raise the left arm towards the ceiling, keeping a straight line through the wrists and shoulders. Keep the head in a neutral position or turn and look towards the left hand. Hold for 30–60 seconds and then switch sides.

Parivrtta Trikonasana >>

1. Revolving Triangle Pose is a variation on Extended Triangle. From *Tadasana*, step the left foot back one leg length and line up the heels. With an exhalation, turn the torso to the right and reach the left hand down to the floor to the outside of the foot; raise the right arm and rotate the right shoulder back. Keep the hips square and look up towards the right hand. Feel the chest expand as the arms stretch away from the midline of the body Bring most of the weight to bear on the left heel and right hand. Hold for 30–60 seconds, then release and switch sides.

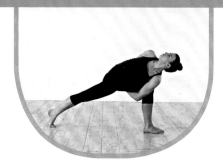

Parivrtta Parsvakonasana
Revolving Side-angle Twist

This pose twists the trunk to create a deep stretch of the muscles surrounding the spine. It also improves your balance.

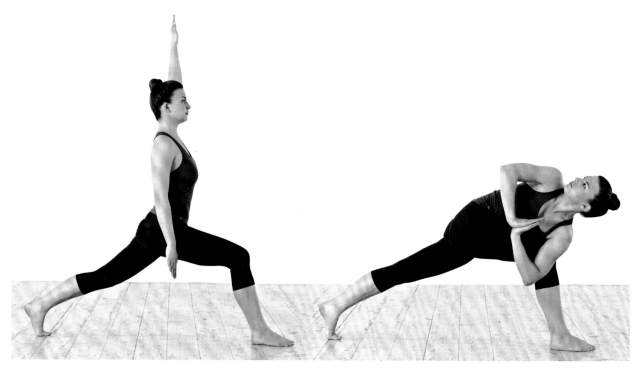

1. From *Tadasana* (see page 86), step the left foot back approximately one leg length. Bend the right knee so that the shin is perpendicular to the floor and align the right thigh parallel to the floor. Inhale and raise the left arm. Lift the left heel off and pivot on the ball of the foot until the insides of both feet are parallel. Keep the left leg active by lifting the thigh and extending through the left heel.

2. Exhale, turn to the right and bring the left arm outside the right knee. Press the arm against the knee and deepen the twist. Now bring the palms together in front of the chest with the elbows in a straight line, and finally turn the head to look up. Hold for 30–60 seconds and release or, if you are able, move on to the next step.

Anatomical Function

- The rear deltoid of the lower arm increases the twist by extending the shoulder, pressing the elbow onto the knee to open the lower half of the chest upwards.

- The pectoralis major and biceps brachii of the upper arm press the upper palm into the lower, which creates more pressure in the lower elbow against the knee to deepen the twist. The oblique abdominals twist the trunk and spine.

- The psoas, pectineus and anterior adductors work together to flex the front hip. The gluteus maximus turns the back hip outwards and to the rear. The quadriceps straighten the back knee.

Benefits

- Strengthens and stretches the legs, knees and ankles.
- Stretches the, spine, chest, lungs and shoulders.
- Stimulates the abdominal organs, improves digestion and aids elimination.

Cautions

- Not recommended for students with high or low blood pressure.
- Students with neck problems should look straight ahead or down at the floor instead of turning the head.

3. Try to fold the left arm through the right leg. Work at bringing the shoulder or armpit to the outside of the right knee. Once you have pushed the left hand through the right leg, reach the left arm behind the back and bind the hands. Grab either the fingers or the right wrist with the left hand. Turn the head to look up. Inhale, come up, then exhale to release the twist. Repeat to the left.

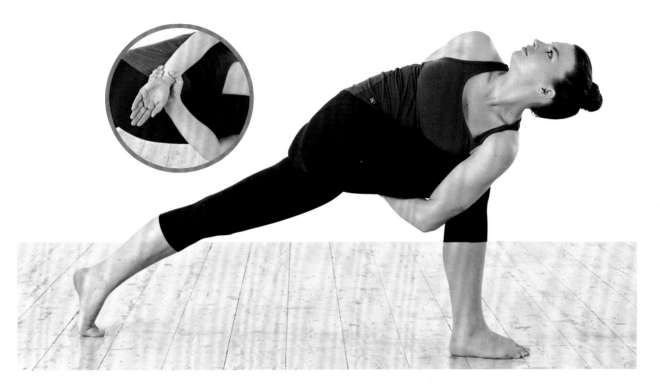

Advanced Variation

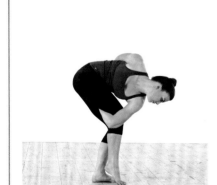

1. With the hands bound, turn the head to look forward and step the left foot forward to meet the right.

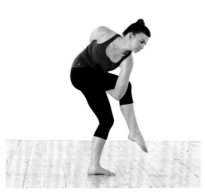

2. Slowly raise the right leg up.

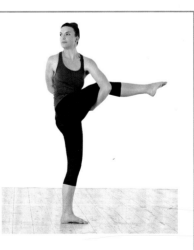

3. Come to a standing position, extend the right leg and look over the right shoulder.

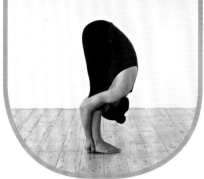

Uttanasana

Forward Bend

This pose helps identify any imbalances or asymmetry in the body, but the main purpose is to give the spine an intense stretch. *Uttanasana* can be used as a resting position between the standing poses. It can also be practised as a pose in itself.

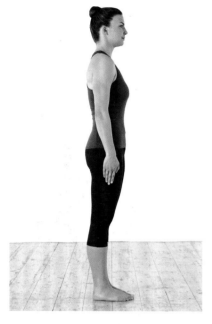

1. Stand in *Tadasana* (see page 86). Exhale and pull in the belly.

2. Fold forward from the hips and reach for both ankles. With each inhalation, lift the hips forward, lengthen the front torso and try to straighten the legs.

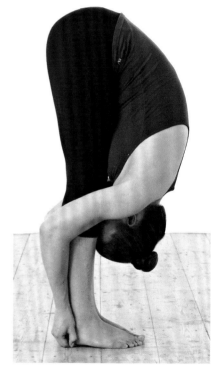

3. With each exhalation, release a little more fully into the pose to bring the belly onto the thighs. Let the head hang and allow the neck to lengthen. The forehead should eventually rest against the knees or shins. Keep drawing the kneecaps up as you lengthen over the legs. Hold the pose for 30–60 seconds.

Anatomical Function

Upper body

- Rectus abdominis muscle contracts to bend the trunk.
- The deltoids draw the shoulders forward and the biceps bend the elbows.

Lower body

- Activating the psoas, pectineus and rectus femoris muscles flexes the hips and lifts the pelvis forward.
- The quadriceps contract and straighten the knees.
- Adductor muscles on the insides of the thighs draw them together.

Benefits

- Stretches the hamstrings, calves and hips.
- Stimulates the liver and kidneys.
- Strengthens the thighs and knees.
- Improves digestion.
- Reduces fatigue and anxiety.

Cautions

- Students with a back injury should perform this pose with bent knees.

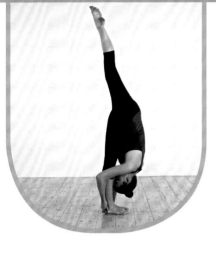

Urdhva Prasarita Eka Padasana

One Leg Raised Up

The standing-splits pose stretches and tones the legs and is also a great preparation for the Handstand Pose.

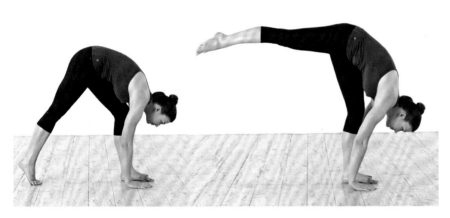

1. From *Tadasana* (see page 86), step the right leg back, then bend forward and bring both hands to the floor either side of the left foot.

2. Take hold of the left ankle and raise the right leg as high as possible with the toes pointed and the knee straight.

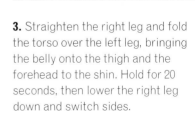

Anatomical Function

Upper body

- Rectus abdominis muscle contracts to bend the trunk.

- The deltoids draw the shoulders forward and the biceps bend the elbows.

Lower body

- Activating the psoas, pectineus and rectus femoris muscles flexes the hips and lifts the pelvis forward.

- The quadriceps contract and straighten the knees.

Benefits

- Tones and stretches the hamstrings, calves and hips.

- Massages the abdominal organs.

- Improves balance.

Cautions

- Not recommended for students suffering from high or low blood pressure.

3. Straighten the right leg and fold the torso over the left leg, bringing the belly onto the thigh and the forehead to the shin. Hold for 20 seconds, then lower the right leg down and switch sides.

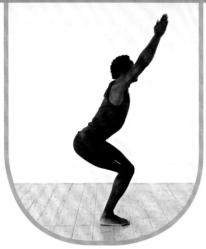

Utkatasana

Chair Pose

This pose relieves stiffness in the shoulders and strengthens the muscles that flex the pelvis, quadriceps and the muscles in the lower back.

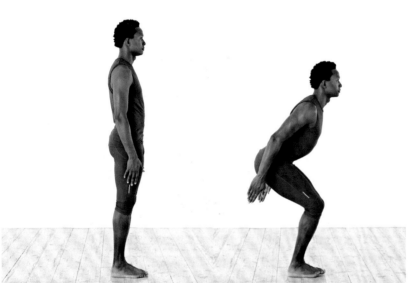

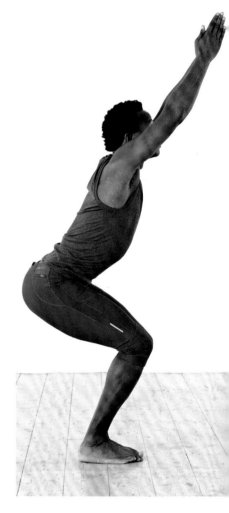

1. Stand in *Tadasana* (see page 86).

2. Bend the knees and shift the torso forward so that the torso and shins are parallel. Keep the inner thighs parallel to each other.

3. Raise the arms over the head. Keep the arms parallel, palms facing inwards, or join the palms. Hold for 30 seconds. To release the pose, inhale and straighten the knees, then exhale to lower the arms to the sides.

Anatomical Function

Lower body

- Hip-flexor muscles keep the femurs in a flexed position.

- The quadriceps muscles keep the knees partially flexed and the adductor muscles draw the knees together.

Lower body

- The lower back is slightly arched by the action of the quadratus lumborum muscle; the psoas protects the lower spine by providing a counterbalance to the action of the lower-back muscles.

- The anterior deltoids raise the arms and the triceps extend the elbows.

Benefits

- Strengthens the ankles, thighs, calves and spine.

- Stretches the shoulders and chest.

- Stimulates the abdominal organs, diaphragm and heart.

Cautions

- Not recommended for those with low blood pressure.

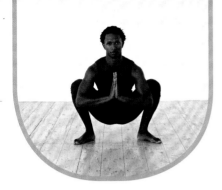

Malasana

Garland or Squatting Pose

Malasana provides deep hip flexion and stretches to the back of the legs, the back and the neck muscles.

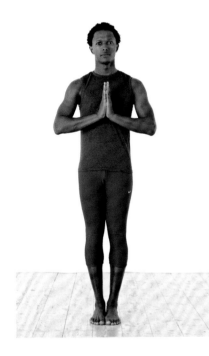

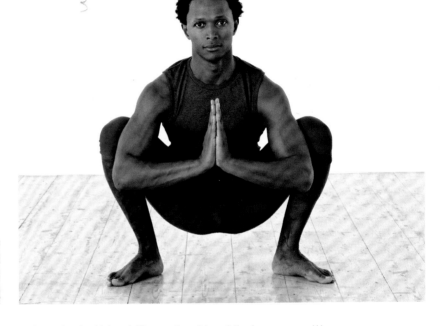

1. Standing in *Tadasana* (see page 86), bring the hands together in front of the chest.

2. Step the feet hip width apart and bend the knees, squatting down, then bring the shoulders inside the thighs and lift the chest to keep the spine straight. Hold for 30–60 seconds. To release, bring the palms to the floor and straighten the knees to slowly come up to a standing position.

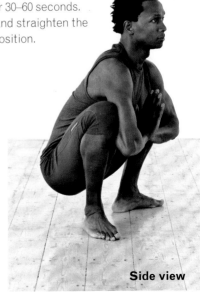

Side view

Benefits

- Stretches the ankles, groin and back torso.
- Tones the abdomen.

Cautions

- Not recommended for students with lower-back problems or knee injuries.

Anatomical Function

- The psoas, pectineus, rectus femoris and sartorius give deep flexion at the hips.
- The quadriceps muscles flex the knees.
- In the lower back, the quadratus lumborum muscle keeps the spine straight.
- The trapezius muscles draw the shoulders down and the biceps bend the elbows.

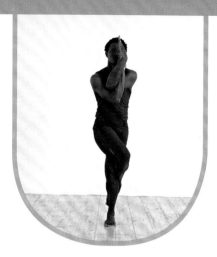

Garudasana

Eagle Pose

This pose is particularly effective for improving balance and coordination, as the balance over one leg and folding and twisting of the arms challenges the way the brain sees the body.

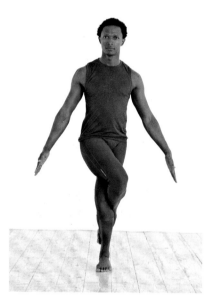

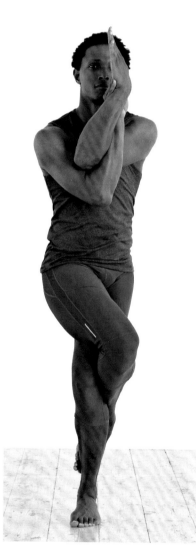

1. Stand in *Tadasana* (see page 86). Bend the knees slightly, lift the right foot and, balancing on the left foot, cross the right thigh over the left. Point the right toes towards the floor, press the foot back and then hook the top of the foot behind the lower left calf. Balance on the left foot.

2. Raise the arms in front of you and cross the left arm over the right, then bend the elbows and bring the backs of the hands to face each other. Cross the wrists and bring the palms together (or as nearly together as you can), lift the elbows up and stretch the fingers towards the ceiling. Hold the pose for 15–30 seconds. Release and repeat with the arms and legs reversed.

Variation

Assume the full pose, then exhale and lean the torso forward, pressing the forearms against the thigh of the top leg. Hold for a few breaths, then come up with an inhalation. Release and repeat on the other side.

Tip

Beginners often find it difficult to hook the raised-leg foot behind the standing-leg calf and then balance on the standing foot. As a short-term option, cross the legs but, instead of hooking the raised foot, press the big toe of the raised-leg foot against the floor to help maintain balance.

Anatomical Function

Upper body

- As for *Vatyanasama*, opposite.

Lower body

- The pose is stabilized by the gastrocnemius/soleus of the calf, which flexes the standing ankle to press the foot down.

- Adductor muscles squeeze the thighs together and the tensor fascia lata and gluteus medius rotate the femurs internally.

Benefits

- Strengthens and stretches the ankles and calves.

- Stretches the thighs, hips, shoulders and upper back.

- Improves the sense of balance.

Cautions

- Students with knee injuries should avoid this pose.

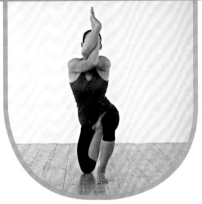

Vatyanasana

Horse Pose

This pose is so called as it is generally considered to resemble a horse's face.

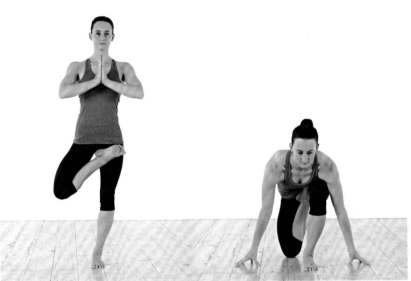

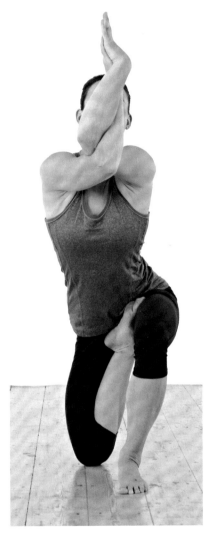

1. From *Tadasana* (see page 86), lift the right foot on top of the left thigh into Half Lotus Pose (see page 142).

2. Slowly bend the left knee and lower the hands and then the top of the right knee to the floor, close to the left foot.

Anatomical Function

Upper body

- The psoas muscle flexes the hips.

- The arms and shoulders are adducted across the chest.

- Eccentric contraction of the deltoid in the upper arm deepens the stretch of the rotator cuff.

Lower body

- Left leg: hip flexion due to contraction of the psoas and pectineus muscles. The quadriceps contract to support the body weight; there is also knee flexion and ankle dorsiflexion.

- Right leg: hip extension due to the gluteus muscles. Knee flexion as the hamstring muscles shorten.

Benefits

- Improves circulation in the hip joints.

- Corrects any deformities to the hip and thigh region and loosens the sacroiliac region.

Cautions

- Not recommended for students with knee, shoulder or wrist problems.

3. Raise the arms and straighten the spine, keeping the back erect. Cross the left arm over the right, then bend the elbows and bring the backs of the hands to face each other. Cross the wrists and bring the palms together (or as nearly together as you can), lift the elbows up and stretch the fingers towards the ceiling. Hold the pose for 15–30 seconds. Release and repeat with the arms and legs reversed.

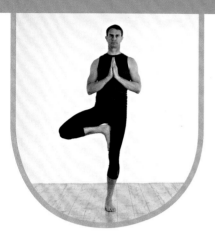

Vrikshasana

Tree Pose

Vrikshasana is considered to be the easier of the one-legged standing poses, as the bones of the upper body are stacked over the standing leg.

Anatomical Function

Upper body

- The erector spinae muscles hold the spine upright.

- The lower trapezius, which spans the back, draws the shoulders downwards.

- The middle trapezius and rhomboids draw the shoulder blades towards the spine and open the front of the chest.

- The biceps bend the elbows.

Lower body

- The gluteus maximus in the buttocks works with the psoas muscle to balance the pelvis from front to back.

- The quadriceps shorten to straighten the left knee.

- The calf muscles, peronei, tibialis anterior and toe flexors work to stabilize the foot.

- The gluteus maximus turns the right hip out, and external rotator muscles in the hip keep the hip turning out.

Benefits

- Strengthens thighs, calves, ankles and spine.

- Improves the sense of balance.

- Relieves sciatica and reduces the effects of flat feet.

Cautions

- Not recommended for students with low blood pressure.

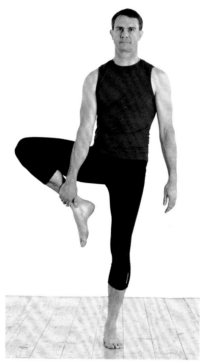

1. Standing in *Tadasana* (see page 86), shift the weight slightly onto the left foot and bend the right knee. Reach down with the right hand and grab the ankle or shin. Place the sole of the right foot on the inside of the left thigh with the toes pointing towards the floor. There should be equal pressure between the sole of the right foot and the inner left thigh.

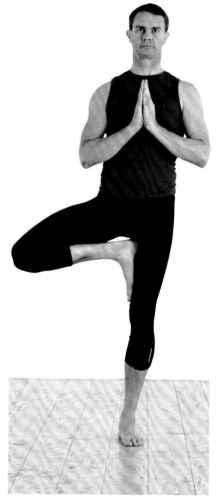

2. Place the hands on the hips, then raise the hands in front of the chest with the palms together. Gaze softly at a fixed point in front of you or focus on the space between the eyebrows. Hold the pose for 30–60 seconds. Release the foot down and switch to the left leg.

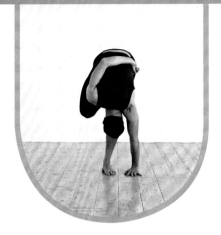

Ardha Baddha Padmottanasana

Half-bound Lotus Forward Bend

In Sanskrit, *ardha* means half, *baddha* means bound or caught, *padma* is lotus and *uttana* is an intense stretch.

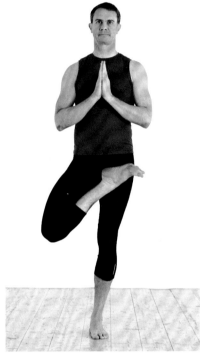

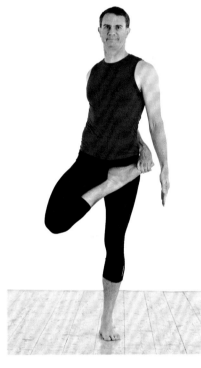

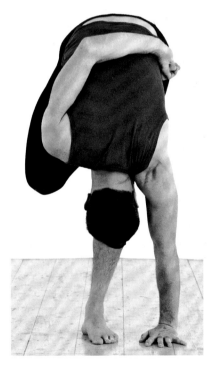

1. From *Tadasana* (see page 86), raise the right leg and bring the foot on top of the left thigh in Half Lotus Pose (see page 142).

2. Reach the right hand behind the back and grab the right foot. Exhale and bend forward.

3. Place the left hand on the floor beside the foot. Inhale and raise the head, then exhale and fold deeper to to rest the forehead or chin against the knee or shin. Hold for 10–15 seconds. To release, bend the left knee and slowly raise the trunk to come up, then release the right foot and lower it to the floor.

Anatomical Function

- Rectus abdominis muscle contracts to bend the trunk; activating the psoas, pectineus and rectus femoris muscles flexes the hips.

- The quadriceps contract to keep the left knee straight; the hamstrings bend the right knee.

- The calf muscles, peronei, tibialis anterior and toe flexors work to stabilize the left foot.

Benefits

- This pose helps stiffness in the knees and increases hip flexibility.

- Helps digestion and eliminates toxins.

Cautions

- Not recommended for students with knee problems.

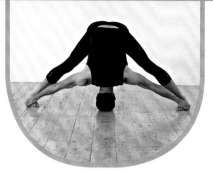

Prasarita Padottanasana
Wide-legged Forward Bend

This pose helps create more symmetry in the body. The body is activated and stretched on both sides and, through regular practice, any imbalances are corrected.

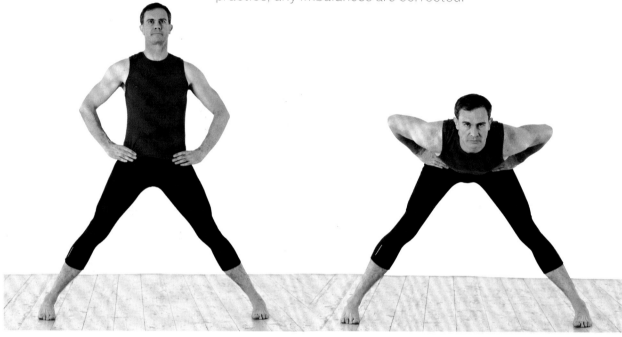

1. Stand with the legs approximately one leg length apart and turn the insides of the feet to face each other. Rest the hands on the hips. Engage the thigh muscles by drawing them up. Inhale, lift the chest and draw the abdomen in slightly.

2. Exhale and fold forward from the hip joints. Bring the torso parallel to the floor.

Anatomical Function

Upper body

- The rectus abdominis muscle bends the trunk forward.

- The lower section of the trapezius draws the shoulders away from the ears to free and lengthen the neck.

- The triceps straighten the arms.

Lower body

- The hips flex, due to the action of the psoas and rectus femoris muscles on the front of the thighs.

- The knees are straightened due to the action of the quadriceps muscles, and the hamstrings are lengthened.

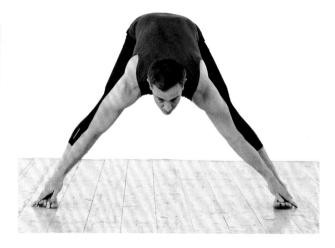

3. Reach for the sides of the feet or the ankles. Inhale and lift the chest, keeping the spine long.

4. Take a few more breaths, then lower the head to the floor by gently pulling against the feet to draw yourself down. The aim is to bring the feet, hands and head into a straight line. Hold for 30–60 seconds. To break the pose, bring the hands onto the hips and then raise the trunk.

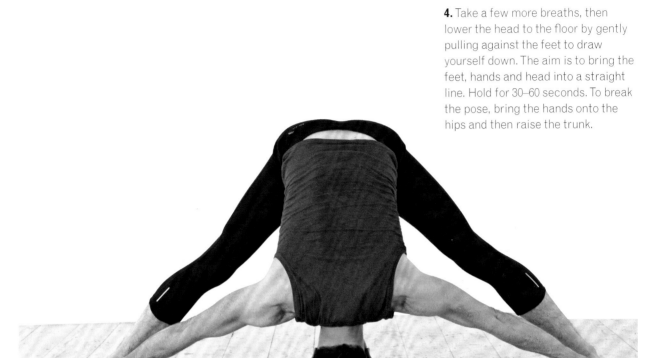

Variation

Assume the full pose, then bring the hands behind the back into a prayer position and press the palms together in *Anjali Mudra* (Salutation Seal). The fingers should be pointing towards the head, ideally between the shoulder blades. Roll the shoulders back and lift the chest, pressing the sides of the palms into the middle of the back. Finally exhale into the forward bend and bring the head close to or onto the floor. If you can't achieve this hand position, simply cross the forearms behind the back and hold each elbow with the opposite hand.

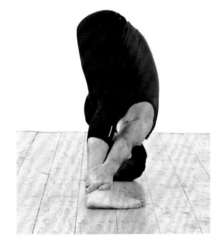

Side view

Benefits

- Strengthens and stretches the inner and back legs and the spine.
- Tones the abdominal organs.
- Relieves mild backache.

Cautions

- Students with lower-back problems should avoid the full forward bend.

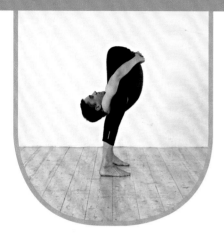

Utthita Tittibhasana

Insect Pose

The full expression of this pose requires a great deal of flexibility in the hips and the hamstrings. If there is any discomfort in the lower back or hamstrings, bend the knees.

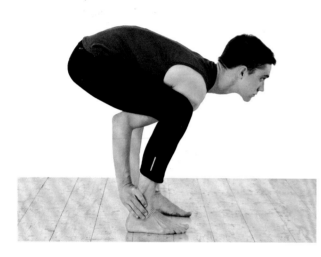

1. Bend the knees and squat with the feet shoulder distance apart. Tilt the pelvis forward and bring the trunk between the legs. Keeping the trunk low, straighten the legs enough to lift the pelvis to about knee height.

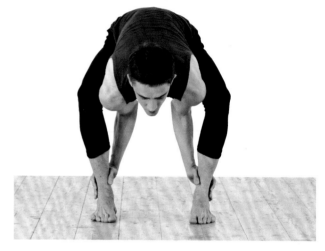

2. Bring the arms through the legs and grab the back of each ankle. Then pull the shoulders through the legs, tucking the shoulders behind the backs of the knees.

Benefits

• Stretches the inner groin and back of the torso.

• Tones the belly.

Cautions

• Not recommended for those with shoulder, elbow, wrist or lower-back injuries.

Anatomical Function

Upper body

• The trapezius and rhomboid muscles are stretched.

• Scapular abduction as the shoulder blades are drawn apart.

Lower body

• The adductor muscles on the inner thighs squeeze the thighs against the upper arms, connecting the upper and lower body.

• The psoas and rectus abdominis muscles flex the hips and bend the trunk.

• The hamstrings straighten the legs.

Tip

Some students have a difficult time lifting into this pose from the floor. Try squatting on a block, so that your feet are off the floor. It will help raise your seat and prepare you for the balance.

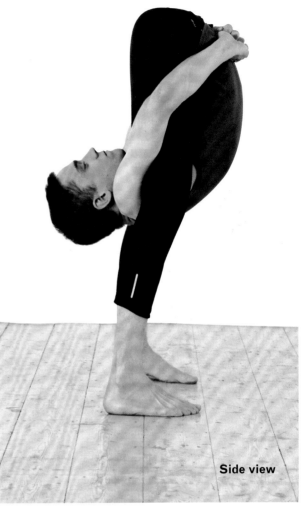

Side view

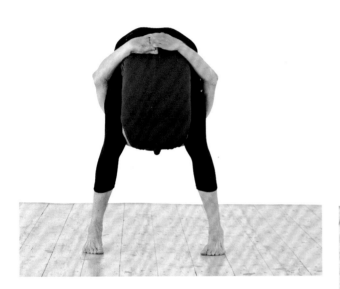

3. Bring the right arm around the back of the right thigh and reach it around the trunk. Bring the left arm around the back of the left thigh, reach it around the trunk and clasp the hands behind the back. Turn the head to look up through the legs towards the ceiling. Keep pulling the shoulders through the legs and straighten the knees.

Stork Pose Variation

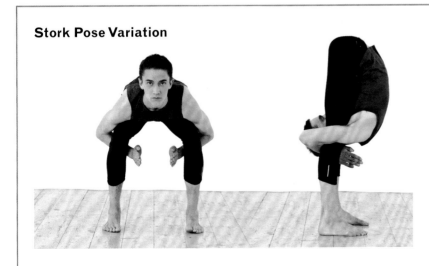

With the feet a little more than hip-width apart, bend the knees and bring the arms behind the back of the legs, then bring the hands through the legs. Bend forward and lower the head. Either place the palms against the ears, interlace the fingers behind the back of head or press the palms together in a prayer position behind the back of the head, as shown here.

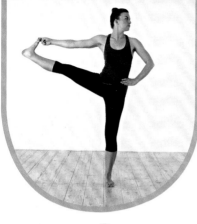

Uttitha Hasta Padangusthasana

Extended Hand to Toe Pose

This pose strengthens the leg muscles, and the balance brings steadiness and poise.

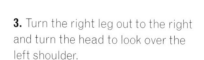

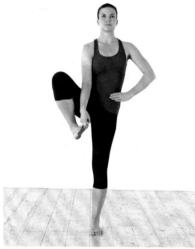

1. From *Tadasana* (see page 86), place the left hand on the left hip and raise the right knee. Hook the big toe of the right foot with the first two fingers of the right hand.

2. Exhale, extend the right leg forward and pull it up.

3. Turn the right leg out to the right and turn the head to look over the left shoulder.

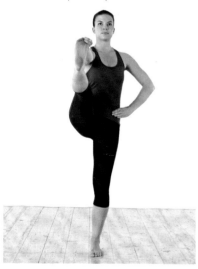

Anatomical Function

Upper body

- The raised arm produces shoulder flexion, while the triceps extend the elbow.

Lower body

- Standing leg: the hamstrings lengthen and the quadriceps shorten to keep the knee straight.
- On the raised leg, hip flexion occurs due to the iliacus, psoas and adductor muscles.
- Ankle dorsiflexion.

Benefits

- Strengthens the legs and ankles.
- Stretches the backs of the legs.
- Improves the sense of balance.

Cautions

- Not recommended for those with ankle or lower-back injuries.

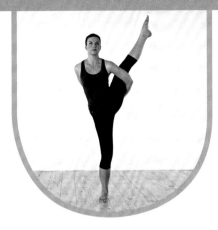

Svarga Dvijasana

Bird of Paradise Pose

This is one of the more difficult poses to do well. It challenges your focus, balance, strength and flexibility.

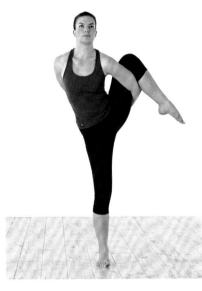

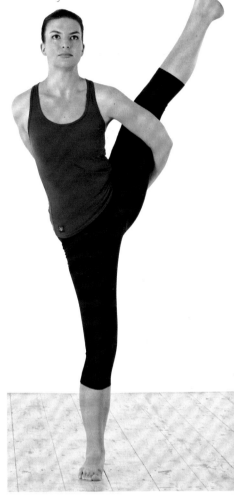

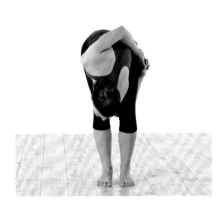

1. Stand with the legs hip width apart. Bend the knees, bring the left shoulder to the left knee and take the left arm through the legs. Now bend the right arm and take it behind the back, keeping the shoulder close to the knee. Bring the left arm behind the back and bind the hands. Keeping the hands bound together, try to straighten the knees and pull the right shoulder through the legs.

2. Move the weight into the right foot and lift the left heel. Slowly raise the left leg, still keeping the hands bound together. At the same time lift the right shoulder and come up to a stand.

3. Keep lifting the shoulder back and try to straighten the left knee, pointing the toes on the left foot.

Variation

Release the hands and keep the left arm wrapped around the left leg. Reach for the outside of the left foot with the right hand and pull the left leg up, bringing it behind the shoulder; try to straighten the knee. The right arm should be behind the head as you pull the left leg up straight. See photograph on page 84.

Benefits

- Strengthens the legs and ankles.
- Stretches the backs of the legs.
- Improves the sense of balance.

Cautions

- Not recommended for those with ankle or lower-back injuries.

Anatomical Function

Upper body

- Shoulder flexion occurs due to the action of the deltoid muscles.

Lower body

- Standing leg and raised leg: as for *Uttista Hasta Padangusthasana*, opposite.
- The quadriceps straighten the knee.

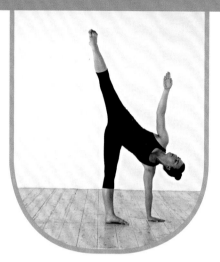

Ardha Chandrasana
Half Moon Pose

In this pose the body weight is on one leg, with one hand extended and one touching the floor. The raised leg acts as a counterbalance. The pose tones the lower spine and nerves connected with the muscles in the legs.

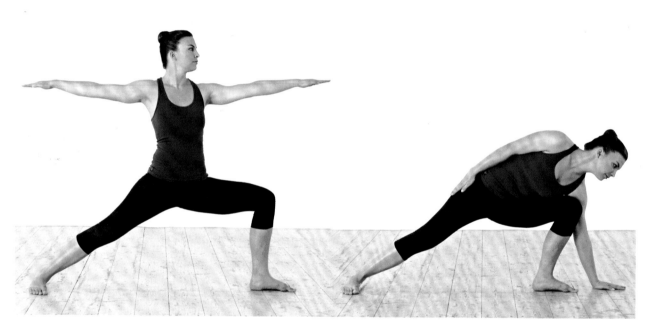

1. Perform *Virabhadrasana II* (see page 88) by turning the left foot forward and bending the knee, with the left arm extended forward and the right arm extended back.

2. Reach the left hand down to the floor beyond the left foot and slightly over to the left.

Anatomical Function

Upper body

- The erector spinae and oblique abdominal muscles bend the trunk over the standing leg.

- The triceps straighten the elbows.

- The anterior deltoids abduct the arms.

- The lower and middle trapezius open the chest and draw the shoulders away from the neck.

Lower body

- The pose is stabilized by the psoas and pectineus muscles, which tilt the hip slightly forward.

- The quadriceps straighten both knees.

- The gluteus medius, gluteus minimus and tensor fascia lata lift the raised leg.

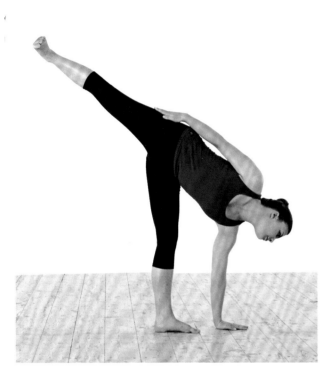

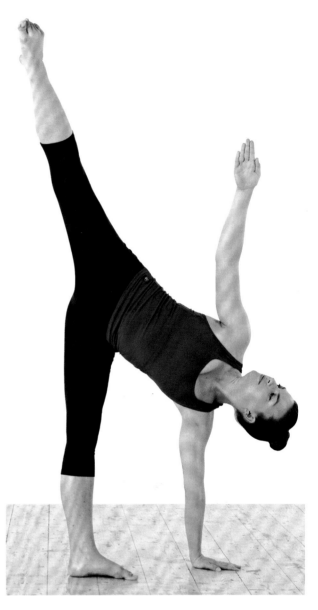

Tip

Beginners can keep the right hand on the right hip and the head in a neutral position, gazing forward. The body's weight is mainly on the standing leg. The left hand is used to assist your balance and can be placed flat on the floor or on the fingertips.

3. Exhale and press the left hand and foot firmly into the floor. Straighten the left leg while raising the right leg until it is at least parallel to the floor. Extend through the right toes to keep the raised leg active and the muscles engaged. Be careful not to lock or hyperextend the standing knee.

4. Rotate the right hip and shoulder upwards and raise the right arm with the fingers extended, turning the head to look up. Hold for 30–60 seconds. Then lower the raised leg to the floor with an exhalation and return to *Virabhadrasana*. Repeat the pose on the right side.

Benefits

- Strengthens the abdomen, ankles, thighs, buttocks and spine.
- The arms are extended away from the body, toning the muscles in the shoulders and arms.
- Improves coordination and sense of balance.

Cautions

- If you have any neck problems, don't turn the head to look upwards.
- Not recommended for those suffering from low blood pressure.

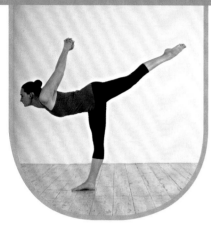

Patan Vrikshasana

Wobbling Tree Pose

This pose helps us to stand correctly on the soles of the feet, tones the stomach muscles and shoulders and brings agility to the body.

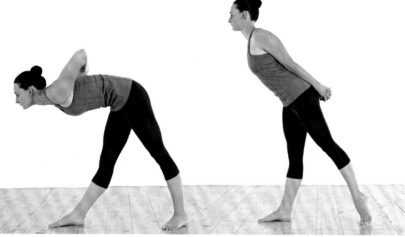

Anatomical Function

Upper body

- The lower trapezius draws the shoulders down to free the neck.
- The erector spinae muscle keeps the spine straight, creating axial extension.
- Infraspinatus and teres minor muscles externally rotate the shoulders.
- The triceps straighten the elbows.

Lower body

- Psoas muscles bends the hip on the right leg.
- Quardriceps straighten both knees.

1. From *Tadasana* (see page 86), step the right foot forward one leg length and line up the heels by turning the left heel 45 degrees in to the right. Interlace the hands behind the the back.

2. Lift the chest forward and bring the weight onto the right foot and slowly raise the left leg up.

Benefits

- Strengthens the spine and shoulders.
- Strengthens the leg muscles.
- Improves balance.

Cautions

- Not recommended for those suffering from high or low blood pressure.

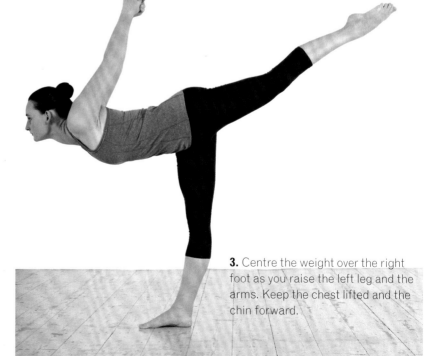

3. Centre the weight over the right foot as you raise the left leg and the arms. Keep the chest lifted and the chin forward.

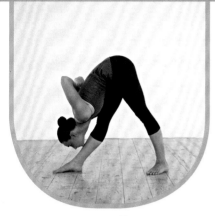

Parsvottanasana

Intense Side-stretch Pose

The pose relieves stiffness in the legs, makes the hips and spine more flexible and tones the abdominal organs.

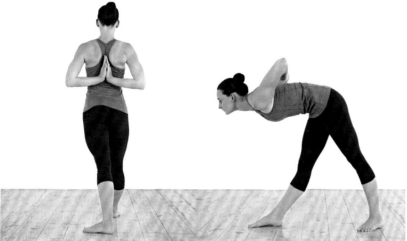

Anatomical Function

Upper body

- The rectus abdominis bends the trunk towards the front thigh.

- The lower trapezius draws the shoulders down to free the neck.

Lower body

- Front leg: the psoas enables the front hip to bend and stabilizes the back hip and leg.

- The quadriceps create knee extension over the legs.

1. From *Tadasana* (see page 86), step the right foot forward one leg length and line up the heels by turning the left heel 45 degrees in to the right. Take the arms behind the back and press the palms together in a prayer position. If you can't do this, fold the arms behind the back and grab the elbows.

2. Ensure that the pelvis is facing forward. Inhale and lift the breastbone, then exhale the torso forward over the right leg until the torso is parallel to the floor. Hold for a few breaths.

3. If you have the flexibility, bring the front of the torso closer to the top of the thigh. Eventually it will rest against the front of the thigh. Hold the maximum position for 15–30 seconds, then come up with an inhalation by pressing actively through the back heel. Break the pose and switch sides.

Benefits

- Stretches the spine, shoulders and wrists (in the full pose), hips and hamstrings.

- Strengthens the legs.

- Stimulates the abdominal organs.

Cautions

- If you have a back injury or high blood pressure, avoid the full forward bend.

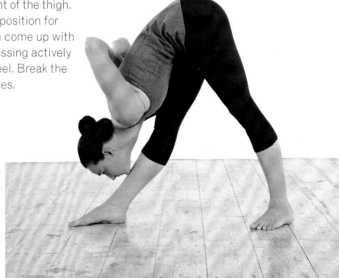

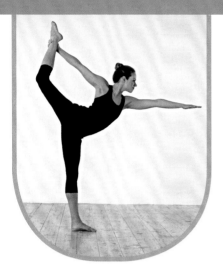

Natarajasana

Dancer Pose

This is an asymmetrical standing backward-bend pose, requiring good balance and concentration. If you practise this pose at home, try holding on to a door handle as you pull the raised leg up as high as you can.

Anatomical Function

Upper body

- The serratus anterior and trapezius upwardly rotate and abduct the shoulder blade. The rotator cuff, anterior deltoid and biceps brachialis create shoulder flexion, adduction and external rotation.

- The forearms supinate.

Lower body

- On the standing leg the action of the psoas muscle creates hip flexion and the quadriceps creates knee extension.

- On the raised leg there is hip extension, knee flexion due to the quadriceps extension, and hamstring contraction and ankle plantar flexion as a result of the action of the gastrocnemius muscles.

Benefits

- Stretches the shoulders and chest.

- Stretches the thighs, groin and abdomen.

- Strengthens the legs and ankles.

Cautions

- Not recommended for those with low blood pressure.

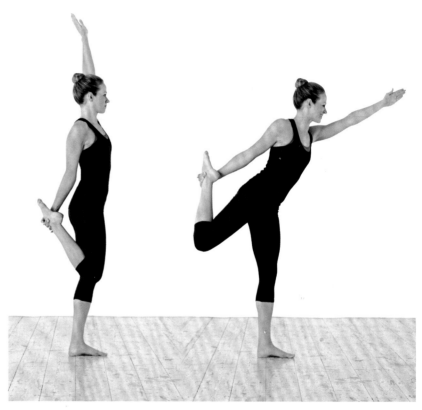

1. Stand in *Tadasana* (see page 86). Inhale, bend the right knee and lift the right foot. With the right palm facing up, reach back and grab the right foot or ankle. If you take hold of the inner part of the foot or shin, you can raise the leg higher. If this isn't possible, hold the outside of the foot.

2. Lift the foot up, away from the torso. Extend the thigh behind you and pull the leg up high.

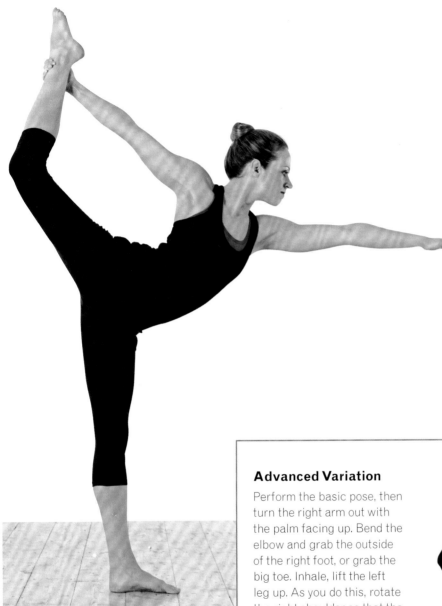

3. Try to straighten the knee and stretch the left arm forward, in front of the torso and parallel to the floor. Hold the pose for 20–30 seconds. Then let go of the foot, place it back on the floor and repeat for the same length of time on the other side.

Advanced Variation

Perform the basic pose, then turn the right arm out with the palm facing up. Bend the elbow and grab the outside of the right foot, or grab the big toe. Inhale, lift the left leg up. As you do this, rotate the right shoulder so that the bent elbow points towards the ceiling. It requires extreme flexibility to externally rotate and flex the shoulder joint in this way. Reach the left arm over the head and grab the foot. Hold for 20–30 seconds, release and repeat on the other side for the same length of time.

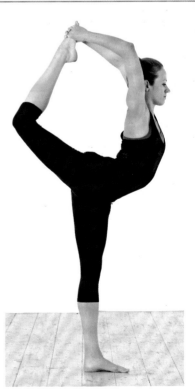

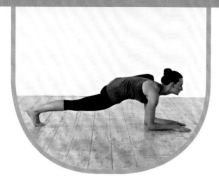

Uttan Pristhasana

Lizard Pose

The Lizard Pose increases hip flexibility, stretches the hamstrings and strengthens the buttocks.

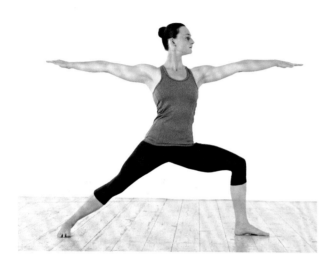

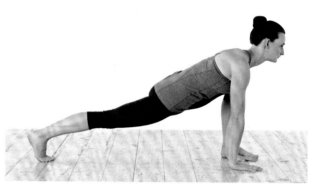

1. Perform *Virabhadrasana II* (see page 88), with the left leg forward and right leg back.

2. Place both hands on the floor inside the left foot. Align the tips of the fingers with the toes. Keep the arms straight and lift the right knee. Look forward.

Benefits

- Strengthens shoulders, arms and wrists
- Creates greater hip flexion.

Cautions

- Avoid if suffering with hip or hamstring problems.

Anatomical Function

Upper body

- The pectoralis major and anterior deltoid muscles stabilize the shoulders.
- The tricep muscles straighten the elbows in step 2; the bicep muscles bend the elbows in step 3.

Lower body

- The psoas muscles are active to flex the left hip and are in neutral to extend the right hip.
- The hamstring muscles bend the left knee and the quadricep muscles sraighten the right knee.

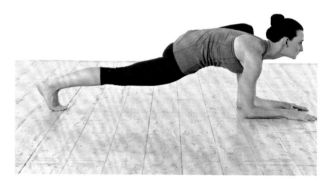

3. If possible, lower the elbows to the floor and line up the elbows with the left heel, so that the upper arms and left shin are aligned and vertical. Hold the pose for 15–20 seconds. To release, lift the elbows and step the right foot back. Repeat the pose on the right side.

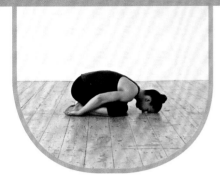

Balasana

Child's Pose

This restorative pose can be practised at any time, especially during a dynamic practice or after an inversion such as Head Stand.

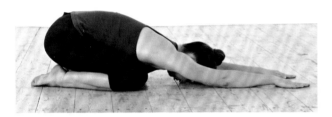

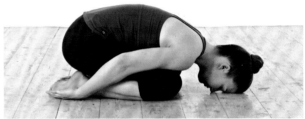

1. Begin by coming to a kneeling position and sit on the heels. Then exhale and bring the torso forward over the thighs and bring the arms forward, with palms resting on the floor.

2. Rest the forehead on the floor and lengthen the spine from the tailbone to the base of the skull. Relax the abdomen onto the thighs and bring the hands beside the feet with the palms facing up.

3.Place the hands on the floor alongside the torso, palms facing up, and relax the shoulders toward the floor.

4.Balasana is a resting pose. Stay anything from 30 seconds to a few minutes.

Benefits

- Gently stretches the hips, thighs and ankles.
- Helps relieve stress and fatigue.

Cautions

- Do not practise during pregnancy.
- If you have a knee injury, avoid unless you have the supervision of an experienced teacher.

Anatomical Function

Upper body

- Spinal flexion. The muscles of the back are passively stretched.

Lower body

- Hip flexion due to the psoas muscle and adduction.
- Knee flexion.
- Ankle plantar flexion.

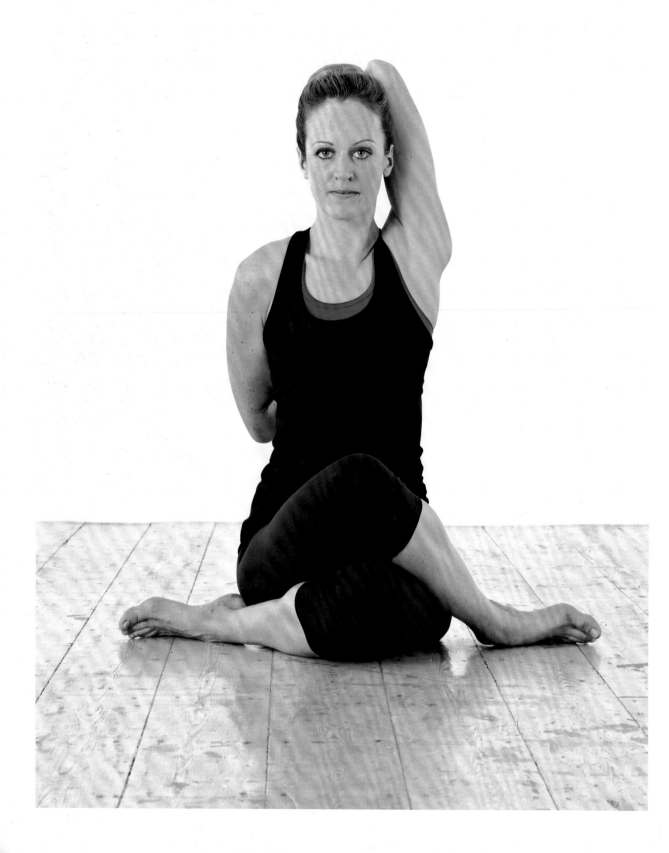

Seated Poses

Most of us spend many of our waking hours sitting on chairs, sofas or in cars, buses and trains. In the same way that bare feet reconnect with the earth through the standing poses, our lower body, hips, pelvic joints and lower spine connect with the earth in sitting poses, removing the need to balance or support the body and leaving the upper body free to extend and release upwards. On a physical level, sitting poses stretch, bend and twist the spine, release the hips and groin and restore natural function to the pelvis and lower back. They give the body the strength and flexibility necessary to sit quietly for long periods and they still the mind, helping to control the senses, taking us to a deeper level of consciousness.

Paschimottanasana 118
Janu Sirsasana 120
Ardha Matsyendrasana 122
Marichyasana I 124
Upavistha Konasana 126
Badhha Konasana 128
Eka Pada Sirsasana 130
Dwi Pada Sirsasana 132
Bharadvajasana 134
Kurmasana 136

Parivrtta Surya Yantrasana 138
Gomukhasana 139
Paripurana Navasana 140
Sukkhasana & Siddhasana 141
Padmasana 142
Hanumanasana 144

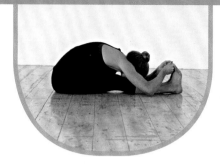

Paschimottanasana

Back-stretch Forward Bend

The spine should lengthen and not be rounded when performing this back-stretching pose.

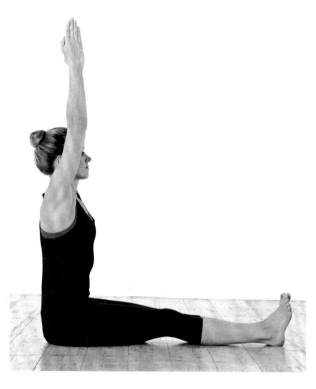

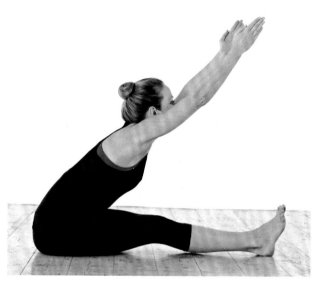

1. Sit on the floor with the legs straight. Flex the ankles and point the toes towards you so that the backs of the knees touch the floor. Bring the palms or fingertips to the floor beside the hips and lift the chest, then inhale and raise the arms.

2. Keep the chest lifted and the front of the torso long. Lift the chin away from the chest, fold forward and bring the belly onto the thighs. The lower belly should touch the thighs first, then the upper belly, then the ribs and the head last.

Benefits

• Calming, helping to relieve stress and mild depression.

• Stretches the spine, shoulders and hamstrings.

• Stimulates the liver, kidneys, ovaries and uterus.

• Improves digestion.

Cautions

• Not recommended for asthma sufferers.

• If you have a back injury, perform this pose only under the supervision of an experienced teacher.

Anatomical Function

Upper body

- The rectus abdominis muscle bends the trunk forward.
- The biceps bend the elbows to deepen the stretch by bringing the torso over the thighs.

Lower body

- The psoas, pectineus, rectus femoris and sartorius muscles flex the hips.
- The adductor muscles draw the thighs together.
- The knees are straightened by the action of the quadriceps, and the hamstrings are stretched.
- Flexing the ankles stretches the calf muscles.

3. Hold the sides of the feet with the hands or wrap the arms around the sides of the feet and keep the knees fully extended; if this isn't possible, bend the knees and bring the belly onto the thighs, but keep the spine straight.

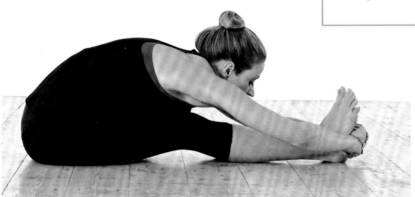

4. With each inhalation, lift and lengthen the front of the torso slightly; with each exhalation release a little more fully into the forward bend. Hold the pose for 60 seconds, then slowly release.

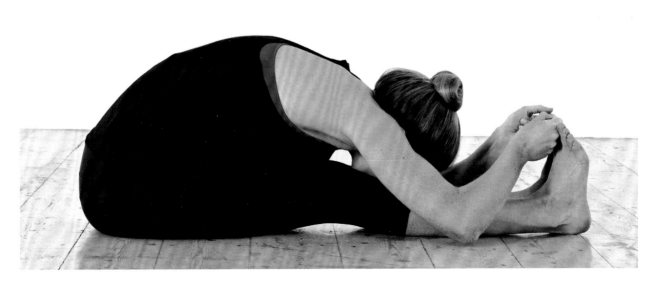

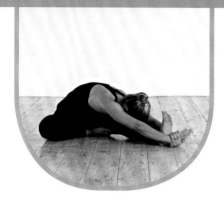

Janu Sirsasana

Head-to-Knee Pose

This is an asymmetrical seated forward-bend pose. The bent leg provides support and leverage while the straight leg is stretched and the hamstrings released by the weight of the torso.

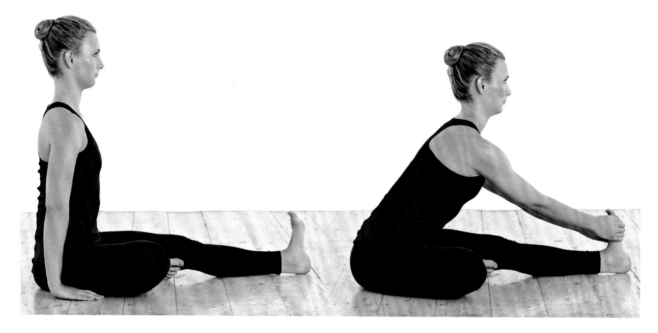

1. Sit on the floor with the legs straight in front of you. Inhale, bend the right knee and draw the heel back towards the groin so that the sole of the right foot is against the inner left thigh. Bring the right knee towards the floor, with the shin at a right angle to the left leg.

2. Exhale and turn the torso slightly to the left, to centre the torso over the left thigh. Keep both sit bones on the floor, reach the right hand to the left foot and lift the front of the torso, then reach the left hand to the outside of the left foot.

Benefits

- Stretches the spine, shoulders, hamstrings and groin.
- Stimulates the liver and kidneys.
- Tones the abdominal organs and improves digestion.
- Is therapeutic for high blood pressure.

Cautions

- If you have a knee injury, don't flex the injured knee completely and support it on a folded blanket.

Anatomical Function

Upper body

- The rectus abdominis bends the trunk over the straight leg.

- The biceps of both the upper arms bend the elbows, which bring the torso deeper into the stretch. There is scapular abduction and upward rotation, shoulder flexion and adduction.

Lower body

- The hip of the straight leg is flexed by the action of the psoas, pectineus, rectus femoris and sartorius muscles.

- The quadriceps hold the leg straight, so the knee extends and there is ankle dorsiflexion.

- On the bent leg there is hip flexion, due to the psoas muscle's external rotation and abduction; knee flexion is due to the hamstrings. There is also ankle plantar flexion.

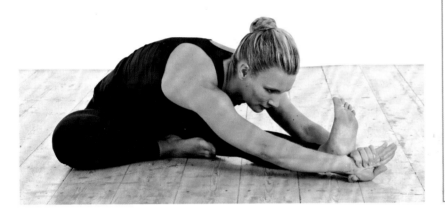

3. With the arms fully extended, exhale and extend forward, lengthening the front torso. As you descend, bend the elbows out to the sides and lift them away from the floor.

4. Lengthen forward into a comfortable stretch. The belly should touch the thighs first, the head last. Stay in the pose for anything from one to three minutes. Inhale to come up and release the pose. Repeat over the right leg.

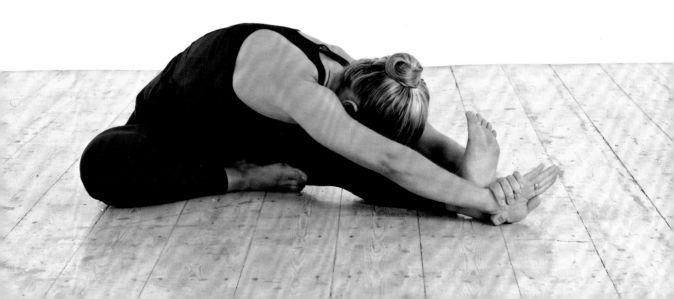

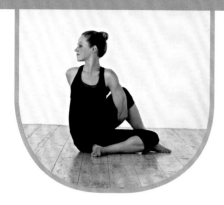

Ardha Matsyendrasana

Half Spinal Twist

Traditional texts say that *Ardha Matsyendrasana* increases appetite, destroys most deadly diseases and awakens *kundalini*.

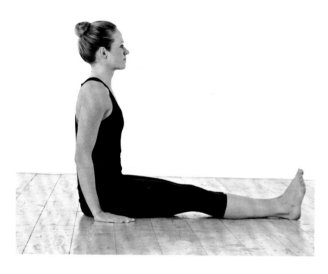

1. Sit on the floor with the legs straight out in front of you.

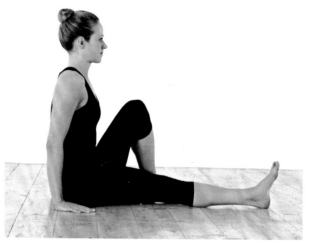

2. Bring the right foot outside the left knee, keeping the right knee upright. Press the right foot to the floor and straighten the spine.

Benefits

- Stimulates the liver and kidneys.
- Stretches the shoulders, hips and neck.
- Stimulates the digestive fire in the belly.
- Relieves menstrual discomfort, fatigue, sciatica and backache.

Cautions

- If you have a back or spine injury, perform this pose only with the supervision of an experienced teacher.

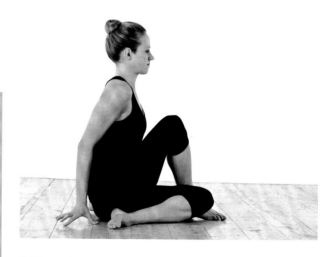

3. Place the right hand behind the right buttock. Bend the left knee and bring the heel beside the right buttock.

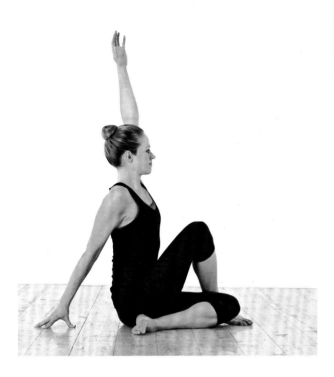

> ### Anatomical Function
>
> **Upper body**
> - There is spinal rotation due to the erector spinae muscles.
> - Front arm: rhomboids are active to hold the scapulae over the ribcage. The arm externally rotates the arm while the deltoids laterally abduct the arm against the raised leg. Biceps flex the elbow.
> - Back arm: the shoulder extends and the arm externally rotates. The elbow is flexed in the bind due to the biceps.
>
> **Lower body**
> - Deep hip flexion with the top leg, which internally rotates. Knee flexion.
> - Hip flexion with the bottom leg, which also adducts.
> - Knee flexion is due to the action of the hamstrings.

4. Inhale and raise the left arm, then place the left arm on the outside of the right thigh. Pull the front torso and inner right thigh together. Exhale and twist to the right.

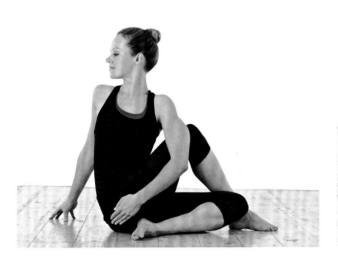

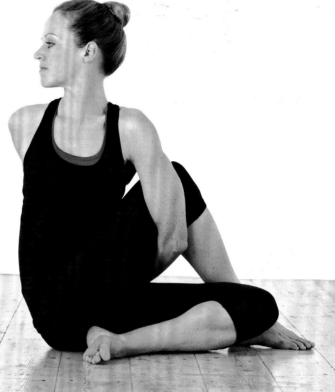

5. Continue twisting the torso by turning the head to the right and looking over the shoulder. Try to keep both sit bones on the floor. With every inhalation lift a little more through the breastbone; twist a little more with every exhalation.

6. If possible, reach the left arm under the right thigh and the right arm behind the back and bind the hands. Distribute the twist evenly through the length of the spine for 30–60 seconds. Release the pose and switch sides.

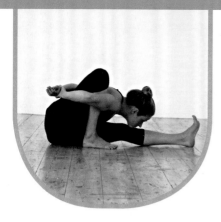

Marichyasana I

Pose of the Sage Marichi

Legend has it that Marichi was the great-grandfather of Manu, the Vedic Adam, and the 'father' of humanity.

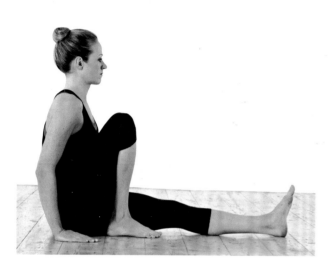

1. Sit with the legs straight. Raise the right knee and bring the heel as close to the right buttock as possible. Keep the left leg straight, pressing the back of the knee to the floor and pointing the toes towards you. Keep the left knee upright and press the inner thigh against the side of the torso.

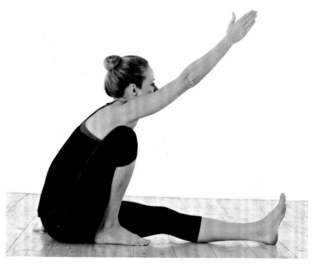

2. Inhale and raise the right arm and lift the trunk forward, reaching towards the right foot. Then exhale, wrap the right arm around the right shin and reach the hand behind the back. The left hand will press against the outside of the left thigh or buttock.

Benefits

- Stretches the spine and shoulders.
- Stimulates abdominal organs such as the liver and kidneys.
- Improves digestion.

Cautions

- Not recommended for asthma sufferers.
- Not recommended during pregnancy.

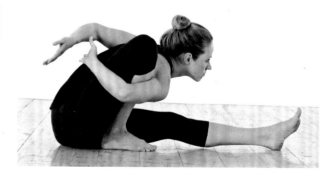

3. Reach the left arm around behind the back and clasp the left wrist in the right hand. Inhale and lift the chest, then exhale and extend the torso forward.

Anatomical Function

Upper body

- Quadratus lumborum and erector spinae muscles round the back.

- Tricep muscles straighten the elbows.

- The pectoralis and the subscapularis muscles turn the shoulders inwards.

Lower body

- Hip flexion on the straight leg is due to the psoas, pectineus, rectus femoris and sartorius muscles.

- The quadriceps keep the knee straight.

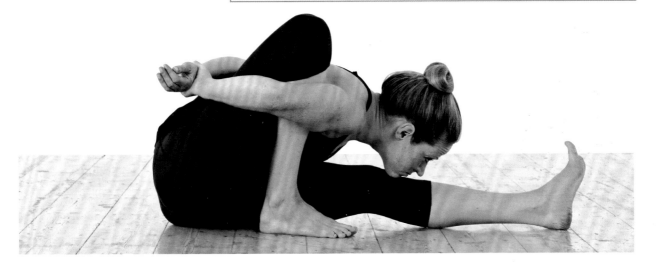

4. Lower the torso over the left leg. Keep the front torso long. Draw the shoulders away from the ears and actively down the back. Hold for 30–60 seconds, then come up as you inhale. Repeat on the other side.

Marichyasana III Twisted Variation

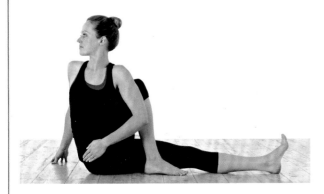

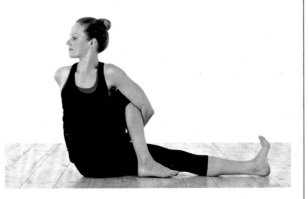

1. With the right knee raised and left leg straight, twist the torso to the right and bring the left arm outside the right thigh.

2. Wrap the left arm around the right knee and reach the right arm behind the back to grab the left wrist. Lift the trunk and twist, looking over the right shoulder.

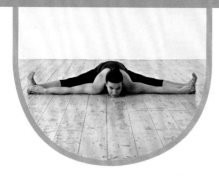

Upavistha Konasana

Wide-angle Seated Forward-bend Pose

This symmetrical deep forward bend focuses on the stretch on the upper hamstrings and lower back. When the quadricep muscles contract to straighten the knees, a powerful force is transmitted on the lower back.

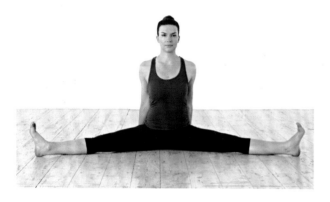

1. Sit with the legs straight, then open the legs wide to form a right angle. Place the hands on the floor behind the hips and push the buttocks and pubic bone forward, widening the legs further.

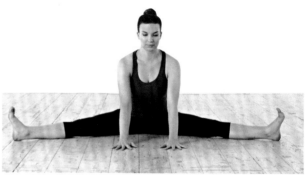

2. Press the backs of the knees into the floor. Extend through the heels and press through the balls of the feet.

Benefits

- Stretches the insides and backs of the legs.
- Stimulates the abdominal organs.
- Strengthens the spine.
- Releases the groin.

Cautions

- If you have a lower-back injury, sit up high on a folded blanket and keep the torso relatively upright.

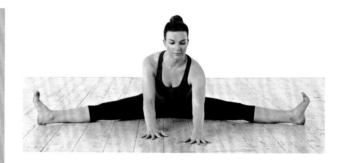

3. Inhale, lift the chest and straighten the torso. Now walk the hands forward between the legs, keeping the arms straight. The emphasis is on moving from the hip joints and maintaining the length of the front of the torso.

4. Keep walking the hands forward and bring the front of the torso to the floor. Eventually the spine will flatten and the shoulders and the abdomen will touch the floor, once full axial extension is achieved. Hold for up to 30 seconds, then walk your hands in towards you and raise the trunk to exit the pose.

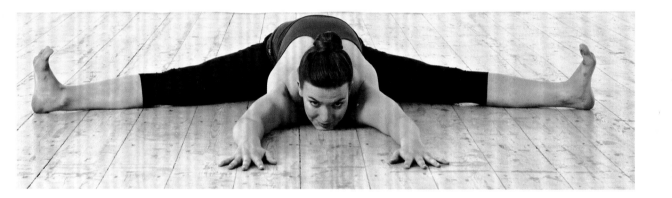

Variation

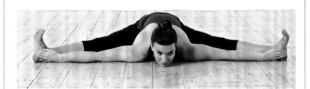

From the final position described in step 4, reach for the insides of the feet with both hands or wrap the index and middle fingers around the big toes. Gradually draw the chest, shoulders and belly down to the floor.

Anatomical Function

Upper body

- Axial extension in the spine by the spinal extensors.

- The biceps and anterior deltoids at the front of the shoulder and the pectoralis major in the chest contract and then relax as the muscles in the back stretch.

- The posterior deltoids at the back of the shoulder stretch the shoulders to deepen the pose.

- The triceps straighten the elbows.

Lower body

- The quadriceps straighten the knees.

- The psoas muscles flex the hips.

- The tibialis anterior along the outside shin creates ankle dorsiflexion, and the peroneus muscles evert the ankles to open the soles of the feet.

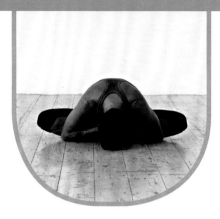

Badhha Konasana

Bound Angle Pose

This pose opens up the hip and groin area and gives a good stretch to the hamstrings and the spine.

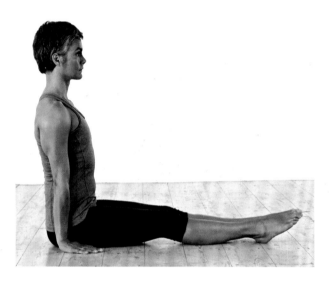

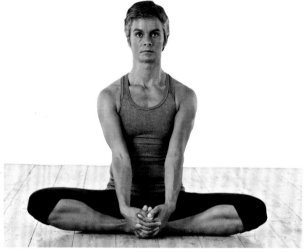

1. Begin by sitting with the legs straight out in front of you. Exhale, bend the knees and pull the heels towards the pelvis. Clasp both hands around the feet.

2. Bring the heels as close to the groin as you comfortably can and press the soles of the feet together. Keeping the back straight, draw the knees towards the floor without forcing them down.

Benefits

- Stimulates the abdominal organs, ovaries, prostate gland, bladder and kidneys.
- Stimulates the heart and improves general circulation.
- Stretches the inner thighs, groin and knees.
- Soothes menstrual discomfort and sciatica.
- Practice of this pose until late in pregnancy is said to help ease childbirth.

Cautions

- If you have a groin or knee injury, perform this pose with a blanket supporting the outer thighs.

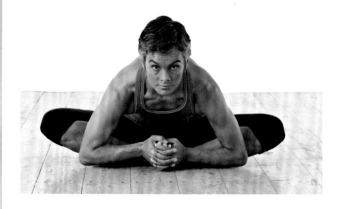

3. Inhale, lift the breastbone and bring the elbows in front of the shins.

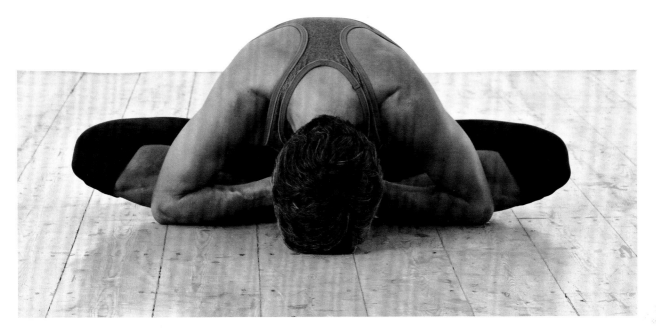

4. Inhale and lift the chest forward, lengthening the spine and keeping the chin away from the chest. You can push the elbows into the shins to help bring the trunk down towards the floor.

5. In the final pose, the chest will rest on the feet and the forehead and elbows will rest on the floor. Stay in this pose for at least 30 seconds.

Anatomical Function

Upper body
- Mild spinal flexion gradually increasing towards axial extension.

Lower body
- Hip flexion, external rotation and adduction, due to the action of the quadratus femoris, piriformis and superior and inferior gemellus.

- Knee flexion occurs through the action of the hamstrings.

- Ankle dorsiflexion and foot supination.

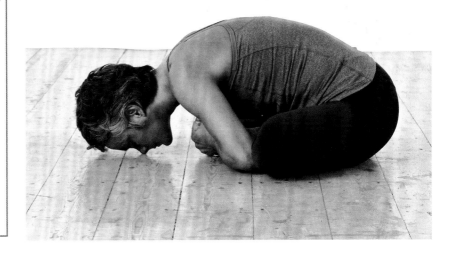

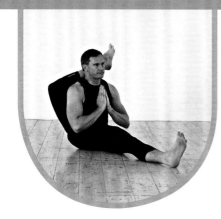

Eka Pada Sirsasana

One-Foot-Behind-the-Head Pose

This strenuous pose requires a lot of practice to master. It strengthens the back and neck and fully stretches the hamstrings. The abdominal muscles are contracted, which increases digestive power.

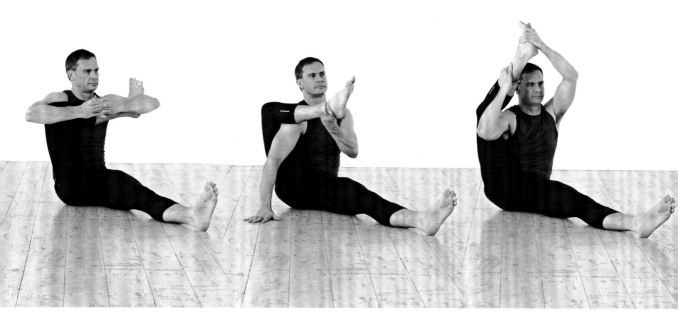

1. Sit with the legs straight. Begin by cradling the right leg: raise the right leg and bend the knee, then bring the foot to the inside of the left elbow and wrap the right arm around the right knee. Draw the shin into the chest, keeping the shin horizontal. Carefully move the knee from left to right to loosen the right hip.

2. Now raise the right leg and bend the knee, turning it slightly to the side. Take hold of the right foot with the left hand, bring the right arm under the right knee.

3. Take hold of the right shin with the right hand. Raise the right foot higher, leaning forward and using the right arm to push the right leg further behind the right shoulder. Release the right hand from the right ankle, then bow the head and carefully lift the foot behind the head.

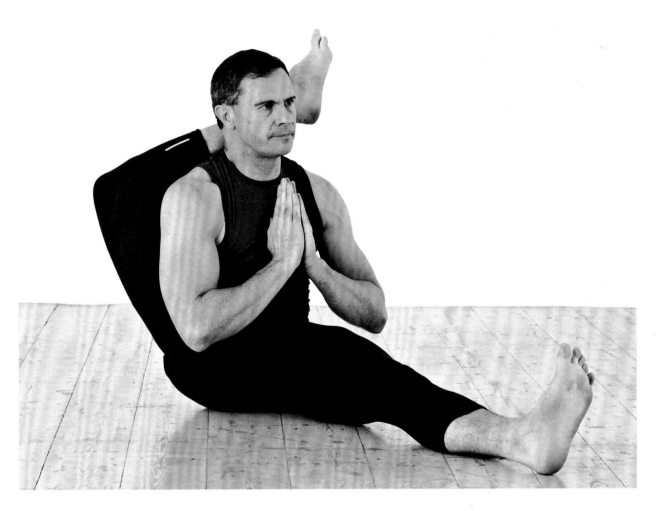

4. Use the muscles in the neck to keep the leg behind the head and try to lift the head up, so that the gaze is forward. When the foot stays in place, bring the hands together in front of the chest into a prayer position and try to straighten the spine. Hold for 15–60 seconds, breathing deeply. To break the pose, take hold of the right foot with both hands, lowering the head to release the leg to the floor. Repeat the pose with the left leg.

Benefits

- Massages the internal organs and improves digestion.
- Relieves constipation.
- Tones the reproductive organs.

Cautions

- Not advisable for anyone suffering from a slipped disc, sciatica or a hernia.

Anatomical Function

Upper body

- There is cervical extension in the spine, due to spinal extensors to counter the position of the legs and arms.
- The rotator-cuff muscles enable the shoulders to abduct and rotate internally to keep the leg back.
- The elbows are flexed, due to bicep action.

Lower body

- The psoas muscle brings the right hips into deep flexion. The legs are adducted and internally rotate, due to the pectineus and adductor muscles.
- The right knee is flexed, due to the hamstrings and the ankles being in dorsiflexion.
- The quadriceps straighten the left leg.

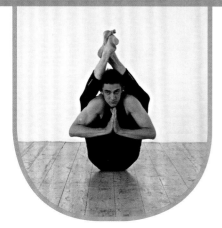

Dwi Pada Sirsasana

Two-Legs or Feet-Behind-the-Head Pose

In *Eka Pada Sirsasana*, one leg is placed behind the head. Here both legs are placed behind the head, as in *Yoga Nidrasana* (see page 152), but the body is vertical and balances on the sit bones. This is a very advanced pose and requires a great deal of practice and patience to master.

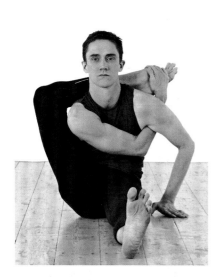

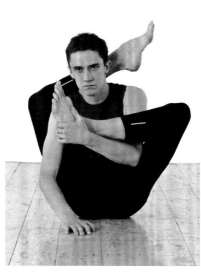

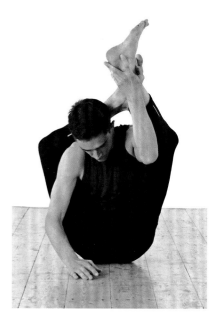

1. Perform *Eka Pada Sirsasana* (see page 130), lifting the right foot behind the head and resting it on the back of the neck.

2. Now inhale and raise the left leg, taking hold of the foot with the left hand while the right hand is on the floor for support.

3. Lift the left foot behind the head and cross it over the right ankle. Release the hand and lift the head to keep the foot from slipping.

Benefits

- Massages the internal organs and improves digestion.
- Relieves constipation.
- Tones the reproductive organs.

Cautions

- Not advisable for anyone suffering from a slipped disc, sciatica or a hernia.

Anatomical Function

Upper body

- There is cervical extension in the spine.
- The rotator-cuff muscles enable the shoulders to abduct and rotate internally to keep the legs back.
- The elbows are flexed due to bicep action.

Lower body

- The psoas muscle brings the hips into deep flexion. The legs are adducted and internally rotate, due to the pectineus and adductor muscles.
- The knees are flexed, due to the hamstrings and the ankles being in dorsiflexion.

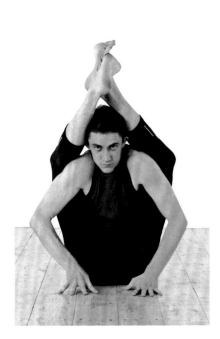

4. Place the hands on the floor and begin working the legs further behind the shoulders by pushing the arms against the backs of the thighs and pulling the shoulders forward.

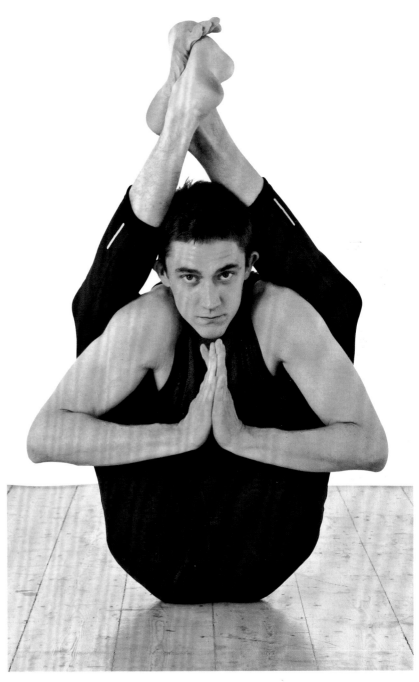

5. Inhale, balance on the sit bones and bring the palms together in front of the chest in a prayer position. To stop yourself rolling backwards, push the feet upwards as if to straighten the knees. Hold the pose for 10–30 seconds or as long as you can. To release, bring the hands to the floor and release the ankles and lower the legs to the floor.

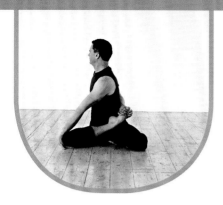

Bharadvajasana

Bound Half-Lotus Spinal Twist

This pose is named after Bharadvaja, one of the seven great Seers. This spinal twist gently massages the internal organs, with special emphasis on the digestive system.

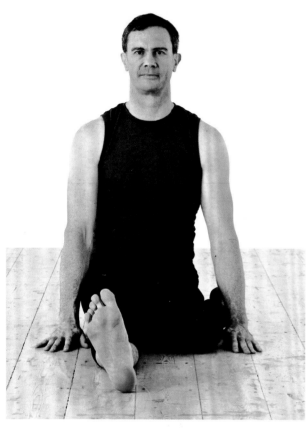

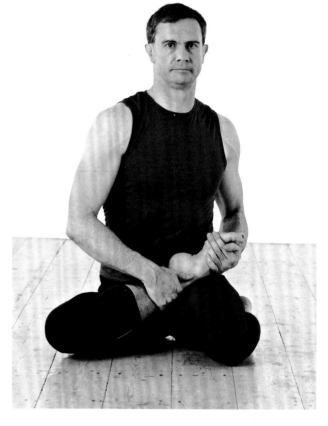

1. Sit on the floor with the legs straight. Bend the left knee and bring the foot alongside the left buttock.

2. Take the right shin with both hands and lift the right foot onto the left thigh in the Half Lotus Pose.

Tip

If you're unable to bring the right leg into a Half Lotus, rest the sole of the foot against the inside of the left thigh, then bring the left hand across to the right knee and reach the right hand behind the back to the inside of the left thigh.

Anatomical Function

Upper body

- Axial extension and rotation of the spine: the erector spinae muscle keeps the spine straight.
- Shoulder extension and adduction on the right shoulder.

Lower body

- Knee flexion: the hamstrings flex the knees.
- Hip flexion and extension due to the action of the psoas muscle.

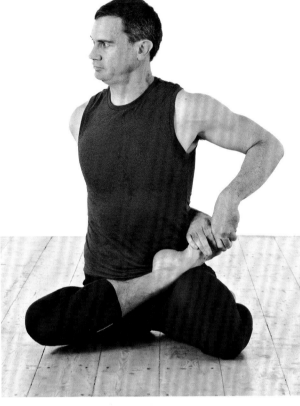

3. Reach the right hand behind the back and grab the right foot. If you can't reach, take the left hand behind the back and pull your right hand to the right foot. Try to keep both sit bones on the floor.

4. Place the left hand on the right knee or under the outside of the knee with the palm facing down. Inhale and lift the breastbone to lengthen the front of the torso. Exhale and twist the torso to the right, keeping the left buttock on or very close to the floor. Hold the pose for 30–60 seconds, then release and switch sides.

Benefits

- Stretches the spine, shoulders and hips.
- Massages the abdominal organs.
- Relieves lower backache, neck pain and sciatica.
- Improves digestion.
- Recommended in the second trimester of pregnancy to strengthen the lower back.

Cautions

- Not recommended for those suffering from high or low blood pressure.
- Avoid during menstruation.

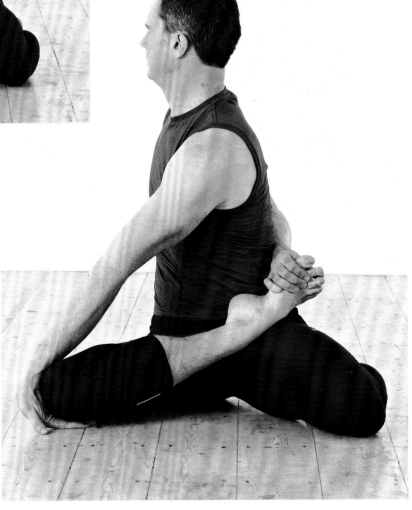

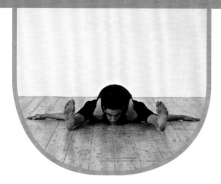

Kurmasana

Tortoise Pose

This pose prepares the yogi for the fifth stage of the yogic path, *pratyahara* or sense withdrawal. Just as the tortoise withdraws into his shell, so the yogi withdraws from sense objects.

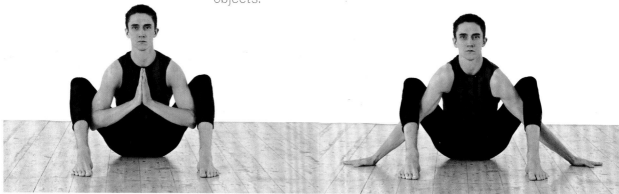

1. Sit with the legs straight, and the feet shoulder width apart. Raise the knees and bring the shoulders inside the knees. Bring the palms togther in front of the chest.

2. Take the right arm under the right leg and the left arm under the left leg, with the palms on the floor and fingers pointing back.

Anatomical Function

Upper body

- The trapezius and rhomboid muscles are stretched.

Lower body

- The psoas and rectus abdominis muscles flex the hips and bend the trunk.

- The adductor muscles on the inner thighs squeeze the thighs against the upper arms, connecting the upper and lower body.

- The hamstrings straighten the legs.

3. Begin to straighten the knees by sliding the heels forward, keeping the knees close to the shoulders.

Benefits

- Tones the spine.

- Stimulates the abdominal organs.

- Strengthens the abdominal muscles.

Cautions

- Do not attempt this pose during pregnancy.

4. Press the backs of the knees against the backs of the arms. Try to straighten the knees and bring the chest and shoulders to the floor. Hold this pose for 30–60 seconds, then raise the knees to release the arms from under the legs.

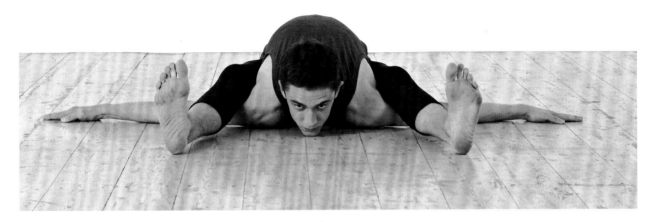

Advanced Variation: Supta Kurmasana

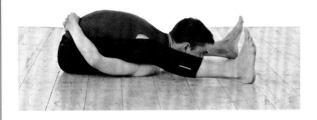

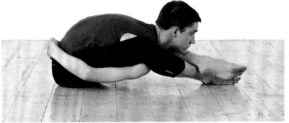

1. Bend the knees and turn the wrists so that the palms face up, then bring the arms behind the back and interlace the fingers.

2. Raise the knees a little higher, bring the feet together and cross one ankle over the other.

3. Insert the head between the feet and bring the forehead to the floor.

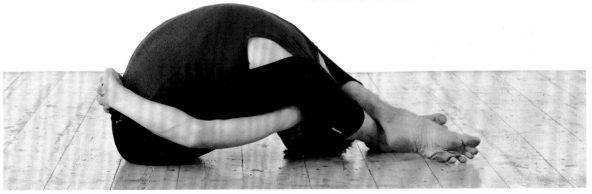

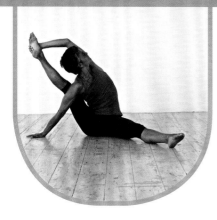

Parivrtta Surya Yantrasana

Compass Pose

This pose is a great preparation for placing the leg behind the head in poses such as *Eka Pada Sirsasana* (see page 130).

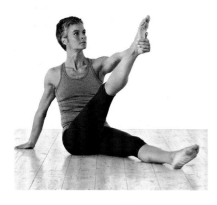

1. Sit with the legs straight, then raise the right leg and bend the knee. Take hold of the top of the foot with the left hand and move the right knee behind the right shoulder.

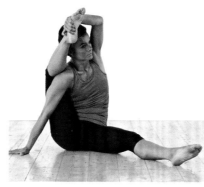

2. Use the right arm against the back of the right thigh to work the knee further back and bring the right hand down to the floor, approximately 15 cm (6 in) away from the right hip, with the fingers pointing to the right.

Anatomical Function

Upper body

- Left shoulder flexion and internal rotation, stretching the teres major, latissimus dorsi, pectoralis major and subscapularis.

- The triceps straighten the right elbow.

Lower body

- The quadriceps straighten the knees.

- The adductor muscles squeeze the right thigh against the upper right arm.

- The psoas combines with the rectus abdominis along the trunk to bend the trunk and the right hip.

Benefits

- Tones the abdomino-pelvic organs.
- Stretches the hamstrings.

Cautions

- Do not attempt to straighten the raised leg if you have hamstring problems.
- Not advisable for anyone suffering from a slipped disc.

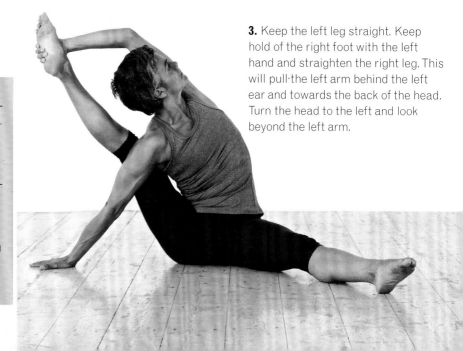

3. Keep the left leg straight. Keep hold of the right foot with the left hand and straighten the right leg. This will pull the left arm behind the left ear and towards the back of the head. Turn the head to the left and look beyond the left arm.

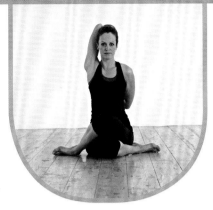

Gomukhasana

Cow Face Pose

In Sanskrit, *Go* means cow and *Mukha* means face. This pose resembles the face of a cow. The pose stretches the leg muscles, opens the chest and shoulders and straightens the spine.

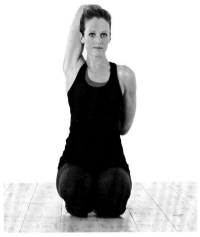

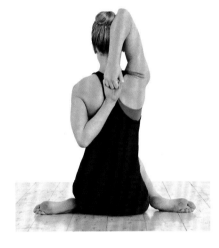

1. The pose can be practised sitting on the heels, as shown above, or with the knees crossed. To cross the knees, sit with the legs straight, then cross the right leg over the left, stacking the knees, and bring the heels beside the thighs. Sit evenly on the sit bones. Inhale and reach the left arm behind the back. Bend the elbow and turn the palm to face away, with the fingers pointing upwards. If necessary, reach the right arm behind the back to grab the left elbow and gently pull it in towards the middle of the back.

2. Now inhale, raise the right arm and reach back to clasp the fingers on the left hand. Move the right elbow behind the head.

3. Stay in this pose for about one minute, then release the arms, uncross the legs (if not sitting on the heels) and switch sides. Remember that whichever crossed leg is on top, the opposite arm is the one that is raised.

Anatomical Function

Upper body

- Raised arm: the serrratus anterior and rhomboids rotate the shoulder blade upwards; lateral rotation and flexion of the shoulder are due to the infraspinatus and teres minor. Biceps create elbow flexion.

- Lower arm: downward rotation and adduction of the shoulder blade, due to the lower trapezius and rhomboids. Internal rotation and adduction of the shoulder are the action of the subscapularis.

Lower body

- Hip and knee flexion.

Benefits

- Stretches the ankles, hips and thighs, shoulders, armpits and triceps, and chest.

Cautions

- Not recommended for those with neck or shoulder problems.

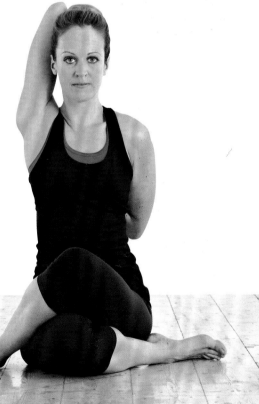

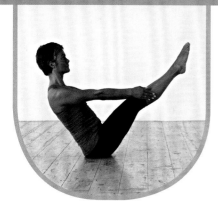

Paripurana Navasana

Boat Pose

This posture resembles the shape of a boat. If it isn't possible to stretch the arms alongside the legs, keep the hands on the floor beside the hips or hold onto the backs of the thighs.

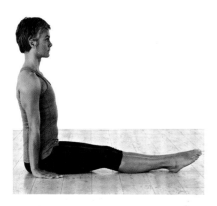

1. Sit on the floor with the legs straight in front of you. Press the hands on the floor and lift the chest. Keep the spine straight and feel the weight shifting onto the sit bones.

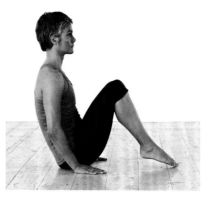

2. Inhale and raise the legs 45–50 degrees relative to the floor. Straighten the knees and point the toes. If this isn't possible, keep the knees bent, perhaps lifting the shins parallel to the floor.

Anatomical Function

Upper body

- Shoulder flexion through activation of the anterior deltoids; rhomboid and trapezius muscles draw the shoulders down.

- Tricep muscles extend the elbows.

Lower body

- Hip flexion due to the psoas major and rectus femoris.

- Rectus abdominis bends the trunk. Adduction of the legs; knee extension due to the quadriceps.

3. Stretch the arms alongside the legs, parallel to each other and the floor. Spread the shoulder blades across the back and lengthen through to the fingertips. At first stay in the pose for 10–20 seconds. Gradually increase this to one minute. Exhale and lower the legs to the floor.

Benefits

- Strengthens the abdomen, hip flexors and spine.

- Stimulates the kidneys, thyroid and prostate glands and intestines.

- Improves digestion.

- Tones the abdominal organs.

Cautions

- Not recommended for those suffering from low blood pressure.

- Avoid during pregnancy.

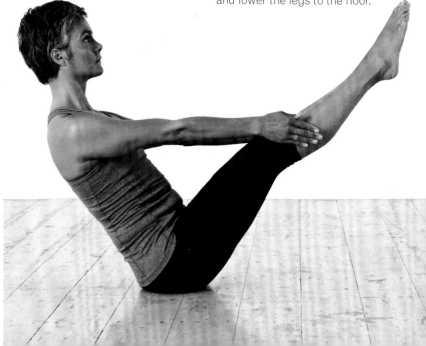

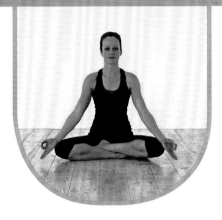

Sukkhasana and Siddhasana

Easy Pose and Adept's Pose

Ideal alternatives to *Padmanasana*, these poses are recommended for *pranayama* practice and meditation. The crossed legs and erect spine keep the mind alert while the body is rested.

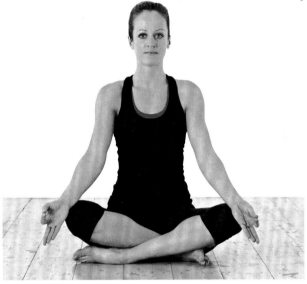

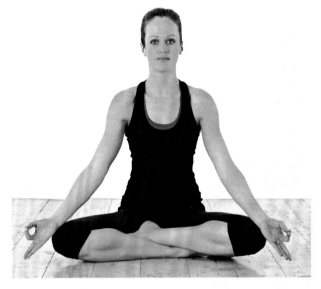

1. From a sitting position with the legs straight, cross the legs so that each foot is under the opposite knee and the sides of the feet rest on the floor. There should be a comfortable gap between the feet and the pelvis.

2. Place the hands on top of the knees with palms facing up or assume a *mudra* (see page 224) with the hands. Draw the tail bone towards the floor and straighten the spine.

3. You can sit in this position for any length of time, but if you practise this pose regularly, alternate the legs so that the same one doesn't always sit on top of the other.

1. From a comfortable sitting position with the legs straight, bend the right knee and bring the heel in towards the groin.

2. Then bend the left knee, lift the foot and tuck it behind the calf of the right leg. The right foot should tuck behind the left calf so that the tops of both feet disappear

3. Sit with the spine straight and place the backs of the hands on top of the knees with palms facing up, or assume a *mudra* (see page 224) with the hands.

Anatomical Function

Upper body

- Axial extension of the spine: the erector spinae muscle keeps the spine straight.

Lower body

- Knee flexion: the hamstrings flex the knees.
- Hip flexion due to the action of the psoas muscle.

Benefits

- Stimulates the pelvis, spine, abdomen and bladder.
- Stretches the ankles and knees.

Cautions

- Not recommended for anyone with an ankle or knee injury.

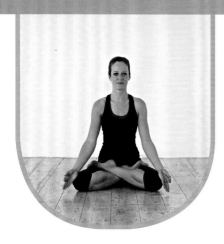

Padmasana

Lotus Pose

Padmasana is the ultimate sitting position for meditation and *pranayama* practice. It is also used in variations of *Sirsasana* (see page 182) and *Sarvanghasana* (see page 186). The pose brings flexibility to the knees and ankles, but is more difficult to master than it appears, requiring hip flexibility. Many find it difficult to hold for long periods.

1. Sit on the floor with the legs straight. Bend the right knee, take hold of the outside of the right foot with the left hand and lift the shin from underneath with the right hand. Carefully lift the right foot on top of the left thigh with the heel close to the left hip.

2. Now take the left leg and lift it on top of the right. To do this, hold the left shin and foot from underneath in both hands. Carefully slide the left leg over the right and bring the left heel towards the right hip. Lift the breastbone and straighten the spine. The hands can be placed with palms facing up on top of the knees as in *Jnana mudra*, with the thumbs and first fingers touching. In the beginning, hold the pose for only a few seconds and release. *Padmasana* should balance both sides of the body, so it is important to alternate the legs.

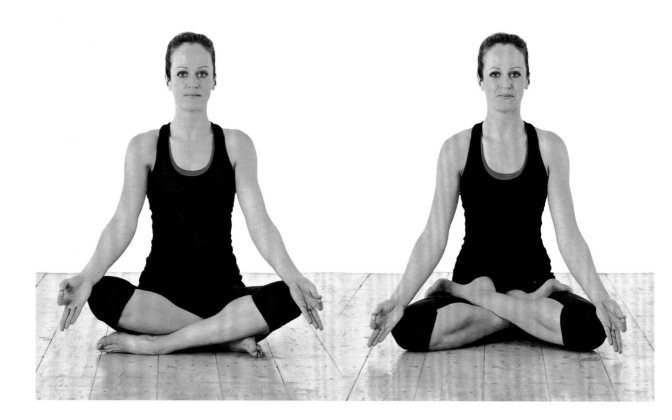

Badha Padmasana: Bound Lotus Variation

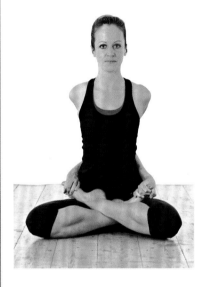

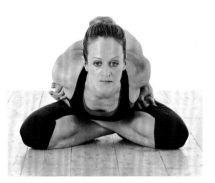

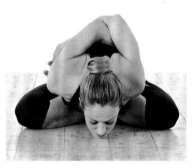

1. From *Padmasana*, lean forward and reach the right arm behind the back and grab the top of the right foot. Then reach the left arm behind the back and grab the top of the left foot.

2. With both arms crossed behind the back and holding the respective feet, begin to bend forward.

3. Bring the chin or forehead to the floor, keeping both sit bones on the floor.

Anatomical Function

Upper body

- Axial extension of the spine: the erector spinae muscle keeps the spine straight.

Lower body

- Knee flexion: the hamstrings flex the knees.
- Hip flexion due to the action of the psoas muscle.

Benefits

- Calming.
- Stimulates the pelvis, spine, abdomen and bladder.
- Stretches the ankles and knees.
- Eases menstrual discomfort and sciatica.
- Consistent practice of this pose until late into pregnancy is said to help ease childbirth.
- Traditional texts say that *Padmasana* destroys all disease and awakens *kundalini*.

Cautions

- Not recommended for anyone with an ankle or knee injury.
- *Padmasana* is considered to be an intermediate to advanced pose. Do not perform it without sufficient prior experience or the supervision of an experienced teacher.

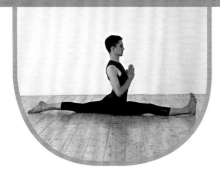

Hanumanasana

Front Splits

This pose, in which the legs are split forward and back, mimics the monkey chief Hanuman's famous leap from the southern tip of India to the island of Sri Lanka.

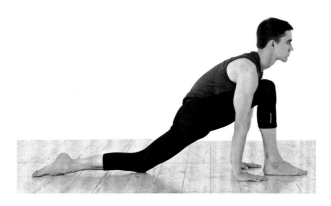

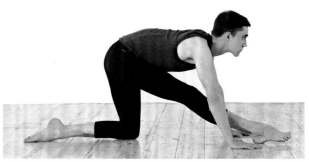

1. Kneel on the floor and place the hands on either side of the knees. Lift the right knee and slide the right heel forward, then carefully slide the left knee back.

2. Try to avoid leaning too far forward. Keep an even stretch in the legs by walking the hands towards the hips and lifting the trunk upright. Keep the weight in the hands and gradually lower the seat down towards the floor with each exhalation.

Anatomical Function

Upper body

• The Erector spinae muscles extend the spine and keep it straight.

• When the arms are raised, the anterior deltoids are active and the triceps straighten the elbows. There is adduction of the arms as the palms press together.

• There is upward scapular rotation, abduction and elevation due to the action of the upper trapezius.

Lower body

• On the front leg, the hip is flexed, the thigh is internally rotated and adducting.

• The knee extends, due to shortening of the quadriceps, and the ankle is dorsiflexed.

• On the back leg the hip extends and the thigh internally rotates.

• As well as knee extension, the ankle is plantar flexed.

Tip

To progress in this pose, place a towel under the front heel and use it to glide the heel gently forward.

Benefits

• Stretches the thighs, hamstrings and groin.
• Stimulates the abdominal organs.

Cautions

• Not recommended for anyone with a groin or hamstring injury.

3. When both legs are on the floor, bring the hands together in front of the chest into a prayer position. This is a difficult pose to master and must be practised every day, switching sides.

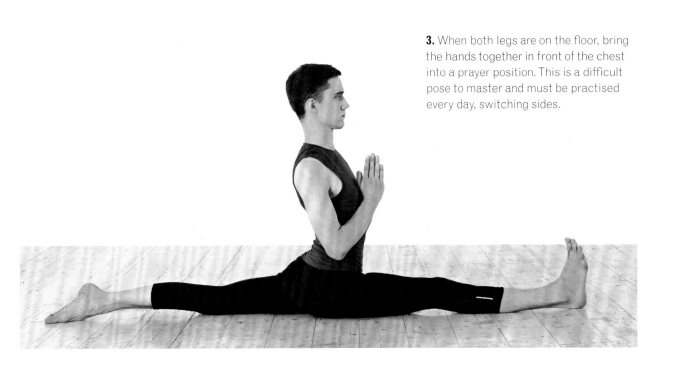

4. Inhale and raise the arms over the head. Hold the pose for 15–30 seconds, then lower the hands to the floor to release the pose. Repeat with the left leg forward and right leg back.

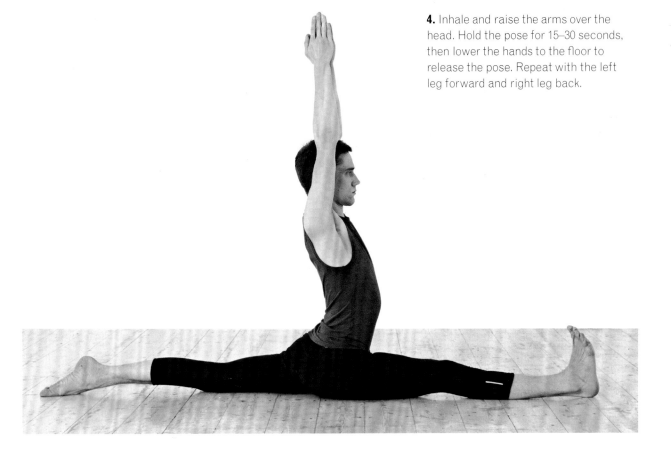

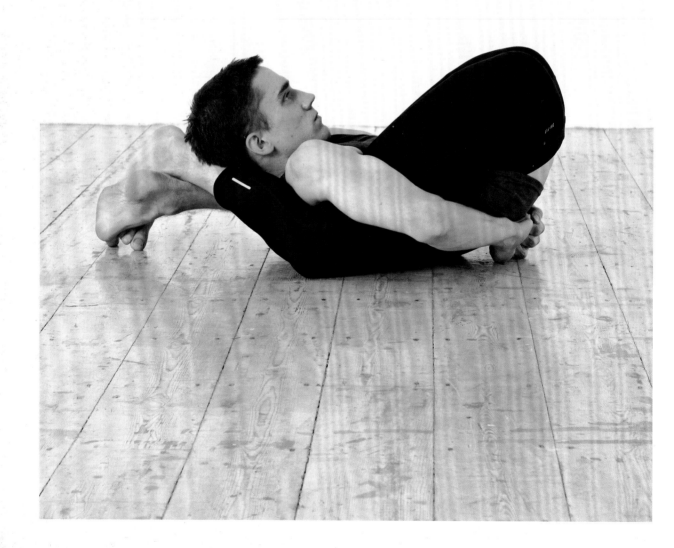

Supine Poses

In supine poses we are lying facing up. As they are performed on the back, most of the supine poses have the lowest centre of gravity, allowing the body to move freely through its full range of motion, fully supported by the earth. Physically, the supine poses engage the body's anterior musculature, stretching us forward and back, up and down and from side to side, to lubricate the joints and open the chest, as we move towards the fundamental supine pose – *Savasana* – to conclude our *asana* practice, when we can experience true stillness and allow the postural muscles to relax.

Matsyasana 148
Supta Virasana 150
Yoga Nidrasana 152
Savasana 153

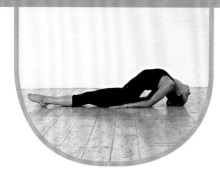

Matsyasana

Fish Pose

Traditional texts state that *Matsyasana* is the 'destroyer of all diseases'. A symmetrical supine back-bending pose, Fish Pose is traditionally performed with the legs in *Padmasana* (see page 142). Since the Lotus Pose is beyond the capacity of many students, here we'll work with the legs straight and pressed against the floor.

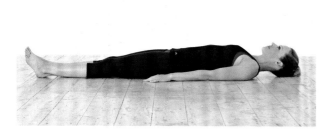

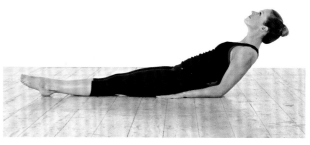

1. Lie on your back with the legs straight and arms by your sides, palms facing down. Inhale, lift the pelvis slightly off the floor and slide the hands, palms facing downwards, under the buttocks. Rest the buttocks on the backs of the hands and don't lift them off. Tuck the elbows close to the sides of the torso.

2. Inhale and press the forearms and elbows firmly against the floor. Press the shoulder blades into the back and, with another inhale, lift the upper torso and head off the floor.

Benefits

- Stretches the deep hip flexors (psoas) and the muscles between the ribs (intercostals).
- Stretches and stimulates the muscles of the belly and the front of the neck.
- Stretches and stimulates the organs of the belly and throat.
- Strengthens the muscles of the upper back and the back of the neck.

Cautions

- Not recommended for those suffering from high or low blood pressure, or for those with a tendency to migraine.
- Avoid if you have a serious lower-back or neck injury.

Anatomical Function

Upper body

- Spinal extension is activated by the psoas major.
- Scapular downward rotation and adduction are due to the trapezius, rhomboids and latissimus dorsi.
- Shoulder extension and adduction due to the triceps; elbow extension, forearm pronation.

Lower body

- Hip flexion and adduction due to the psoas and iliacus muscles.
- Knee extension due to the quadriceps.

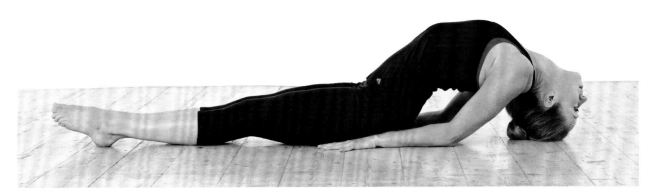

3. Then release the head back down, but keep the upper torso off the floor. Depending on how high you can arch the back and lift the chest, either the back of the head or the crown will rest on the floor. There should be a minimal amount of weight on the head. Stay for 15–30 seconds, breathing smoothly. With an exhalation, lower the torso and head to the floor. Draw the thighs up into the belly and squeeze.

Advanced Variation: Bound Fish

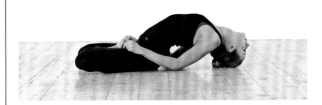

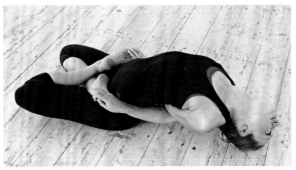

1. Lie on your back, bring the legs into the Lotus Pose and pull the thighs close together. Then press the forearms and elbows into the floor and lift onto the crown of the head, with the back arched.

2. Bring the right hand behind the lower back and reach for the right foot. Then bring the left hand behind the back and reach for the left foot. Pull the elbows close together.

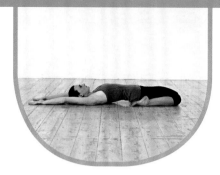

Supta Virasana

Reclining Hero Pose

Supta means lying down and *vira* means a hero or warrior. This pose stretches the abdominal organs and the pelvic region and helps relieve aching, tired legs.

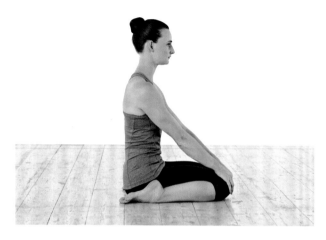

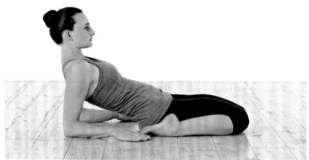

1. Kneel on the floor with the knees together. Separate the feet so that they are wider than the hips and bring the seat to the floor.

2. Place the hands on the floor beside the hips and slowly begin to lower the back towards the floor. First lean onto the hands, then the forearms and elbows, and gradually release the spine, shoulders and back of the head down.

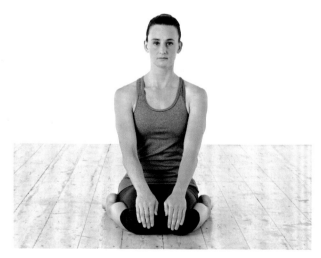

Front view

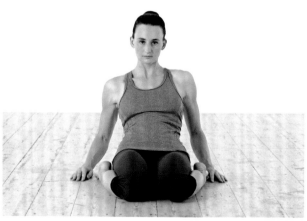

Front view

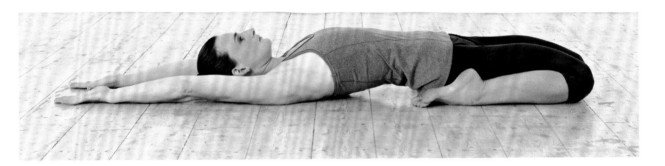

3. Lengthen the lower back and lower it towards the floor, then lay the arms and hands on the floor, with the palms facing up. Check that the knees are still together, as they tend to separate as you lower yourself. Inhale and raise the arms overhead, towards the floor, palms facing up.

You may hold the pose like this or grab each elbow. Hold the pose for 30–60 seconds. To come out, press the forearms against the floor and come onto the hands. Then use the hands to lift yourself up.

Benefits

- Stretches the abdomen, thighs and deep hip flexors (psoas), knees and ankles.

- Strengthens the arches.

- Relieves tired legs.

- Improves digestion.

- Helps relieve menstrual pain.

Cautions

- If you have any serious back, knee or ankle problems, avoid this pose unless you have the assistance of an experienced instructor.

Anatomical Function

Upper body
- The deltoid muscles raise the arms over the head.

- The triceps straighten the arms.

Lower body
- Hip extension through action of the psoas muscles. Internal rotation and adduction.

- Knee flexion and adduction through action of the gracilis and adductor magnus.

- Ankle plantar flexion.

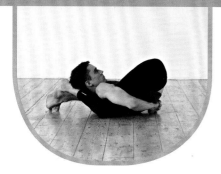

Yoga Nidrasana

Sleeping Yogi Pose

Nidra means sleep and *yoga nidra* is the state between sleep and wakefulness. Here the legs are crossed at the ankles behind the neck and the hands are clasped behind the back.

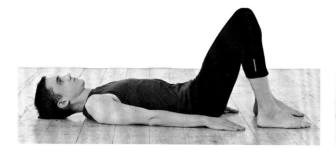

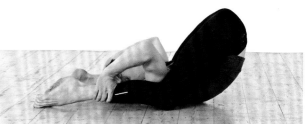

1. Lie flat on the back on the floor and bend both knees. Bring both legs over the head and bring the knees beside the shoulders.

2. Grab hold of the backs of the ankles with each hand and lift the shoulders, using both arms to move the legs back. Take the right leg and begin to move it behind the back of the neck as in *Eka Pada Sirsasana* (see page 130). Lift the left leg and move it behind the neck under the right leg and cross the ankles.

Anatomical Function

Upper body

- Cervical extension in the spine.

- The shoulders abduct and rotate internally to keep the legs back. The elbows are flexed due to the biceps.

Lower body

- The psoas brings the hips into deep flexion. The legs are adducted and rotated internally due to the pectineus and adductor muscles.

- The knees are flexed due to the hamstrings; the ankles are in dorsiflexion.

3. Lift the shoulders and keep working the legs further behind the back of the neck, as you pull the arms through the legs further and clasp the hands behind the back. Try to breathe normally and hold the pose for at least 30 seconds.

Benefits

- Stretches the spine and shoulders.

- Stimulates abdominal organs such as the liver and kidneys and improves digestion.

Cautions

- Not recommended for asthma sufferers.

- Not recommended during pregnancy.

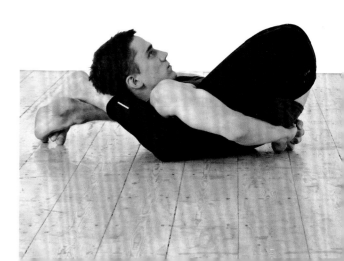

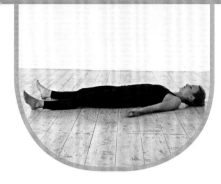

Savasana

Corpse Pose

This is conscious relaxation. Invigorating and refreshing to both the body and mind, this seemingly easy pose is one of the most challenging for the yogi, as it is hard to keep the mind still while remaining motionless and fully conscious at the same time.

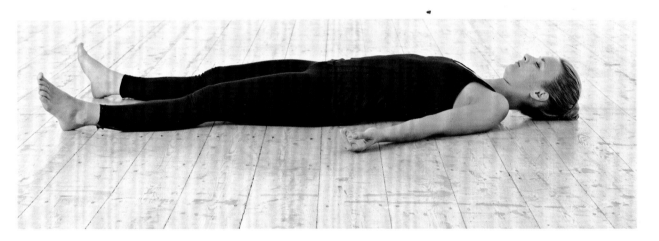

1. Lie flat on your back like a corpse. Keep the hands away from the thighs with the palms facing up. Turn the feet out and separate the legs. In *Savasana* it is important to place the body in a neutral position.

2. Relax the whole body completely. Slow the breathing down. It should be soft and slow. In addition to quieting the physical body, it's also necessary to pacify the sense organs. Relax all the features of the face – cheeks, lips, eyes and brow, especially between the eyebrows. Close the eyes. If you wish, place an eye bag or folded cloth over the eyes.

3. Stay in the pose for at least 5 minutes after your *asana* practice. Ideally you should stay in *Savasana* for 10–15 minutes. To exit, begin to move the fingers and toes. Inhale and raise the arms over the head, then stretch the legs away. Draw the knees to the chest and roll on one side, preferably the right. Take two or three breaths. With another exhalation press the hands against the floor, lift the torso and sit up.

Benefits

- In this pose, the body is completely at rest. Deep conscious relaxation is different from sleep – which tends to happen in this pose.

- *Savasana* invigorates and refreshes the body and the mind. Steady, smooth and deep breathing while the body is still soothes the nerves and calms the mind. For the body's nerves, this is the best antidote to the stresses of modern life.

Cautions

- If you have a chesty cough, lie on your right side with your knees bent.

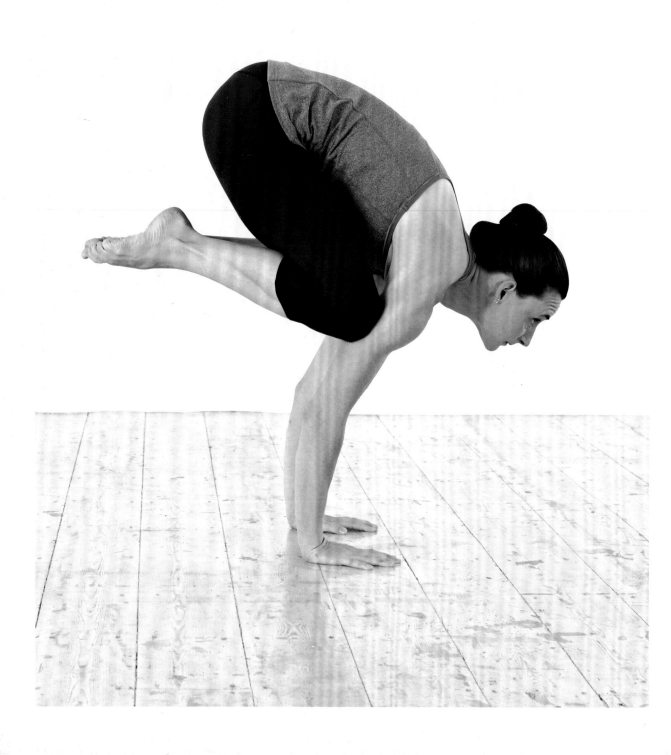

Balancing Poses

Finding stillness in a balancing pose requires the practitioner to be completely focused and in the present moment. The weight-bearing action stimulates the bones and strengthens the wrists, arms, legs and spine. As well as improving balance and coordination, these poses increase stamina. The concentration required to maintain the balancing pose leads to a steady mind. In order for the pose to be held for longer, the breath must be fully integrated into the pose, leading to more efficient breathing. On a deeper level, the balance and focus required to hold these poses lead to greater awareness in our daily lives.

Pincha Mayurasana 156
Adho Mukha Vrikshasana 158
Beerasana 160
Kakasana 162
Parsva Kakasana 164
Mayurasana 166
Tittibhasana 168
Galavasana 170
Vasisthasana 172
Vishvamittrasana 174
Astavakrasana 176
Chaturanga Dandasana 177
Urdhva Mukha Svanasana 178
Ardho Mukha Svanasana 179

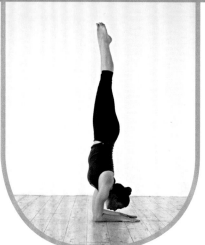

Pincha Mayurasana

Feathered Peacock Pose

In this pose the trunk and the legs are lifted off the floor and the body balances on the forearms and palms, resembling a peacock starting its dance.

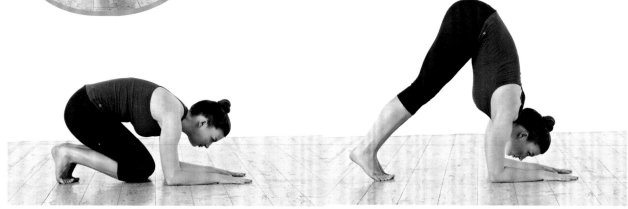

1. Kneel on the floor, with the toes tucked under, and lower the elbows and forearms to the floor. The forearms should be shoulder width apart and parallel to each other. Spread the fingers out and press the palms firmly to the floor.

2. Now lift the knees and straighten the legs, then walk the feet towards the elbows and lift the hips. Lift the shoulders forward and keep the chest lifted.

Tip

To prevent the elbows from sliding away from each other in this pose, buckle a strap and loop it over the upper arms, just above the elbows. Alternatively, place a block between the forearms and squeeze the insides of the forearms against it.

Anatomical Function

Upper body

- Extension of the cervical spine. The erector spinae slightly arches the back, countered by the rectus abdominis. The quadratus lumborum stabilizes the lower back.

- In the shoulders there is scapular upward rotation, elevation and abduction using the serratus anterior.

- Shoulder flexion and adduction due to the action of the anterior deltoids and biceps.

- Elbow flexion is due to the biceps. The triceps prevent you from falling on your face.

Lower body

- The psoas and gluteals stabilize the pelvis to prevent swaying.

- Knee extension due to the quadriceps.

Benefits

- Strengthens the shoulders, arms and back.
- Stretches the shoulders and neck, chest and belly.
- Improves the sense of balance.

Cautions

- Avoid this pose if you have a back, shoulder or neck injury, or if you have a heart condition, high blood pressure or a tendency to headaches.

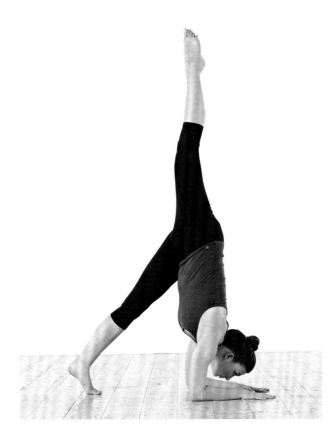

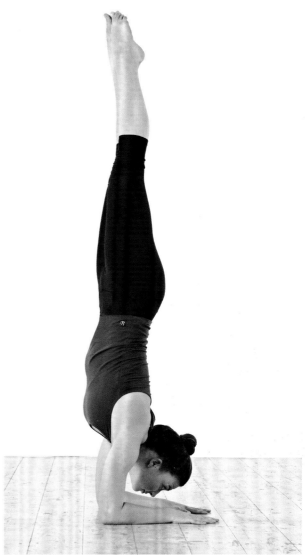

3. Inhale and raise one leg, keeping it straight. Exhale and swing the other leg up. If that is not possible, bend the knee, lift the heel and hop off the back foot.

4. Stay in the pose for 10–15 seconds. Gradually work up to one minute. Take one foot down at a time with an exhalation. We tend to kick up with the same leg all the time, so remember to alternate the legs.

Advanced Variations

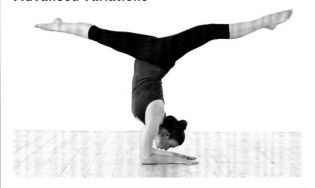

Try bringing one leg forward and the other leg back.

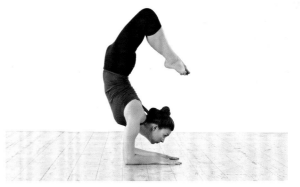

In this variation the knees are bent and the back is arched to bring the feet over the head.

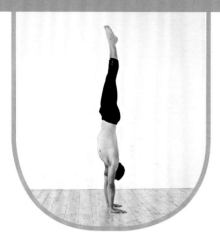

Adho Mukha Vrikshasana
Downward Facing Tree Pose

The Handstand is more about confidence, courage and concentration than it is about balance. Initially it is advisable to practise the pose against a wall in order to develop the strength and momentum required to raise the legs and to prevent falling.

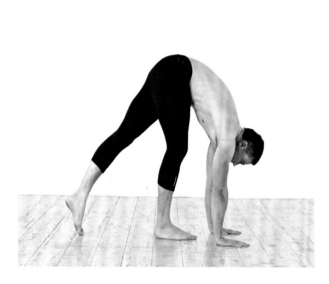

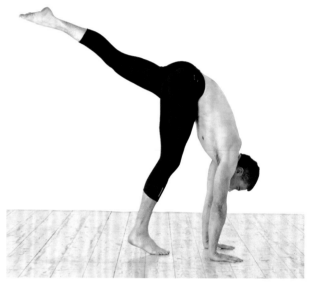

1. Begin by bringing both hands to the floor, shoulder width apart, roughly 30 cm (12 in) away from the wall. Keep the arms straight and look down at the space between the hands. Move forward, bring the shoulders over the wrists and straighten the elbows.

2. Inhale and raise one leg up, then exhale and swing the other leg up. Bring the legs to the wall. Check that the shoulders are still aligned over the wrists and ensure that the spine isn't arching by pulling the belly in.

Benefits

- Strengthens the shoulders, arms and wrists.
- Stretches the belly.
- Improves the sense of balance.
- Strengthens the lower back.

Cautions

- Avoid if you have wrist, shoulder or neck injury, if you have a heart condition or high blood pressure or if you suffer from headaches.
- Do not practise this pose during menstruation.

Anatomical Function

Upper body

- Spinal extension: the rectus abdominis and erector spinae hold the trunk solid.
- Shoulder flexion: anterior deltoids flex the shoulders over the head. The lower trapezius draws the shoulders down.
- Elbow extension is due to the action of the triceps.

Lower body

- Hip extension: the psoas and gluteus maximus stabilize the hips and balance the pelvis.
- The quadriceps create knee extension.
- Ankle plantar flexion: the peroneus longus and brevis evert the ankles.

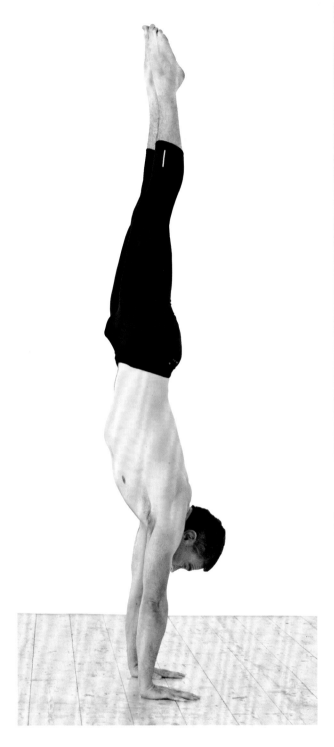

Lotus Variation

1. Come in to the handstand. Fold the right foot across the left thigh into half Lotus, then carefully try to move the foot up towards the left hip.

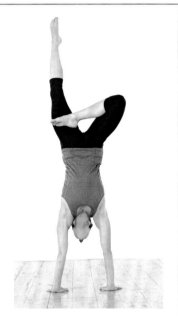

2. Keeping your balance, fold the left foot across the right shin. Try to push the knees closer towards each other and push the feet higher up the thighs.

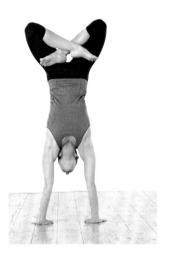

3. Press the hands into the floor and keep the elbows straight. Lift the shoulders and slowly raise the knees up. Wrist, shoulders, hips and knees should be in a straight line.

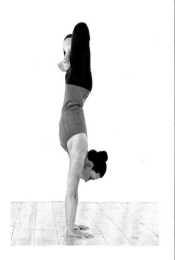

SIDE VIEW

3. Gradually lift one leg away from the wall and then the other. Once you have mastered the pose with both feet off the wall, try it in the middle of the room. Lay some cushions or bolsters out along a mat in case you lose your balance. Hold for 10–15 seconds and release.

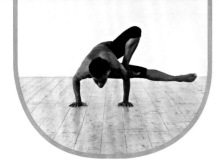

Beerasana
Dragonfly Pose

Beerasana, or Dragonfly Pose, is also known as the Hummingbird Pose. This arm-balancing pose strengthens the upper body and core muscles, as well as being a hip-opening exercise.

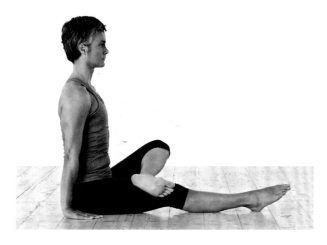

1. Sit with the legs straight in front of you, then cross the left leg over the right, with the left shin resting high up the right thigh.

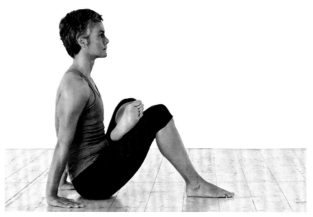

2. Bend the right knee and slide the right heel towards the right buttock.

Anatomical Function

Upper body

- The serratus anterior muscle draws the shoulder blades forward, stretching the middle trapezius and rhomboids.
- The pectoralis major and anterior deltoid muscles stabilize the shoulders.
- The lower trapezius, which spans the back, presses down on the shoulder blades.
- The infraspinatus and teres minor turn the humerus outwards to refine shoulder stability.
- The biceps muscles bend the elbows.

Lower body

- The hamstring muscles bend the left knee.
- The adductor muscles squeeze the left foot into the upper left arm to link the upper and lower extremities.
- The psoas and rectus abdominis muscles combine to flex the left hip.
- The quadriceps straighten the right knee.
- There is plantar flexion of the right ankle by the action of the gastrocnemius and soleus muscles.

Benefits

- Strengthens the arms and wrists.
- Stretches the upper back.
- Strengthens the abdominal muscles.
- Opens the groin.
- Tones the abdominal organs.

Cautions

- Not recommended for anyone suffering from carpal tunnel syndrome, as it may aggravate the problem.
- Do not attempt this pose during pregnancy.

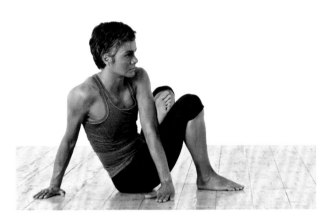 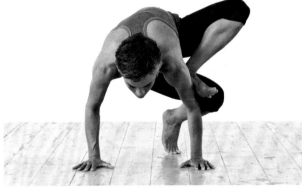

3. Turn to the right and bring both palms to the floor on your right side. The hands should be approximately shoulder width apart. Place the left foot on the back of the left arm, above the elbow.

5. Once you've lifted yourself up, straighten the right leg. You should be able to rest the right leg on the back of the left arms if the left foot is high up the back of the left arm, but this takes practice. To come out of the pose, bend the right knee and bring the right foot back to the floor.

4. Bring the weight into the hands as you lift your seat off the floor. Bend the left elbow, making a shelf with the back of the left arm for the left foot to rest on. Keep the right knee pressing against the left ankle to keep the foot from slipping.

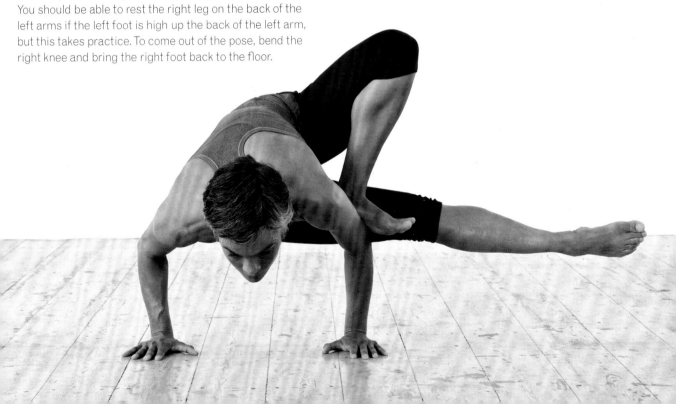

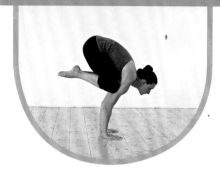

Kakasana
Crow Pose

The Crow Pose looks harder than it is – it requires more coordination, concentration and awareness than muscular strength in the upper arms. As you hold the pose the chest is immobilized so that you can only breathe abdominally.

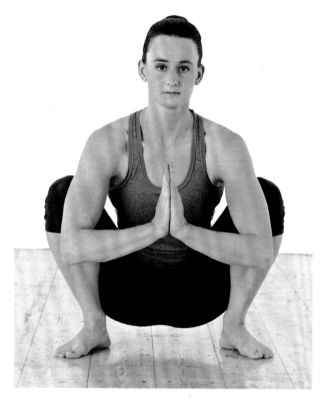

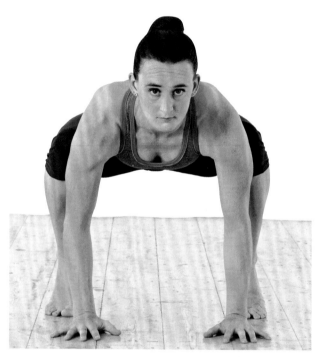

1. Come into a squatting position with the feet apart and the heels on the floor. Separate the knees and lean the torso forward, bringing the upper arms between the knees.

2. Bring your palms to the floor and spread out the fingers. Bend the elbows and lean the shins on the back of the upper arms, making a shelf for the shins to sit on.

Benefits

- Strengthens arms and wrists.
- Stretches the upper back.
- Strengthens the abdominal muscles.
- Opens the groin.
- Tones the abdominal organs.

Cautions

- Not recommended for anyone suffering from carpal tunnel syndrome, as it may aggravate the problem.
- Do not attempt this pose during pregnancy.

Anatomical Function

Upper body

- The serratus anterior muscle draws the shoulder blades forward while the pectoralis and deltoid muscles stabilize the shoulders.

- The lower trapezius, which spans the back, presses down on the shoulder blades.

- The tricep muscles straighten the elbows.

Lower body

- The hamstring muscles bend the knees.

- The adductor muscles squeeze the knees into the upper arms to link the upper and lower extremities.

- The psoas and rectus abdominis muscles combine to flex the trunk and hips.

3. Inhale and look forward, raising the heels and seat, and begin bending the elbows, bringing your weight onto the backs of the arms. Exhale and lift your weight forward, so that the elbows are aligned over the wrists and the feet begin to lift off the floor, one at a time or both together. Once you feel steady, bring the heels closer to the buttocks and point the toes.

4. Keep breathing and hold the pose for 20–30 seconds. To release, exhale and slowly lower the feet to the floor, back into a squat.

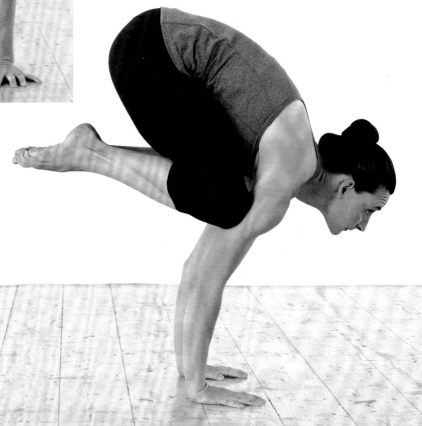

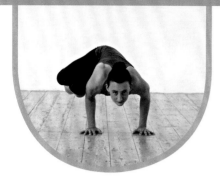

Parsva Kakasana
Side Crow Pose

In *Parsva Kakasana* both legs are resting on the back of one arm and the trunk is twisted to one side.

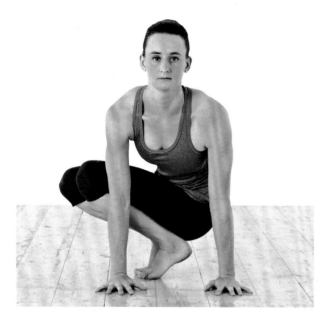

1. Come into a squat position with the knees together. Keep the knees and feet facing forward, but turn the torso to the left and place both hands on the floor beside you.

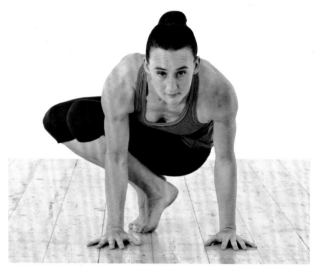

2. Make sure that the side of the left thigh is against the back of the right arm. Then inhale and slowly raise the buttocks and bend the ellbows.

Benefits

- Strengthens the arms and wrists.
- Stretches the upper back.
- Strengthens the abdominal muscles.
- Tones the abdominal organs.

Cautions

- Not recommended for anyone suffering from carpal tunnel syndrome, as it may aggravate the problem.
- Do not attempt this pose during pregnancy.

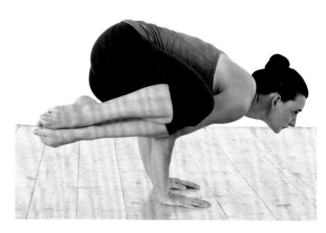

3. Bending the elbows makes a shelf for the side of the left thigh to sit on. Keep the knees together and lift the feet off the floor.

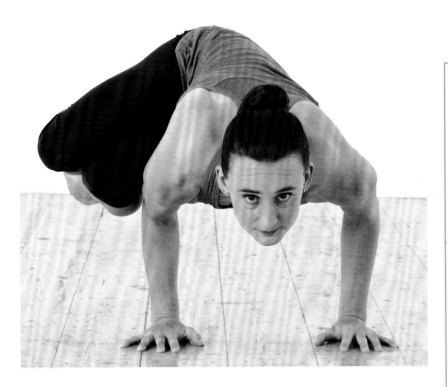

Anatomical Function

Upper body

- The serratus anterior muscle draws the shoulder blades forward while the pectoralis and deltoid muscles stabilize the shoulders.

- The lower trapezius, which spans the back, presses down on the shoulder blades.

- The tricep muscles straighten the elbows.

Lower body

- The hamstring muscles bend the knees.

- The adductor muscles squeeze the knees into the upper arms to link the upper and lower extremities.

- The psoas and rectus abdominis muscles combine to flex the trunk and hips.

4. Exhale and lift the legs on to the back of the right arm. Keep the elbows over the wrists. Hold for 20–30 seconds, then release the feet to the floor by bending the elbows. Repeat on the right side.

Variation

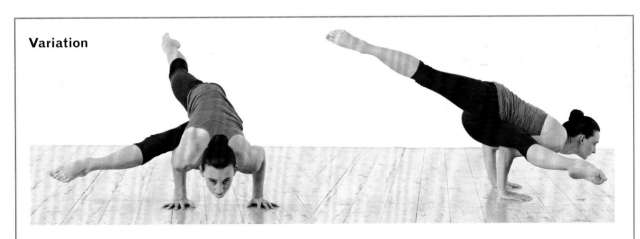

When you become more competent in the pose and your balance is steady, try splitting the legs. Extend the lower leg forward and the upper leg back.

SIDE VIEW

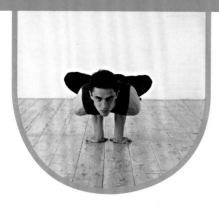

Mayurasana

Peacock Pose

In Hindu lore the peacock is a symbol of immortality and love. This *asana* tones the abdominal region. The pressure from the elbows stimulates blood circulation in the abdominal organs, improving digestion and stomach ailments, removing toxins in the body.

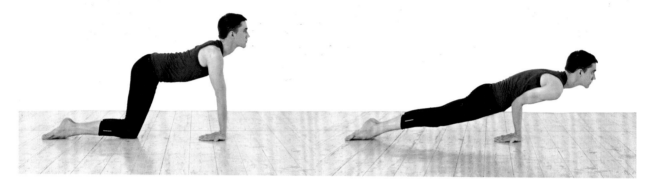

1. Kneel on the floor with the knees apart. Bring the palms to the floor in front of you and turn the hands so that the fingers point towards the knees. Try to bring the elbows together so that the little fingers touch.

2. Bend the elbows and rest the chest against the back of the upper arms, with the elbows pressing against the abdomen, towards the navel. Bring more weight into the hands and wrists as you lift the knees and straighten both legs. Keep them straight.

Anatomical Function

Upper body

- In the spine there is cervical extension; thoracic flexion and lumbar extension – the erector spinae, quadratus lumborum and rectus abdominis muscles hold the trunk solid.

- Scapular abduction due to the action of the serratus anterior and pectoralis major and minor. Rotator cuff and deltoids protect the shoulder joint.

- There is elbow flexion as the biceps and triceps keep the elbows at right angles.

- Forearm pronation due to the supinator.

- Wrist dorsiflexion.

Lower body

- The hips extend and adduct due to the action of the hamstrings, adductor magnus and gluteus maximus.

- Knee extension due to the quadriceps.

- Ankle plantar flexion due to the soleus muscle.

Tip

If necessary, use a strap to keep the elbows from slipping apart. Position it just above the elbows. If you can't quite manage the full pose as described in step 3, support the feet on a block (positioned on its side).

Benefits

- The pose strengthens the wrists and forearms.
- The abdomen is toned.
- Strengthens the back torso and legs.

Cautions

- Don't practise this pose if you have any wrist or elbow injuries.

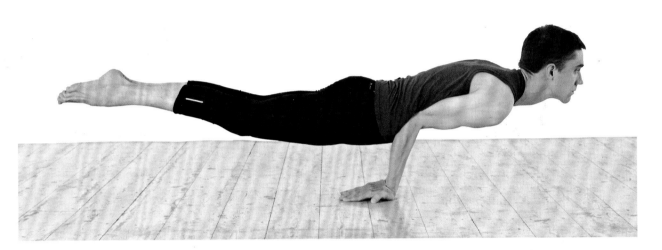

3. Exhale and raise the legs off the floor, either together or one at a time. Move the weight slightly forward and hold the torso and legs parallel to the floor with the feet together. Hold at first for about ten seconds.

Gradually increase the hold to 30 seconds as you gain more experience and strength in the pose. To release, lower the knees and feet to the floor, and lift the torso off the arms.

Advanced Variation: Padma Mayurasana

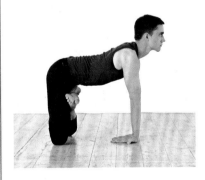

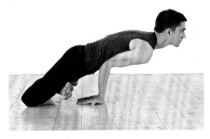

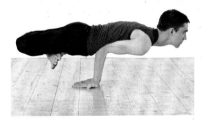

1. Come in to the Lotus Pose and lift onto the knees. Bring the palms to the floor and rotate the wrists so the fingers point towards the knees.

2. Bend the elbows and lower the chest onto the back of the arms.

3. Move the body weight forward so that the knees lift off the floor and balance on the hands.

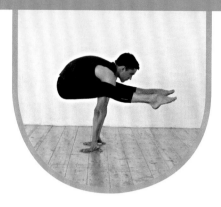

Tittibhasana

Firefly Pose

This pose is related to *Kurmasana* (Tortoise Pose, see page 136) and is also similar to *Kakasana* (Crow Pose, see page 162). It strengthens the upper body, the quadriceps and psoas muscles, and the wrists.

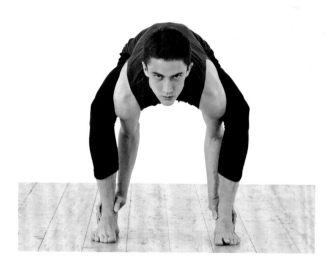

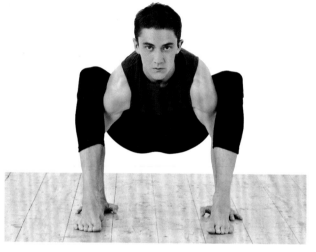

1. Bend the knees and squat with the feet shoulder distance apart. Tilt the pelvis forward and bring the trunk between the legs. Keeping the trunk low, straighten the legs enough to lift the pelvis to about knee height. Bring the arms through the legs and grab the back of each ankle.

2. Now pull the shoulders through the legs, tucking the shoulders behind the backs of the knees. Place the hands palms down on the floor behind the heels, fingers pointing forward.

Benefits

• Stretches the inner groin and back of the torso.

• Strengthens the arms and wrists.

• Tones the belly.

• Improves balance.

Cautions

• Not recommended for those suffering from shoulder, elbow, wrist or lower-back injuries.

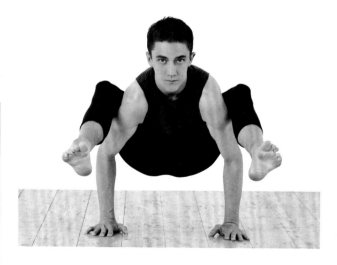

3. Press the hands into the floor and slowly begin to shift the weight onto the backs of the arms. The feet should begin to lift off the floor as you bring more weight onto the hands. Keep the thighs as high up the arms as possible.

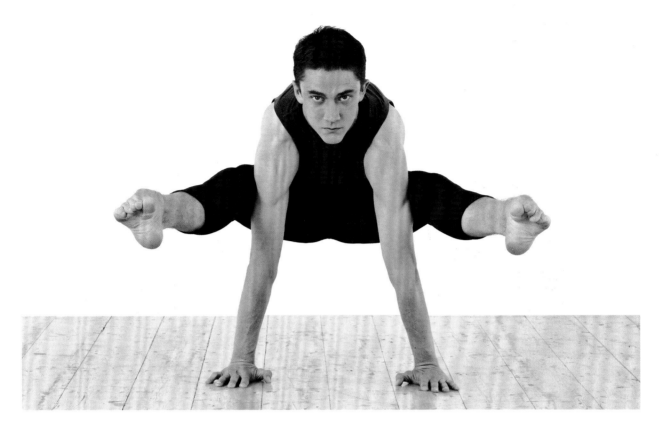

4. Inhale and straighten the legs, keeping the pelvis high to bring the legs parallel to the floor. Straighten the arms as much as possible. Without tensing the neck, lift the head and gaze forward. Breathe slowly and hold the pose for 15 seconds or longer, then release the feet to the floor with an exhalation.

Variation

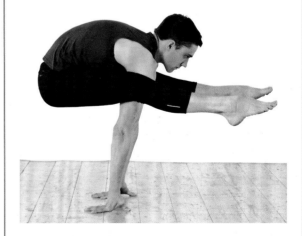

In this variation the hands are turned so that the fingers are pointing back, and the weight is on the fingers and thumbs – but note that the palms are raised.

Anatomical Function

Upper body

- The trapezius and rhomboid muscles are stretched.

- The arms are straightened due to the triceps.

- The adductor muscles on the inner thighs squeeze the thighs against the upper arms, connecting the upper and lower body.

Lower body

- The psoas and rectus abdominis muscles flex the hips and bend the trunk.

- The gastrocnemius and soleus muscles flex the ankles.

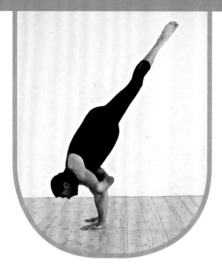

Galavasana

Pose of the Sage Galava

This pose is named after the sage Galava. It requires a reasonable amount of hip flexibility so is an intermediate level pose. It strengthens the wrists, increases core strength and opens the hips. The pressure of the foot against the abdomen massages the abdominal organs.

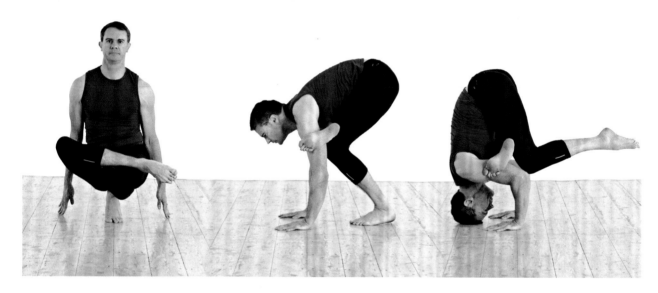

1. From a standing position, raise the right leg and bend the knee. Place the side of the right shin above the left knee, so that the knee is at a 90-degree angle. Now bend the left knee and bring the hands to the floor.

2. Bring the hands to the floor in front of the left shin, keeping them shoulder width apart, and fold the trunk forward so that the right shin is pressing against the backs of both arms. Try to tuck the right knee into the right armpit, bring the right shin to the left armpit and wrap the right toes around the left arm.

3. Bend the elbows and shift the weight forward onto the back of both arms. The backs of the arms should form a shelf for the right shin to sit on. If necessary, lower the forehead to the floor.

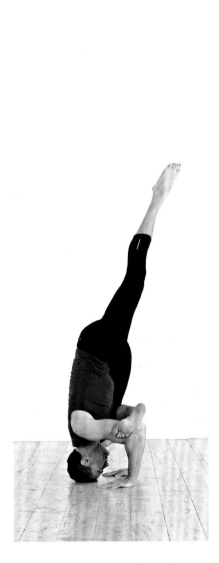

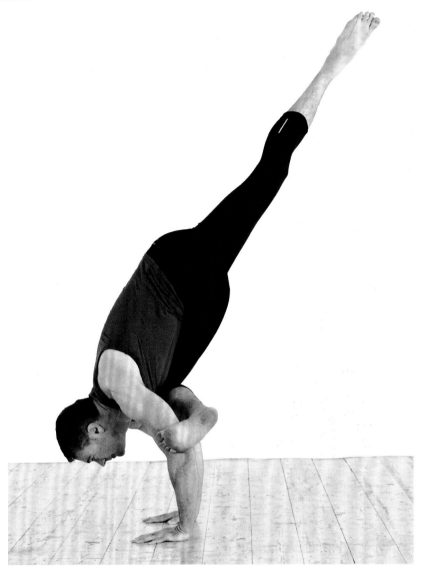

4. As the weight moves forward, lift the left foot off the floor. Slowly straighten the left leg and raise it a little higher.

5. Slowly straighten the arms and raise the head off the floor. Extend the left leg as high as possible. Hold the pose for 15 seconds, then lower the left foot to the floor and release the right foot down. Repeat the pose on the other side.

Benefits

• Strengthens the arms and wrists.

• Tones the belly and spine.

Cautions

• Don't do this pose if you have any wrist or lower-back injury.

Anatomical Function

Upper body

• The erector spinae, quadratus lumborum and rectus abdominis muscles hold the trunk solid.

• Scapular abduction involves the rotator cuff and deltoids.

• The biceps and triceps keep the elbows at right angles.

Lower body

• Front leg: this is rotated outwards by the psoas, sartorius and the deep external rotators in the thigh; the hamstrings bend the knee.

• Back leg: the gluteus maximus presses the hip forward and tilts the pelvis to extend the thigh. The quadriceps straighten the knee.

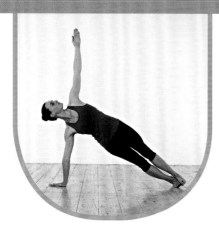

Vasisthasana

Side Plank Pose

Vasistha means 'most excellent, best, richest'. It is the name of several well-known sages in the yoga tradition.

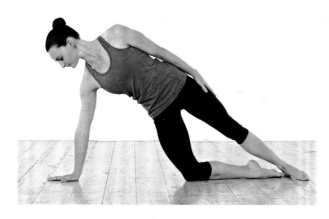

1. Bring the right hand and knee to the floor and straighten the left leg. Place the left hand on the side of the left thigh.

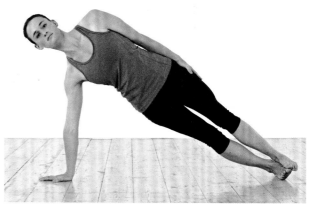

2. Press into the floor with the right hand and lift the right knee off the floor. Stack the left foot on top of the right. Strengthen the thighs and align the body into one long diagonal line from the heels to the crown of the head.

Benefits

- Strengthens the arms, belly and legs.
- Stretches and strengthens the wrists.
- Stretches the backs of the legs (in the full variation described opposite).
- Improves the sense of balance.

Cautions

- Students with wrist, elbow or shoulder injuries should avoid this pose.

Anatomical Function

Upper body
- Spine: the erector spinae and rectus abdominis muscles stabilize the spine.
- Top arm: shoulder abduction involves the deltoid muscle.
- Lower arm: elbow extension involves the triceps.

Lower body
- Hip in neutral extension and adduction.
- Knee extension due to quadriceps action.
- Ankle dorsiflexion involves the tibialis anterior.

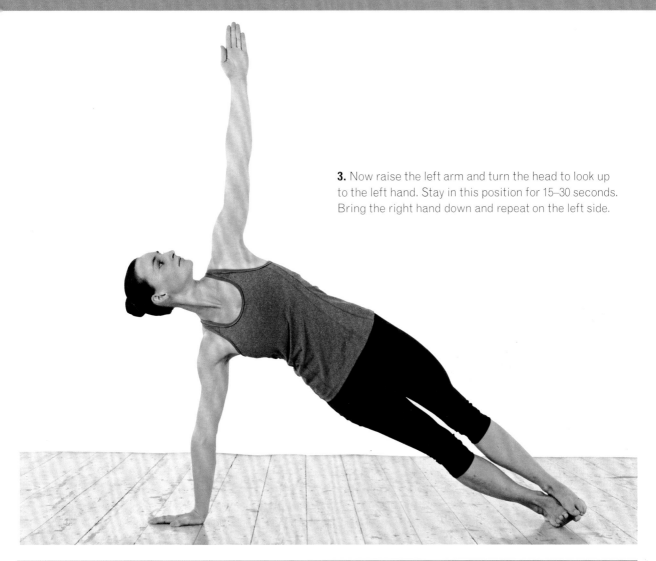

3. Now raise the left arm and turn the head to look up to the left hand. Stay in this position for 15–30 seconds. Bring the right hand down and repeat on the left side.

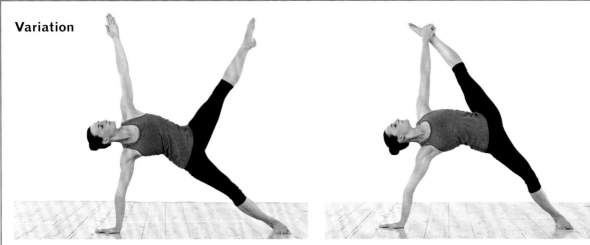

Variation

1. Raise the left leg up as high as possible.

2. Raise the left leg further and grab the heel or toe of the foot and take the leg out to the left. Press the inside of the left foot to the floor for balance.

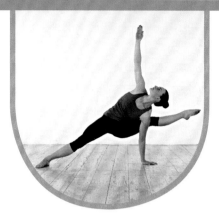

Vishvamittrasana

Pose of the Sage Vishvamitra

This pose strengthens the hands, abdominal organs and thighs.

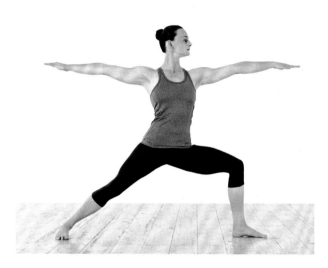

1. Perform *Virabhadrasana II* (see page 88) by turning the left foot forward and bending the knee, taking the right leg back and extending the arms.

2. Lean forward and bring the left shoulder inside the left knee, placing the hands on the floor on either side of the left foot.

Anatomical Function

Upper body

- The serratus anterior muscle draws the shoulder blades forward, stretching the middle trapezius and rhomboids.

- The pectoralis major and anterior deltoid muscles stabilize the shoulders.

- The lower trapezius, which spans the back, presses down on the shoulder blades.

- The infraspinatus and teres minor turn the humerus outwards to refine shoulder stability.

- The tricep muscles straighten the elbows.

Lower body

- The hamstring muscles bend the knees.

- The adductor muscles squeeze the knees into the upper arms to link the upper and lower extremities.

- The psoas and rectus abdominis muscles combine to flex the trunk and hips.

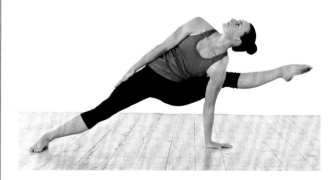

3. With the left elbow slightly bent, bring the weight of the left leg onto the back of the arm. Press the right foot into the floor. The left foot should lift off the floor. Place the right hand on the right thigh and straighten the left leg.

4. Inhale and raise the right arm up, then turn the head to look up to the right hand. Hold the pose for up to 30 seconds and exhale and bend the knee to release the foot to the floor. Repeat the pose on the other side.

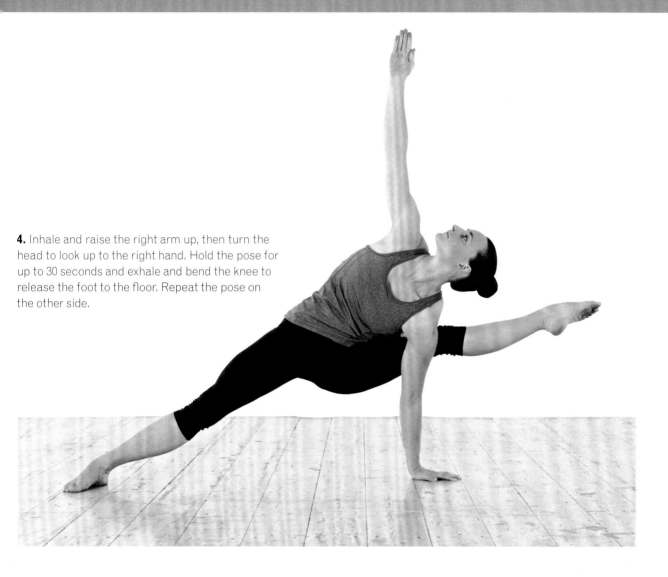

Advanced Variation

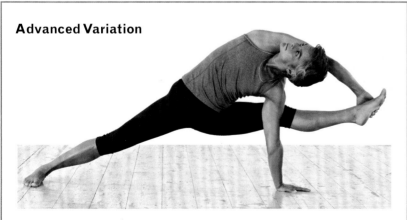

Reach the right hand across and take hold of the left foot, then raise the right arm over the head, keeping hold of the foot, and straighten the left leg. Keep your balance by pressing the right foot and left hand into the floor.

Benefits

- Strengthens the arms and wrists.
- Stretches the upper back.
- Strengthens the abdominal muscles.
- Opens the groin.
- Tones the abdominal organs.

Cautions

- Not recommended for anyone suffering from carpal tunnel syndrome, as it may aggravate the problem.
- Do not attempt this pose during pregnancy.

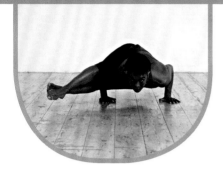

Astavakrasana

Eight-limbed Pose

This arm-support pose has a similar effect on the spine to *Parsva Kakasana* (Side Crow, see page 164), but with less rotation.

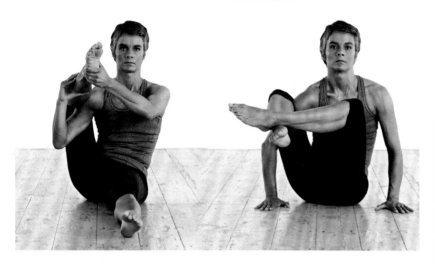

1. Sit on the floor with the legs straight. Raise the right leg and take hold of the foot with the left hand. Lift the right knee back and bring the leg onto the back of the right arm.

2. Place the hands on the floor. Press the knee against the shoulder and cross the left ankle over the right. Press the hands into the floor and contract the anus slightly. Exhale and lift the bottom off the floor.

Anatomical Function

Upper body

- Extension of the cervical spine and rotation, due to internal oblique and erector spinae muscles.

- Shoulder flexion and adduction; the rotator cuff and deltoid muscles protect the shoulder.

- Elbow flexion due to the action of the biceps.

Lower body

- Hip flexion and adduction due to the action of the psoas major and iliacus, pectineus, adductor longus and brevis.

- Knee extension due to the quadriceps.

- Ankle dorsiflexion due to the tibialis anterior.

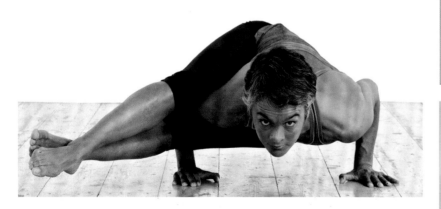

3. With the right leg supported on the shoulder, exhale and bend the elbows. Lean the torso forward; at the same time, straighten the knees and extend the legs out to the right, parallel to the floor. Look at the floor or look ahead. Hold for 30–60 seconds. Then straighten the arms slowly, lower the seat to the floor and uncross the ankles. Repeat the pose for the same length of time to the left.

Benefits

- Strengthens the wrists and arms.

- Tones the abdominal organs.

Cautions

- Avoid this pose if you have any wrist, elbow or shoulder injuries.

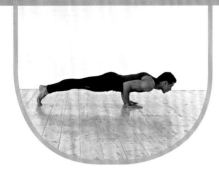

Chaturanga Dandasana

Four-limb Staff Pose

This pose is commonly used as a transition pose during dynamic *Vinyasa* practice.

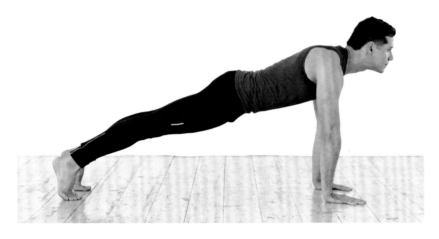

1. Start in a high press-up position with the arms straight and the shoulders over the wrists. With an exhalation, slowly lower the torso parallel to the floor with the elbows bent at 90 degrees and the upper arms parallel to the floor.

Anatomical Function

Upper body

- The erector spinae, quadratus lumborum and rectus abdominis muscles hold the trunk solid.

- Scapular abduction due to the rotator cuff and deltoids.

- The biceps and triceps keep the elbows at right angles.

Lower body

- Hips are in neutral extension and adduction due to the hamstrings and adductor magnus.

- Knee extension is due to the quadriceps.

Benefits

- Strengthens arms, wrists and abdominal muscles.

Cautions

- Avoid if suffering any wrist or shoulder injury.

2. Keep the breastbone lifted and the space between the shoulder blades broad. Tuck the elbows beside the torso and push them towards the heels. Lift the head to look forward and hold the pose for anything from 10 to 30 seconds. Release with an exhalation: either lay yourself lightly down onto the floor or push strongly back to *Adho Mukha Svanasana* (Downward-facing Dog, see page 179).

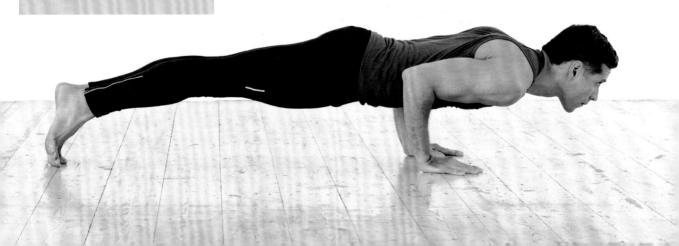

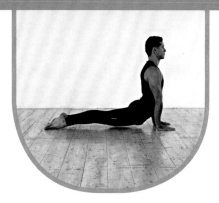

Urdhva Mukha Svanasana

Upward-facing Dog

A symmetrical backward-bending, arm-support pose, *Urdhva Mukha Svanasana* is one of the positions in the traditional Sun Salutation sequence (see page 209).

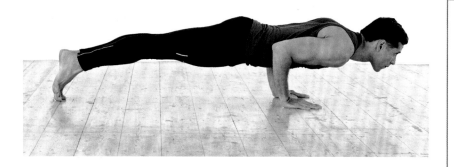

1. From *Chaturanga Dandasana* (see page 177), inhale and lift the chest forward and straigthen the arms, rolling onto the tops of the feet.

Anatomical Function

Upper body

- Spinal extension: the erector spinae muscles arch the back.
- Shoulder extension and adduction enabled by the posterior deltoid.
- Triceps enable elbow extension.
- Forearm pronation from the pronator quadratus and teres.

Lower body

- Hip extension and adduction enabled by the hamstrings and adductor magnus.
- Knee extension due to the quadriceps.
- Ankle plantar flexion due to the soleus muscle.

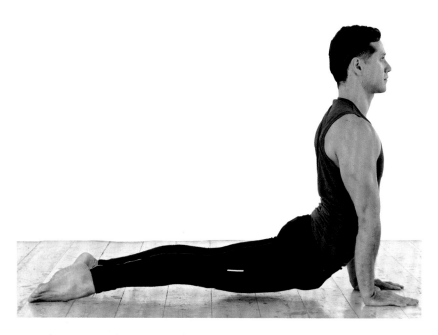

2. Inhale and lift the torso up and straighten the arms, raising the knees off the floor. Keep the thighs firm and turned slightly inwards. Roll the shoulders back and lift the chest, looking straight ahead. Release back to the floor or lift into *Ardho Mukha Svanasana* (Downward-facing Dog) with an exhalation.

Benefits

- Strengthens the spine, arms and wrists.
- Stretches the chest and lungs, shoulders and abdomen.
- Firms the buttocks.

Cautions

- Not recommended for anyone suffering from carpal tunnel syndrome, as it may aggravate the problem.

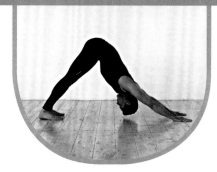

Ardho Mukha Svanasana

Downward-facing Dog

This is one of the poses in the traditional Sun Salutation sequence. It's also an excellent yoga *asana* all on its own. In dynamic practice this is a transitory pose as well as a restorative one.

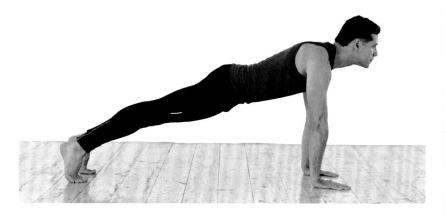

1. Come onto the floor on the hands and knees with the knees directly below the hips and the hands slightly in front of the shoulders. Spread the palms, index fingers parallel, and tuck the toes under. Exhale and lift the knees off the floor, straightening the legs.

Benefits

- Energizes the body.
- Stretches the shoulders, hamstrings, calves, arches and hands.
- Strengthens the arms and legs.
- Beneficial for high blood pressure, asthma, flat feet and sciatica.

Cautions

- Not recommended for anyone suffering from carpal tunnel syndrome.
- Pregnancy: do not do this pose late-term.

Anatomical Function

Upper body

- Scapular upward rotation and shoulder flexion: the anterior deltoids lift the shoulders and arms over the head.
- Elbow extension: the triceps straighten the elbows.
- Forearm pronation due to the pronator quadratus and teres.
- Wrist dorsiflexion.

Lower body

- Hip flexion involving the psoas, pectineus, sartorius and rectus femoris.
- Knee extension due to the quadriceps. The hamstrings, gastrocnemius and soleus muscles are stretched.
- Ankle dorsiflexion due to the tibialis anterior.

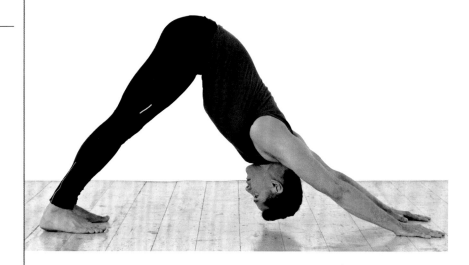

2. Exhale and lift the hips away from the shoulders and lengthen the spine. Press the hands firmly into the floor, rotate the forearms out and draw the shoulders away from the wrists. Lengthen the backs of the legs by pressing the heels towards the floor and lift the tops of the feet towards the shins. Stay in this pose for 1–3 minutes. Then bend the knees to the floor with an exhalation and rest in Child's Pose (see page 115).

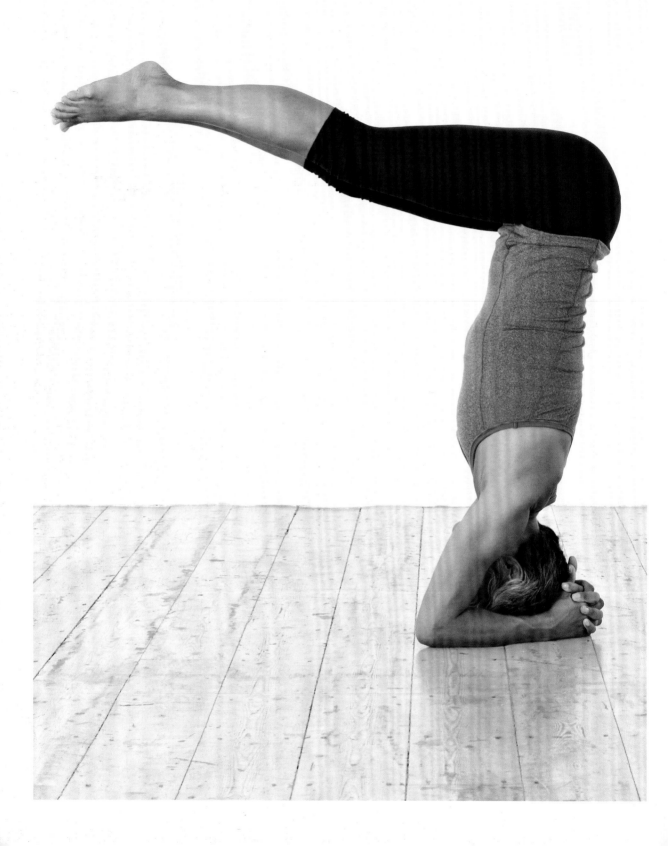

Inverted Poses

Turning our world upside down enables us to remain grounded and present. The inverted poses energize and stabilize the body. On a physical level, inversions are a boon to our circulatory and endocrine systems. By reversing our relationship to gravity we allow fresh, oxygenated blood to circulate and replace stagnant blood in the veins and arteries. Psychologically, inversions are a great way to clear the mind and bring a renewed sense of balance and focus.

Sirsasana 182
Sirsasana Variations 184
Sarvanghasana 186
Halasana 188

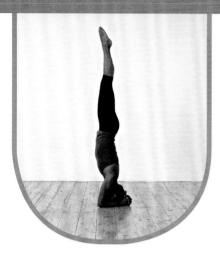

Sirsasana

Head Stand Pose

Sirsasana is a symmetrical inversion usually performed at the end of the practice. It is the king of the poses and is said to bring the most benefits.

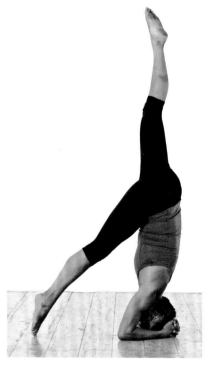

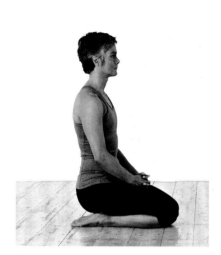

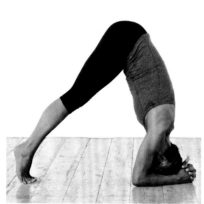

1. Kneel on the floor. Bring the forearms to the floor and grab the elbows, ensuring they are shoulder width apart.

2. Release the elbows, interlace the fingers and press the forearms on the floor. Bring the crown of the head to the floor. Open the palms and place the back of the head into the open palms. Inhale and lift the knees off the floor. Straighten the legs and walk the feet closer to the elbows.

3. Exhale and raise one leg up and then the other. If necessary bend the knee of the leg that is on the floor and lighly push off with the foot to hop up. Rotate the upper thighs slightly inwards and actively press the heels towards the ceiling (straightening the knees if you bent them to come up).

Anatomical Function

Upper body

- Spine: the erector spinae stabilizes the trunk. The rectus abdominis draws the abdomen and ribcage in.

- Scapular upward rotation due to the action of the serratus anterior. Shoulder flexion and adduction involve the anterior deltoids and trapezius muscles.

- Elbow flexion due to the biceps.

Lower body

- Hip extension involves the hamstrings, adductor magnus and gluteus maximus. The psoas muscle balances the pelvis to keep it straight.

- Knee extension due to the quadriceps.

- Ankle dorsiflexion due to the tibialis anterior.

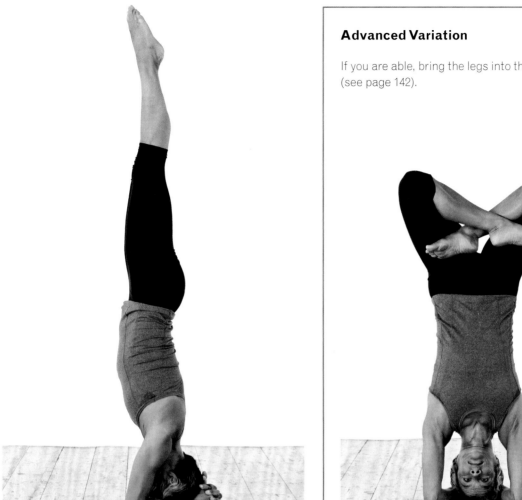

Advanced Variation

If you are able, bring the legs into the Lotus Pose
(see page 142).

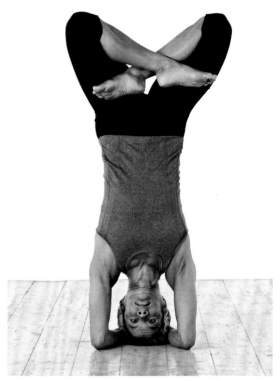

4. Keep the weight evenly balanced on both forearms.
Keep the tailbone lifted and lift the shoulders away from
the ears. Once the legs are straight, press up through the
balls of the feet. Ideally hold the pose for three minutes –
or longer for more advanced students – but it is important
to build up gradually. Don't strain to hold the pose.
Release by bringing one foot down at a time and rest in
Balasana, Child's Pose (see page 115), for a few breaths.

Benefits

- Helps relieve stress and mild depression.
- Stimulates the pituitary and pineal glands.
- Strengthens the arms, legs and spine.
- Tones the abdominal organs.
- Brings fresh blood to the lower extremities and brain.

Cautions

- Do not practise if you have a back or neck injury, a heart
  condition or high blood pressure.
- Avoid during menstruation.
- if you are experienced in this pose and become pregnant,
  you can practise it during pregnancy.

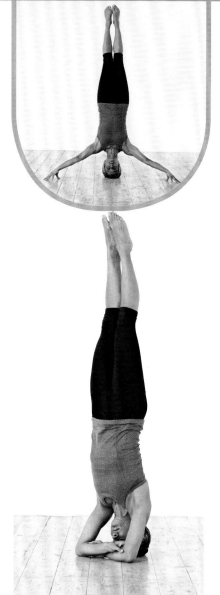

Sirsasana Variations
Head Stand Variations

These poses are recommended for those with an advanced practice, who are experienced in holding the head stand (see page 182) for long periods and would like to try some variations.

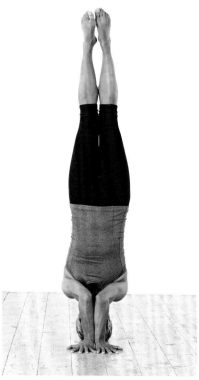

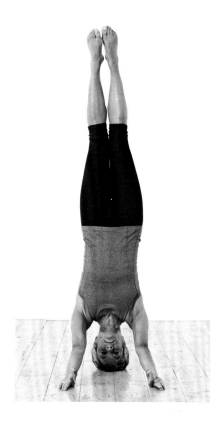

From *Sirsasana*, the arms can be folded in front of the head. First release the right arm from behind the head and bring it in front of the forehead. Then carefully bring the left arm from behind the head and fold the left arm over the right, pressing the elbows and forearms into the floor for support.

From *Sirsasana*, the hands can be placed on the floor in front of the forehead with the palms facing down and fingers pointing away from the head. Try to bring the elbows to touch, or as close together as possible.

From *Sirsasana,* the arms are extended forward, shoulder width apart and with the palms facing up. Press the backs of the hands into the floor to keep your balance.

Benefits

- Stimulates the pituitary and pineal glands.
- Strengthens the arms, legs and spine.
- Tones the abdominal organs.

Cautions

- These poses are only recommended for experienced practitioners.

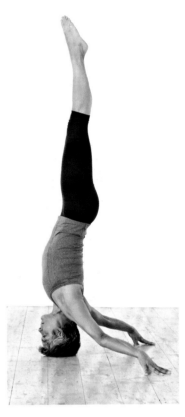

Side view

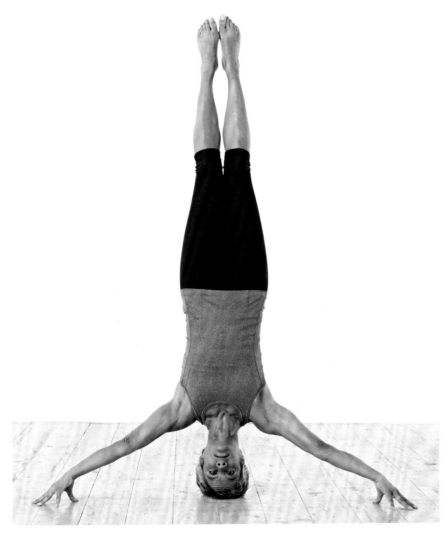

From *Sirsasana*, the arms move out to the side. The palms can be flat on the floor or, as in this example, the balance is on the head and fingertips. This requires concentration and practice.

Anatomical Function

Upper body

- Spine: the erector spinae stabilizes the trunk. The rectus abdominis draws the abdomen and ribcage in.

- Scapular upward rotation due to the action of the serratus anterior. Shoulder flexion and adduction involve the anterior deltoids and trapezius muscles.

- Elbow flexion due to the biceps.

Lower body

- Hip extension involves the hamstrings, adductor magnus and gluteus maximus. The psoas muscle balances the pelvis to keep it straight.

- Knee extension due to the quadriceps.

- Ankle dorsiflexion due to the tibialis anterior.

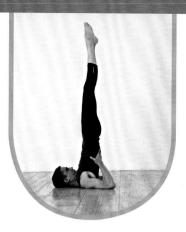

Sarvanghasana

Shoulder Stand Pose

This pose is a restorative inversion, usually done towards the end of the practice, as a counterpose after the head stand.

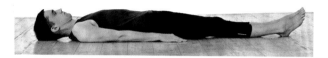

1. Lie on your back with the legs straight and the arms by your side, palms facing down.

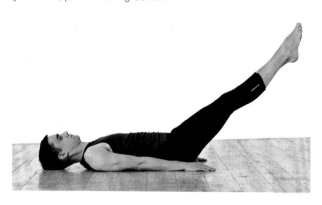

2. Press the backs of the arms and palms into the floor, exhale and raise both legs.

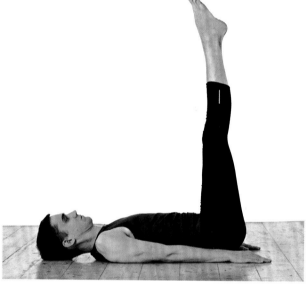

3. Bring the legs to a right angle with the body. Press the arms down as you exhale and lift the buttocks and lower back off the floor.

Benefits

- Stimulates the thyroid and prostate glands and abdominal organs.
- Stretches the shoulders and neck.
- Tones the legs and buttocks.
- Helps relieve the symptoms of the menopause.
- Reduces fatigue and alleviates insomnia.

Cautions

- Avoid if you are suffering from high blood pressure or have a neck injury.
- Avoid during menstruation.
- If you are experienced in this pose and become pregnant, you can practise it during pregnancy.

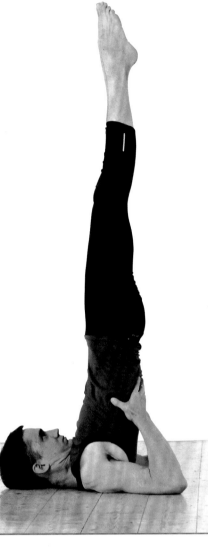

Anatomical Function

Upper body

- Spine: cervical and upper thoracic flexion; lower thoracic and lumbar extension.

- Scapular adduction, downward rotation and elevation due to the rhomboids and levator scapulae.

- Shoulder extension and adduction due to the triceps, teres major and posterior deltoid; elbow flexion due to the biceps; forearm supination. The erector spinae and rectus abdominis muscles lift the trunk.

Lower body

- Hip extension is activated by the gluteus maximus and psoas muscles, which support the pelvis; adduction is activated by the adductor magnus and gracilis muscles.

- Knee extension is activated by the quadriceps.

- Ankle dorsiflexion.

4. Now bend the elbows and bring the palms behind the ribcage. The backs of the upper arms and shoulders should be resting on the floor. Walk the hands up the back towards the shoulder blades without letting the elbows slide much wider than shoulder width apart. Soften the throat and tongue. Firm the shoulder blades against the back and move the breastbone towards the chin. Actively press the backs of the upper arms and the tops of the shoulders into the floor and try to lift the upper spine. Keep the legs straight and perpendicular to the floor by tightening the backs of the thighs.

5. Beginners should stay in the pose for about 30 seconds. Add five to ten seconds every day until you can comfortably hold it for three minutes, then gradually build up to five minutes. To break the pose, exhale and bend the knees into the torso; release the spine carefully, keeping the back of the head on the floor.

Advanced Variation

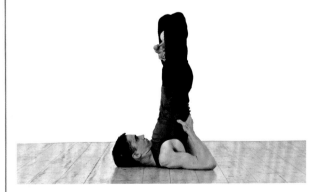

1. If you are able, bring the legs into the Lotus Pose (see page 142).

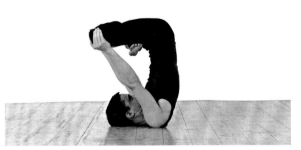

2. Flex the hips and lower the knees down and rest the palms on the knees.

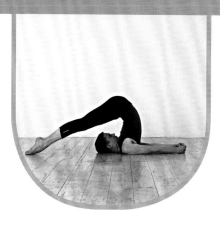

Halasana
Plough Pose

Usually performed immediately after the shoulder stand (see page 186), this pose has beneficial effects on the cardiovascular system as well as on the flow of cerebrospinal fluid.

Anatomical Function

Upper body

- There is scapular adduction, downward rotation and elevation due to the rhomboids and levator scapulae; and elbow flexion due to the biceps.

Lower body

- Hip flexion due to the psoas and pectineus muscles, and adduction due to the adductor longus and brevis.

- Knee extension occurs due to the quadriceps.

- Ankle dorsiflexion due to the tibialis anterior.

Benefits

- Stimulates the abdominal organs and the thyroid gland.

- Stretches the shoulders and spine.

- Reduces stress and fatigue.

Cautions

- Do not practise this pose during menstruation.

- Avoid if you have a neck injury.

- If you suffer from asthma or high blood pressure, practise *Halasana* with the legs supported on props.

- If you are experienced with this pose and become pregnant, you can continue to practise it late into pregnancy.

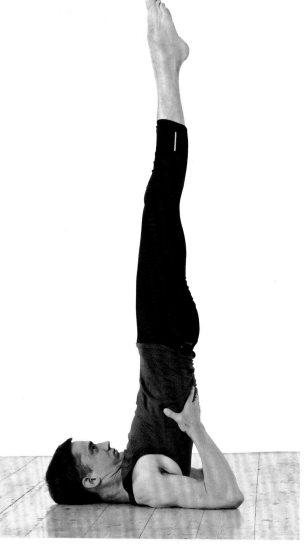

1. From *Sarvangasana*, exhale and bend from the hip joints, slowly lowering the toes to the floor above the head. As much as possible, keep the torso perpendicular to the floor and the legs fully extended.

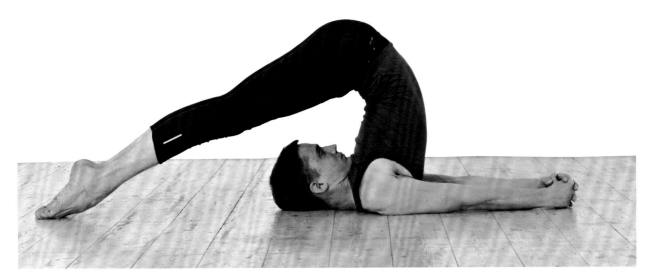

2. With the toes on the floor, lift the tailbone towards the ceiling. Draw the chin away from the breastbone and soften the throat. You can continue to press the hands against the back, lifting the hips up towards the ceiling as you press the backs of the upper arms down. Or you can release the hands away from the back and stretch the arms out behind you on the floor, opposite the legs. Clasp the hands and press the arms actively down on the support as you lift the thighs towards the ceiling. *Halasana* is usually performed after *Sarvangasana* for anything from one to five minutes. To exit the pose bring the hands onto the back again, lift back into *Sarvangasana* with an exhalation, then roll down onto the back. Alternatively, simply roll out of the pose on an exhalation.

Advanced Variation

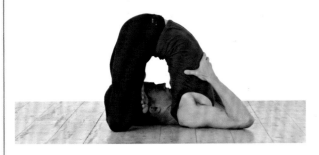

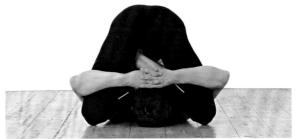

1. If you are able, bring the legs into the Lotus Pose (see page 142) and lower the knees to the floor, keeping the back supported.

2. Wrap the arms around the backs of the thighs and draw the knees to the floor.

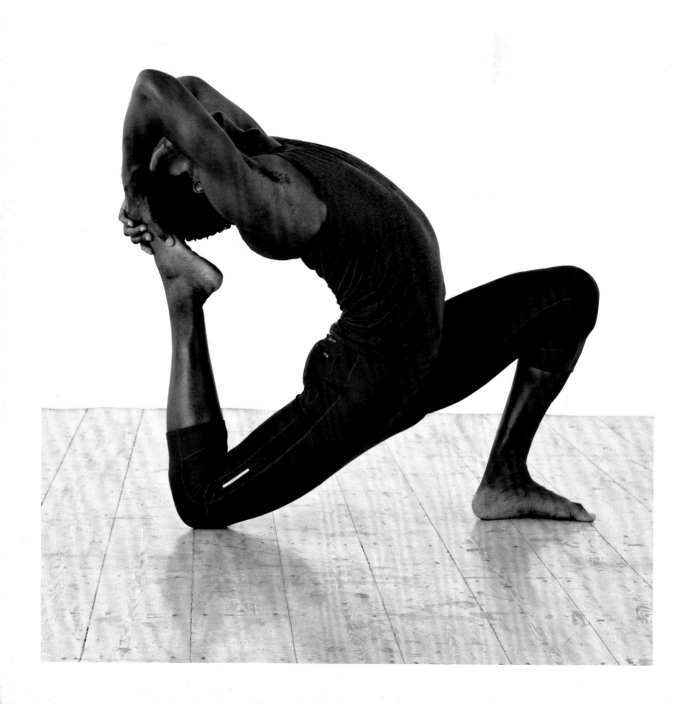

Back-bending Poses

Energizing and extroverting, back-bending *asanas* are expansive, enabling us to open our hearts and turn our bodies out to fully embrace life. Back-bending creates space in the chest for the breath to move more freely, encouraging inhalation – not only creating a lighter sense of being, but giving us the resources to deal with whatever the universe has in store for us.

Urdhva Dhanurasana 192
Ustrasana 194
Kapotasana 196
Eka Pada Raja Kapotasana I 198
Eka Pada Raja Kapotasana II 200
Dhanurasana 202
Ashva Sanchalasana 204
Salabhasana 206
Bhujanghasana 208
Surya Namaskara 209

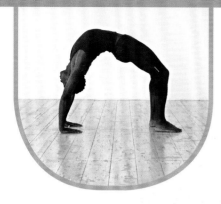

Urdhva Dhanurasana

Upward-facing Bow Pose

Also known as *Chakrasana* or Wheel Pose, this is an invigorating back bend. It opens the chest and heart centre (*Anahata chakra*). This expansion in the heart centre brings vitality. Bending backwards turns the body out to face the world and helps you to see things from a different perspective – an action associated with embracing life.

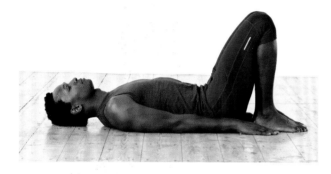

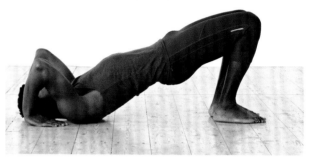

1. Lie on the floor and raise the knees, bringing the feet to the floor, with the heels as close to the buttocks as possible.

2. Raise the arms over the head and bend the elbows. Spread the palms on the floor beside the head, with the fingers pointing towards the shoulders. The forearms should be perpendicular to the floor. Pressing the feet actively into the floor, exhale and lift the buttocks. Keep the thighs and inner feet parallel. Take two or three breaths.

Benefits

- Stretches the chest and lungs.
- Strengthens the arms and wrists, legs, buttocks, abdomen and spine.
- Stimulates the thyroid and pituitary glands.
- Counteracts depression.

Cautions

- Avoid this pose if you have a back injurymor suffer from carpal tunnel syndrome orheart disease.
- Avoid if you suffer from headaches.

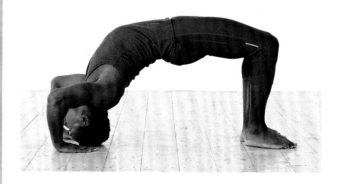

3. Firmly press the hands into the floor and the shoulder blades against the back, and lift yourself up onto the crown of the head. Keep the arms parallel. Take two or three breaths.

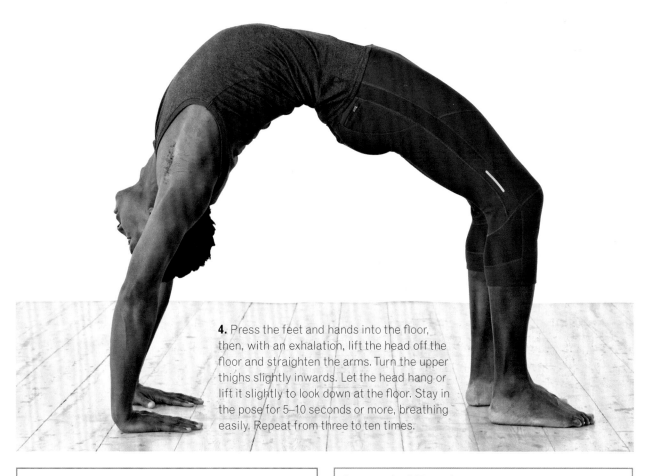

4. Press the feet and hands into the floor, then, with an exhalation, lift the head off the floor and straighten the arms. Turn the upper thighs slightly inwards. Let the head hang or lift it slightly to look down at the floor. Stay in the pose for 5–10 seconds or more, breathing easily. Repeat from three to ten times.

Advanced Variation

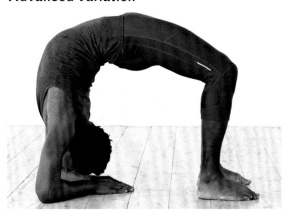

Dwi Pada Viparita Dandasana

From *Urdvha Dhanurasana*, lower the head and then the elbows to the floor. Spread the palms out and lift the heels, then lift the head and try to look back towards the feet. Press the forearms down and lift the shoulders as you lower the heels to the floor.

Anatomical Function

Upper body

- The erector spinae arches the back. The quadratus lumborum works with the psoas muscle and the rectus abdominis to stabilize the lower back.

- Upward rotation and elevation of the shoulder blade due to the action of the serratus anterior.

- Shoulder flexion due to the anterior deltoids and biceps. The rotator cuff and deltoids stabilize the shoulder joint.

- Elbow extension involves the triceps.

- Forearm pronation due to the action of the pronator quadratus and teres.

- Wrist dorsiflexion caused by the wrist extensors.

Lower body

- Hip extension and adduction involve the hamstrings and gluteus maximus.

- Knee flexion involves the quadriceps.

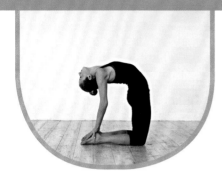

Ustrasana
Camel Pose

Ustrasana is a deep back-bending pose that can be challenging at first. The hands and feet connect the upper and lower appendicular skeleton.

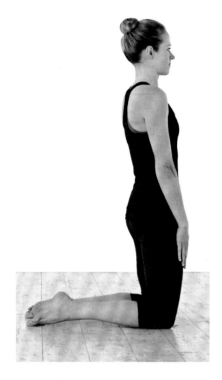

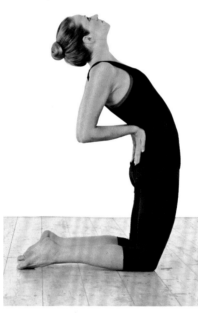

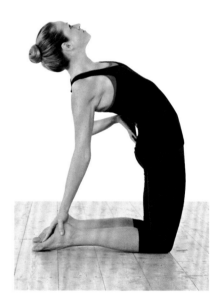

1. Kneel on the floor with the knees hip width apart and thighs perpendicular to the floor. Rotate the thighs slightly inwards. Press the shins and the tops of the feet firmly into the floor.

2. Rest the hands on the back with the palms just above the buttocks, fingers pointing down.

3. Now reach the right hand down to the right heel and the left hand to the left heel. Inhale, lift the chest, roll the shoulders back and down and relax the head back while keeping the thighs perpendicular to the floor.

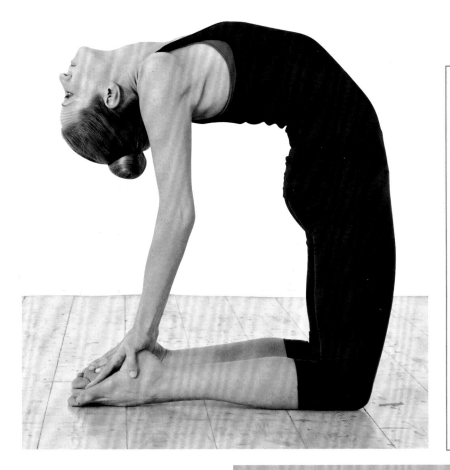

Anatomical Function

Upper body

- Scapular adduction and downward rotation through the action of the rhomboids and trapezius muscles.

- Shoulder extension occurs due to the action of the posterior deltoids at the back of the shoulders and adduction.

- Elbow extension involves the triceps.

- The spine is protected from over-mobilization by the psoas and abdominal muscles.

Lower body

- Hip extension and adduction due to the gluteus maximus and hamstrings.

- Knee flexion and ankle plantar flexion due to the gastrocnemius and soleus muscles.

4. Press the palms firmly against the heels, with the bases of the palms on the heels and the fingers pointing towards the toes. Lift the breastbone and push the pelvis forward, keeping the thighs vertical. Stay in this pose for 30–60 seconds. To exit, bring the hands onto the hips. Inhale and lift the head and torso, then sit back on the heels and bring the forehead to the floor for a few breaths.

Benefits

- Stretches the entire front of the body, the ankles, thighs and groin.
- Stretches the deep hip flexors (psoas).
- Strengthens the back muscles.
- Stimulates the abdominal organs.

Cautions

- Not recommended for those suffering from high or low blood pressure or those with a tendency to suffer from migraines.

- Avoid this pose if you have a serious lower-back or neck injury.

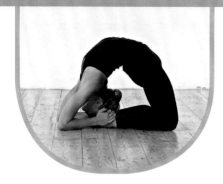

Kapotasana

Pigeon Pose

Kapota means a pigeon or a dove, and this pose resembles a pigeon as it puffs out its chest. It tones the spine, massages and strengthens the heart and stimulates the genital organs, keeping them healthy.

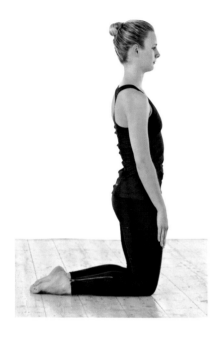

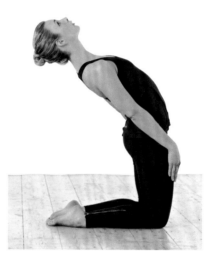

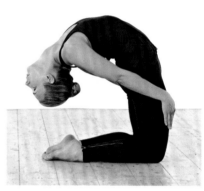

1. Kneel upright, with the knees hip width apart and the hips, shoulders and head aligned above the knees. Place the hands on the front of the thighs.

2. Inhale, tuck the chin towards the breastbone and lean the head and shoulders back as far as you can without pushing the hips forward.

3. Roll the shoulder blades against the back and lift the chest. Keep the chest lifted and gradually release the head back.

Benefits

- Stretches the entire front of the body, the ankles, thighs and groin, abdomen, chest and throat.
- Stretches the deep hip flexors (psoas).
- Strengthens the back muscles.
- Stimulates the abdominal organs and strengthens the heart.

Cautions

- Not recommended for those suffering from high or low blood pressure or those with a tendency to suffer from migraines.
- Avoid if you have a serious low-back or neck injury.

4. Raise the arms over the head towards the floor behind you. Push the hips forward enough to counterbalance the backward movement of the upper torso and head. Keep the thighs as perpendicular to the floor as possible as you drop back. Place the palms on the floor, fingers pointing towards the feet, then lower the crown of the head to the floor.

Anatomical Function

Upper body

- The serratus anterior and upper trapezius muscles upwardly rotate and abduct the shoulder blade.

- The rotator cuff, pectoralis major and anterior deltoids create shoulder flexion, adduction and external rotation.

- The erector spinae extend the torso, which lengthens and stretches the rectus abdominis, which in turn contracts to protect the lumbar spine.

Lower body

- Hip extension: the gluteus maximus presses the hip forward and tilts the pelvis to extend the thigh.

- The hamstrings bend the knees and further extend the hip.

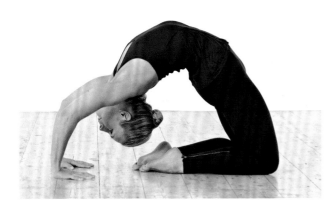

5. Press the palms down, lift the head off the floor and raise the hips, lifting the pelvis as much as possible. Lengthen and extend the upper spine and walk the hands to the feet. As you do so, lower the forearms to the floor. If possible, grip the ankles (or, if you're very flexible, the calves). Draw the elbows towards each other until they're shoulder width apart, then press them firmly on the floor. Extend the neck and place the forehead on the floor. Take a full inhalation to expand the chest. Then, exhaling, press the shins and forearms against the floor, lengthen the tailbone towards the knees and lift the chest. Hold the pose for 30 seconds or longer. Then release and lift the torso back to an upright position. Rest in Child's Pose (see page 115) for a few breaths.

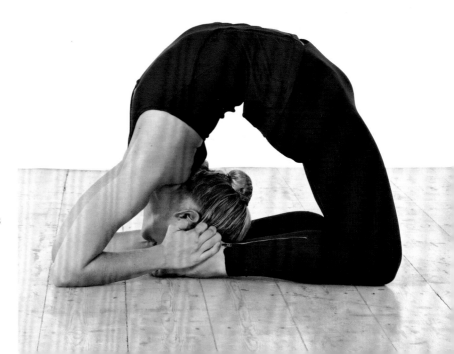

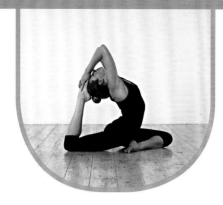

Eka Pada Raja Kapotasana I

King Pigeon Pose I

Rajakapota means the king of pigeons. This is the one-legged Pigeon Pose, in which the chest is pushed forward like that of a pigeon.

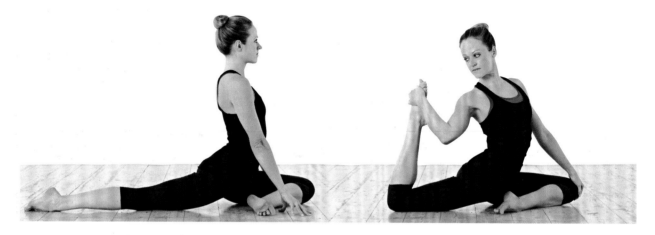

1. Sitting on the floor, bend the left knee and bring the left heel in line with the right hip. Keep the left knee on the floor and press the side of the calf down. Lift the right leg back and straighten it. The thigh, knee and top of the foot should be touching the floor.

2. Place the palms on the waist, push the chest forward, lift the shoulders back and drop the head back. Hold for a few breaths. Now bring the hands to the floor and bend the right knee, lifting the foot towards the head. Keep the right thigh muscles active. Reach back with the right hand and pull the foot towards your shoulder.

Benefits

- Stretches the thighs, groin and psoas, abdomen, chest, shoulders and neck.
- Stimulates the abdominal organs.
- Opens the shoulders and chest.

Cautions

- Do not practise this pose if you have a sacroiliac injury, ankle or knee injury, or tight hips or thighs.

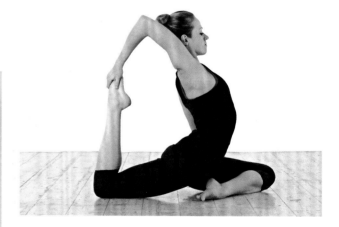

3. Carefully raise the right elbow so that the foot is centred behind the head. Take a few breaths here, then reach the left arm over the head to grab the foot.

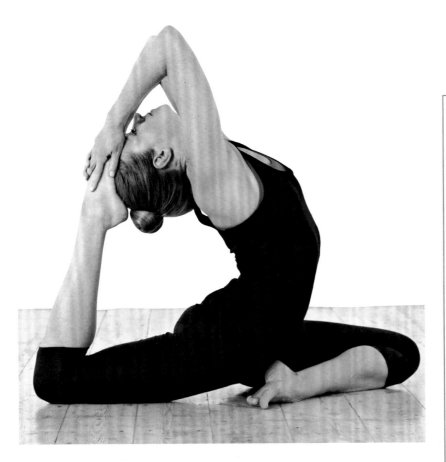

4. Bring the foot to the back of the head and rest the head against the foot. Hold the pose for 10–15 seconds, then release the foot down. Then bring the right leg forward and switch sides, bringing the leftf foot to the back of the head and holding the foot with both hands.

Anatomical Function

Upper body

- Upward rotation of the shoulder blade and abduction and elevation – serratus anterior and upper trapezius muscles; shoulder flexion adduction and external rotation, forearm supination – rotator cuff, pectoralis major, anterior deltoids and biceps muscles.

- The erector spinae extend the torso, which lengthens and stretches the rectus abdominis, which in turn contracts to protect the lumbar spine.

Lower body

- Front leg: hip flexion and external rotation; knee flexion; ankle plantar flexion; foot supination – the front leg is rotated outwards by the psoas, sartorius and the deep external rotators in the thigh; the hamstrings bend the knee.

- Back leg: hip extension, internal rotation and adduction; knee flexion; ankle plantar flexion – the gluteus maximus presses the hip forward and tilts the pelvis to extend the thigh. The hamstrings bend the back knee and further extend the hip.

Intermediate Variation

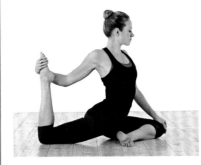

1. Take hold of the right foot with the right hand.

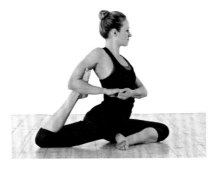

2. Fold the foot inside the right elbow and bind the hands.

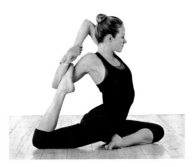

3. Keep the bind and lift the left elbow beind the head.

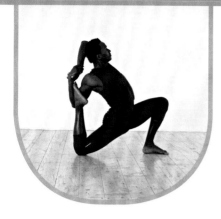

Eka Pada Raja Kapotasana II

King Pigeon Pose II

This is a variation of the one-legged Pigeon Pose (see page 198), in which the back foot is raised and the hands are bound behind the head.

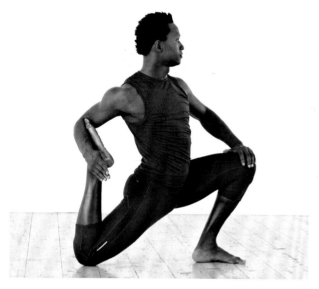

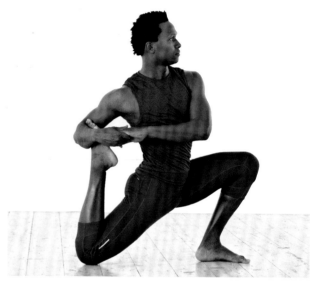

1. Come into a lunge position with the left leg forward and the right leg back, with the knee resting on the floor. Bend the right knee and raise the shin approximately perpendicular to the floor. The body weight will balance on the left foot and right knee. Bring the right foot in towards the right buttock, and fold the foot inside the right elbow.

2. Reach the left hand across the front of the chest and bind the hands. To stabilize the position, push the left knee forward until it extends beyond the left ankle, sinking the right thigh to the floor and releasing the hip down.

Benefits

- Stretches the thighs, groin and psoas, abdomen, chest, shoulders and neck.
- Stimulates the abdominal organs.
- Opens the shoulders and chest.

Cautions

- Do not practise this pose if you have a sacroiliac injury, ankle or knee injury or tight hips or thighs.

Anatomical Function

Upper body

- Upward rotation of the shoulder blade and abduction and elevation; shoulder flexion, adduction and external rotation, forearm supination.
- The erector spinae extend the torso and the rectus abdominis contracts to protect the lumbar spine.

Lower body

- Front leg: hip flexion due to the psoas muscle. Knee flexion is the action of the hamstring muscles.
- Back leg: hip extension, internal rotation and adduction; knee flexion; ankle plantar flexion – the gluteus maximus presses the hip forward and tilts the pelvis to extend the thigh. The hamstrings bend the knee and extend the hip.

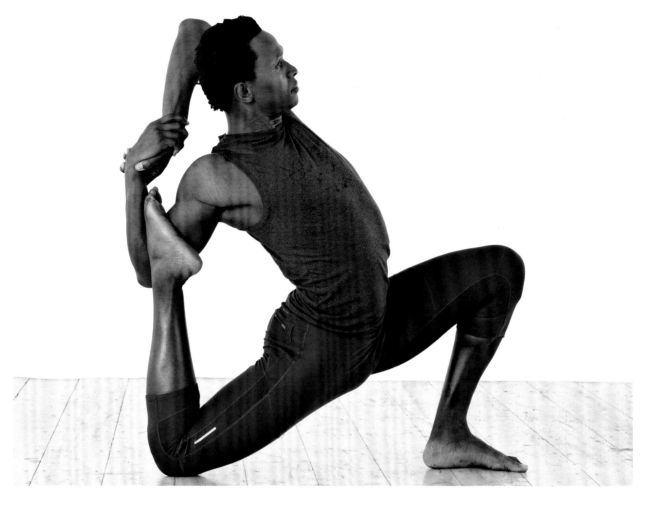

3. Now raise the left elbow over the head and behind it, and bring the right shoulder forward to square the chest and hips to face forward. Hold for about 15–30 seconds, breathing as smoothly as possible.

Exhale and release the right foot, bringing it back to the floor. Repeat the pose with the left leg to the back of the head.

Advanced Variation

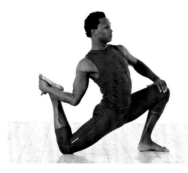

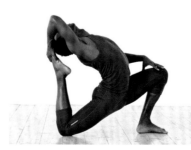

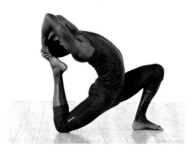

1. Take hold of the right foot with the right hand.

2. Draw the foot into the shoulder and bring the foot to the head.

3. Reach back with the left hand and grab the foot.

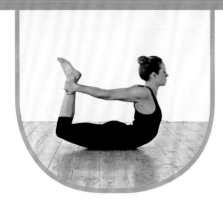

Dhanurasana

Bow Pose

This pose is so called because it resembles an archer's bow. The torso and legs represent the body of the bow and the arms the strings.

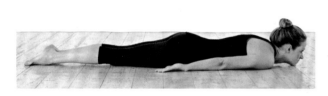

1. Lie on your stomach with the arms alongside the torso, palms facing up.

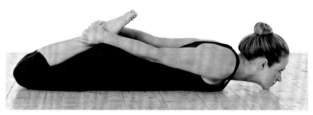

2. Exhale and bend the knees, then reach back with the hands and take hold of the ankles. Keep the knees hip width apart, and no wider, for the duration of the pose.

Benefits

- Stretches the entire front of the body, ankles, thighs and groin, abdomen and chest, throat and deep hip flexors.
- Strengthens the back muscles.
- Improves posture.
- Stimulates the organs of the abdomen and neck.

Cautions

- Not recommended for those suffering from high or low blood pressure, or migraine.
- Avoid if you have a serious lower-back or neck injury.

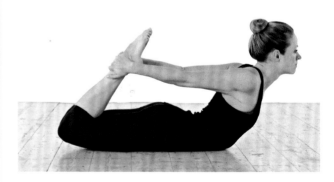

3. Inhale and lift the heels away from the buttocks. Then lift the thighs away from the floor, trying to straighten the legs. This will have the effect of lifting the upper torso and chest off the floor. Keep the back muscles relaxed.

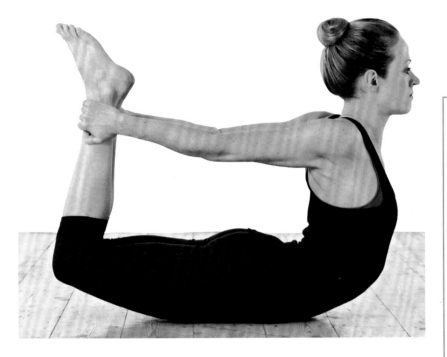

4. As you continue lifting the heels and thighs higher, draw the shoulder blades together to open the chest. Draw the tops of the shoulders away from the ears and look ahead. Hold the pose for 20–30 seconds. Release as you exhale and lie quietly for a few breaths. You can repeat once or twice more.

Anatomical Function

Upper body

- Spinal extension due to the erector spinae and quadratus lumborum muscles.

- Scapular adduction, shoulder extension and internal rotation due to lower trapezius and rhomboids; elbow extension due to posterior deltoids and triceps.

Lower body

- Hip extension and adduction. The hip flexors and rectus abdominis are stretched.

- Knee flexion due to the action of the hamstrings.

- Ankle plantar flexion due to the soleus muscle.

Advanced Variation

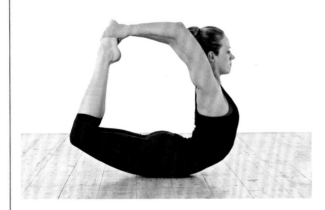

1. Lie on the belly and bend the knees, then raise the arms and reach back to take hold of the tops of the feet or the toes.

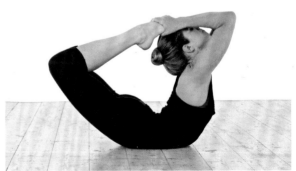

2. Lift the elbows up and bring the feet to the back of the head.

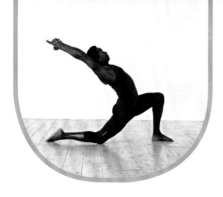

Ashva Sanchalasana

Crescent Moon Pose

This pose opens the chest, stomach, shoulders, arms and hips, and lengthens, arches and opens the spine.

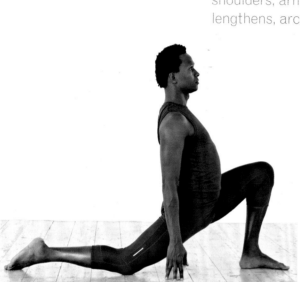

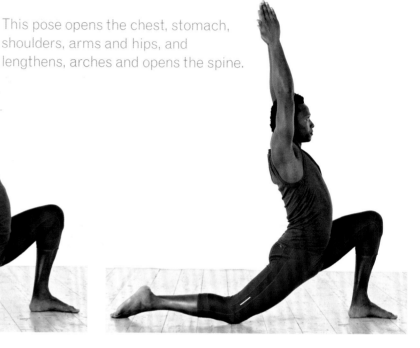

1. Come into a deep lunge with the left knee bent and the right leg stretching back, with the knee on the floor and the arms beside the trunk.

2. Sink the right thigh to the floor and relax the hips down. Inhale, raise the arms over the head and bring the palms togther.

Benefits

- Stretches the chest and lungs.
- Strengthens the shoulders and arms.
- Strengthens the legs, buttocks, abdomen and spine.

Cautions

- Avoid this pose if you have a back or shoulder injury.

Anatomical Function

Upper body

- The erector spinae arches the back. The quadratus lumborum works with the psoas muscle and the rectus abdominis to stabilize the lower back.

- Upward rotation and elevation of the shoulder blades is the action of the serratus anterior. Shoulder flexion is the action of the anterior deltoids and biceps. The rotator cuff and deltoids stabilize the shoulder joint.

- Elbow extension involves the triceps.

Lower body

- Hip extension and adduction involve the hamstrings and gluteus maximus.

- Hip flexion on the front leg is the action of the psoas mucles, and knee flexion involves the action of the quadriceps.

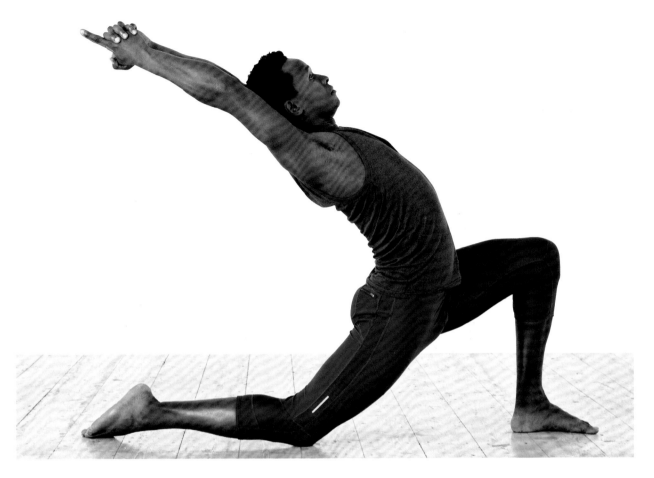

3. Interlace the fingers and cross the thumbs, then reach the arms back behind the head. Move the shoulders from side to side to loosen and lower them down. Imagine reaching towards the right foot with both hands.

Hold the pose for 15–30 seconds. To release, bring the palms to the floor and step the left foot back to come on to the knees, then repeat on the other side by stepping the right foot forwards.

Advanced Variations

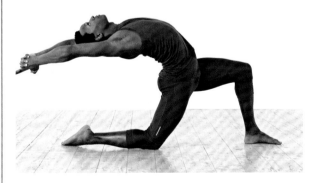

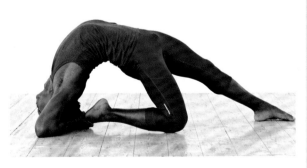

Continue to lift the arms back and arch the spine more, reaching towards the right foot. This is a very advanced pose and requires great flexibility in the spine.

In some cases it is possible to reach for the back foot and hold it. This usually rquires the supervision of an experienced teacher.

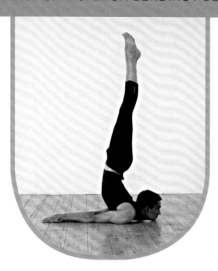

Salabhasana
Locust Pose

An advanced prone back-bending pose, this *asana* strengthens the muscles in the back – the erector spinae, quadratus lumborum and lower trapezius.

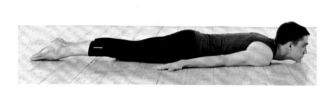

1. Lie on your stomach with legs straight and arms by your side, palms facing down. Stretch the neck and rest the chin on the floor.

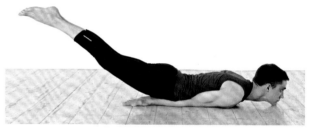

2. Bring the hands together underneath the body, either with the palms flat as shown or the fingers interlaced to make a fist. Inhale and raise the legs up. Press the palms, forearms, upper arms and shoulders firmly into the floor. For many of us, this is as far as we can advance in the pose.

Anatomical Function

Upper body

- Spinal extension due to the erector spinae, which arch the back.

- Scapular downward rotation and adduction due to the lower trapezius and rhomboids. Elbow extension due to the triceps. Pectoralis muscles open the chest.

Lower body

- Hip extension due to the gluteus maximus and adduction due to the adductor muscles.

- Knee extension due to the quadriceps; adduction due to the hamstrings and adductors.

- Ankle plantar flexion due to the soleus muscle.

Benefits

- Strengthens the muscles of the spine, buttocks and backs of the arms and legs.

- Stretches the shoulders, chest, belly and thighs.

- Improves posture.

- Stimulates the abdominal organs.

Cautions

- Not recommended for those with a tendency to headaches.

- Avoid if you have a serious back injury.

- Students with neck injuries should keep their head in a neutral position by looking down at the floor.

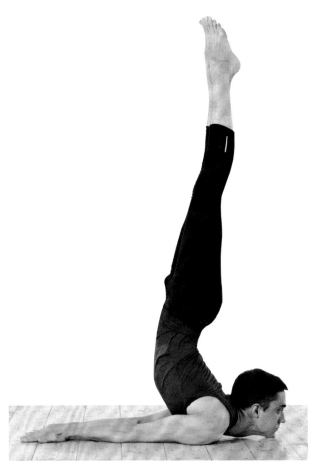

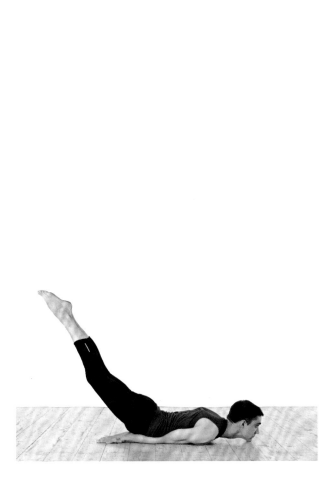

3. Keep pressing the arms into the floor and try to lift the legs higher; lift the thighs, hips and groin off the floor by swinging the legs up.

4. In the full pose, which is very advanced and impossible for many of us, the chest is lifted off the floor with the hips fully extended upwards and the legs pointing up. The pose is held for 10–30 seconds, then the trunk is slowly lowered to the floor and the legs come down one at a time.

Advanced Variation

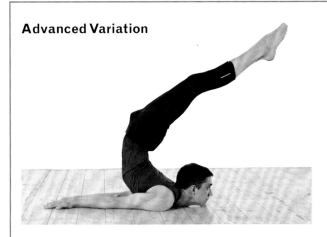

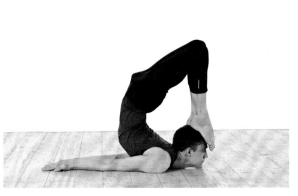

1. If you are able to raise the trunk and legs high enough, the legs can be brought over the head.

2. By bending the knees, the feet can be lowered on top of the head. This is an extremely advanced pose.

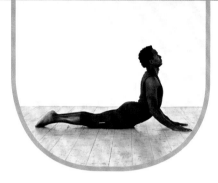

Bhujanghasana

Cobra Pose

In Sanskrit, *bhujanga* means serpent. In this pose, like a serpent about to attack, one lifts the trunk up from the floor and throws the head back.

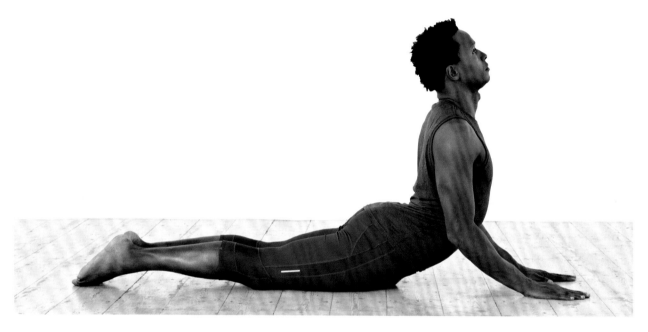

1. Lie on the belly with the legs straight and the tops of the feet on the floor. Spread the hands on the floor under the shoulders. Keep the elbows beside the ribs. On an inhalation, begin to straighten the arms to lift the chest, keeping the pubic bone and the thighs on the floor.

2. Draw the shoulder blades against the back. Lift the breastbone without pushing the front ribs forward. Distribute the back-bend evenly through the spine. Hold the pose for 15–30 seconds, breathing easily. Release back to the floor with an exhalation.

Anatomical Function

Upper body

- The spine extends due to the erector spinae muscles. The lower trapezius draws the shoulders back and down and the pectoralis major opens the chest.

- Elbow extension occurs by the action of the triceps, and forearm pronation due to the pronator quadratus.

Lower body

- Hip extension and adduction are activated by the gluteus maximus; the deep hip flexors stretch the psoas, pectineus and adductor longus muscles.

- Knee extension is due to the quadriceps and ankle plantar flexion due to the soleus muscle.,

Benefits

- Strengthens the spine.
- Stretches the chest and lungs, shoulders and abdomen.
- Firms the buttocks.
- Stimulates the abdominal organs.

Cautions

- Avoid if you have a back injury.
- Avoid during pregnancy.

Surya Namaskara
The Sun Salutation

Surya means sun, which in ancient times represented spiritual consciousness and was worshipped daily, and *namaskara* means salutations. *Surya Namaskara* or 'salutations to the sun' is a dynamic sequence of *asanas*, which are an effective means of warming up the body, stretching, toning and loosening the muscles and joints and the internal organs.

As well as its physical benefits, the Sun Salutation induces greater awareness and prepares the practitioner for spiritual enlightenment. The Sun Salutation is a complete practice in itself, comprising *asana*, *pranayama*, *mantra* and meditation. The 12 *asanas* that make up the sequence (see following pages) generate pranic energy, which activates the psychic channels in the body. The steady rhythmic sequence corresponds with the rhythms of the universe – the 24 hours of the day, the astrological calendar and the biorhythms of the human body.

When to practise
The recommended time to practise *Surya Namaskara* is at sunrise. The solar energy that flows through the *pingala nadi* within the body is vitalized, and with regular practice this *nadi* is regulated, leading to a balanced energy system on both mental and physical levels, and a more fulfilled, energized sense of being.

To complete one full round of *Surya Namaskara*, begin by practising the 12 stages on the right side (to activate *pingala nadi*), stepping the right foot back in step 4 and the right foot forward in step 9, and then complete another 12 stages by stepping the left foot backwards in step 4 and forward in step 9. To increase concentration or for meditational purposes, the cycle can begin on the left side.

At least two rounds and as many as 12 complete rounds should precede any other *asanas*. This ensures that the body is fully prepared for the rest of your *asana* practice. In specific cases 108 rounds are practised for purification purposes and, in modern society, individuals are often sponsored in order to raise money for charitable causes.

A *mantra* is traditionally ascribed to each of the 12 steps of *Surya Namaskara* and can be recited during each round.

1. *Om Mitraya Namaha* – To he who is friendly to all
2. *Om Ravaye Namaha* – To the shining, radiant one
3. *Om Suryaya Namaha* – To the dispeller of darkness
4. *Om Bhanave Namaha* – To he who illumines, the bright one
5. *Om Khagaya Namaha* – To he who is all-pervading,
6. *Om Pushne Namaha* – To he who gives strength
7. *Om Hiranyagarbhaya Namaha* – To the golden cosmic self
8. *Om Marichaye Namaha* – To the Lord of the dawn
9. *Om Adityaya Namaha* – To the son of Aditi, the cosmic Mother
10. *Om Savitre Namaha* – To the Lord of Creation
11. *Om Arkaya Namaha* – To he who is worthy of praise and glory
12. *Om Bhaskaraya Namaha* – To he who leads to enlightenment

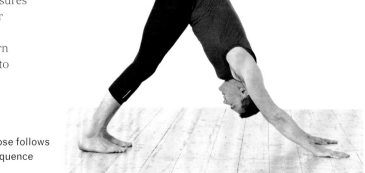

There are twelve stages to *Surya Namaskara*. Each pose follows on from the one before to create a flowing, dynamic sequence that prepares the body for *asana* practice..

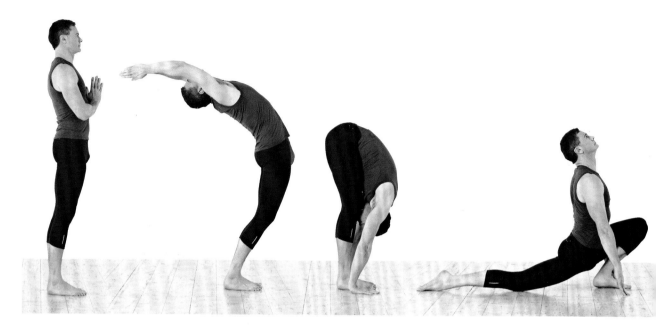

1. Stand with the feet together and the hands in front of the chest in *Pranamasana*, Prayer Pose. Close the eyes and bring the awareness to the right side of the heart, the centre of your physical chest. This is where the spiritual heart lies.

2. Inhale and raise the arms over the head and arch back into *Hasta Uttanasana*.

3. Exhale and bend forward and bring the palms either side of the feet and the head to the knees or shins. This is *Uttanasana*.

4. Inhale and step the right leg back as far as possible and bring the knee to the floor, lowering the right hip and thigh towards the floor. Lift the chest, and tilt the head back. This is *Ashva Sanchalanasana*, the Equestrian Pose.

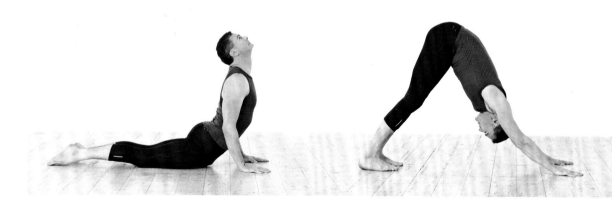

7. Lower the thighs and hips to the floor and inhale and lift the trunk by straightening the elbows, and arch the back as you push the chest forward into Cobra Pose, *Bhujanghasana*.

8. Exhale, tuck the toes under and lift the knees off the floor as you push back into Downward-facing Dog, *Adho Mukha Svanasana*. LIft the hips away from the shoulders and bring the heels to the floor.

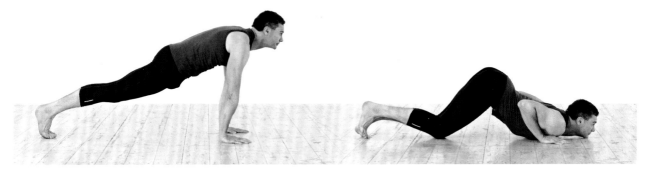

5. Press both palms to the floor and straighten the arms. Tuck the right toes under, lift the knee off the floor and step the left leg back to meet the right. This is *Phalakasana*.

6. Exhale and bring the knees, chest and chin to the floor. The buttocks, hips and abdomen should be raised. This is *Ashtanga Namaskara.*

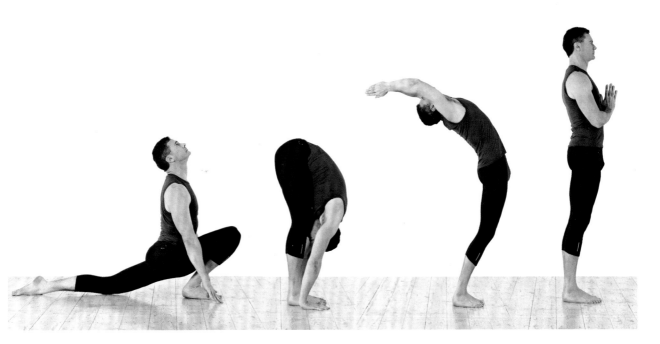

9. Inhale and step the right leg forward as far as possible and assume *Ashva Sanchalanasana*.

10. Exhale and step the left foot forward to meet the right and bend forward and come into *Uttanasana*.

11. Inhale and lift the trunk, then raise the arms over the head and arch back.
12. Exhale and lower the hands into *Pranamasana*.

A Daily Practice Plan

The suggested practice plans opposite are recommended for anyone wishing to develop a daily or regular yoga practice. Through constant practice, spiritual perfection and radiant mental as well as physical health are attained.

The following plans are intended as a guide to developing your own self-practice. Over time you will be able to structure a practice that suits and responds to your own physical and mental needs. For example, you may wish to incorporate more advanced poses into your practice after your strength and flexibility have increased. First and foremost, you must enjoy your practice. Don't let it become a chore or a bore. Remember, it is *your* practice and you should regard it as your own form of creative expression that you can look forward to, so don't make it so challenging for yourself that you approach it with trepidation or dread.

When I practise, little else matters apart from the mat and me. It's a time when I can work through and try to overcome my physical limits and celebrate my physical strengths, as well as analysing any mental obstacles; it is above all, a time when I can explore my own consciousness. Yoga has become a valuable resource, which I am forever applying to other more challenging occurences in my daily life whenever they arise.

It is important to create a practice to suit your lifestyle: it is more benefitial to practise regularly for 30-minute periods rather than sporadically for longer periods, so develop a routine that you can stick to. But remember, as a rule of thumb any *asana* that is performed should be countered with its opposite pose, in order to maintain a healthy spine. Therefore, if you practise a forward bend, counter the pose with a backward bend.

What to include

Traditionally, some poses are considered essential for a complete yoga practice. Always begin your *asana* practice with several rounds of the Sun Salutation (*Surya Namaskara*, see page 86) to prepare the body for *asanas*. If you have time, it is important to include the Head Stand (*Sirsasana*), Shoulder Stand (*Sarvangasana*) and Fish Pose (*Matsyasana*) in your practice, as these poses are believed to have the most physical and mental benefits; as well as at least one forward bend, back-bend and a spinal twist. Conclude your *asana* practice with the Corpse Pose (*Savasana*) for at least five minutes. Relaxing the muscles is as important as developing them and it is this balance of the two that brings optimum health.

Nowadays, the order of the poses varies according to different schools of yoga and traditions. In some cases, there is no particular structure to a class.

Pranayama and meditation practice can be performed separately and earlier in the day, while *asanas* can be practised later. Purification techniques such as *Jala Neti* and *Nauli* should be practised in the morning as part of your daily cleansing regimen.

The tables opposite offer three practice plans to suit the time you have available and your level of experience. Most of the poses can be replaced with an alternative pose from its corresponding *asana* section or modified to suit your ability. If some are too challenging, then omit them. They are provided as a guide for you to explore your *asana* practice. Steps 1–6 form what is more commonly known as *vinyasa*, a flowing sequence leading you from one pose into another in an almost seamless fashion. Remember to hold each pose for at least five breaths or 10–15 seconds.

Below is a quick checklist to enable you to develop and structure your practice. Remember that for all bilateral poses, for example *Virabhadrasana* (Warrior) or *Vasisthasana* (Side Plank), practise on the right side first and then the left. Try to include the following poses if time allows.

- *Surya Namaskara* (Sun Salutation) – at least 2 rounds
- **1 Standing Pose** (for example *Vrkshasana* – Tree Pose)
- **1 Balancing Pose** (for example *Kakasana* – Crow Pose)
- **Head Stand** (*Sirsasana*)
- **Shoulder Stand** (*Sarvanghasana*)
- **Fish Pose** (*Matsyasana*)
- **1 Back-bend** (for example *Dhanurasana* – Bow Pose)
- **1 Forward Bend** (for example *Paschimottanasana* – Forward Bend)
- **1 Seated Pose** (for example *Janu Sirsasana* – Head-to-Knee Pose)
- **1 Twisting Pose** (for example *Ardha Matsyendrasana* – Spinal Twist)
- *Savasana* to conclude the *asana* practice
- *Pranayama* (Several rounds of *Nadi Sodhana*)
- **Meditation**

A 30-minute practice plan

1. Complete 2 full rounds of **Surya Namaskara**

2. From **Pranamasana**, inhale and raise the arms, **Hasta Uttanasana**, exhale, bend forward and bring the hands to the floor and perform **Chaturanga Dandasana**, inhale **Urdhva Mukha Svanasana** and exhale **Adho Mukha Svanasana**

3. Step the right foot forward and perform **Virabhadrasana I and II**, then twist to the right and perform **Parivrtta Parsvakonasana**, then **Uttan Pristhasana**

4. Place the hands to the floor, step the right foot back and perform **Chaturanga Dandasana**, then **Urdhva Mukha Svanasana** and **Adho Mukha Svanasana**

5. Step the left foot forward and perform **step 3** on the left side

6. Jump or step both feet forward and come into **Uttansana**, inhale **Hasta Uttanasana** and exhale **Pranamasana**

Now perform the following poses:

7. **Vrikshasana** on both sides
8. **Utkatasana**
9. **Kakasana**
10. **Sirsasana**
12. **Sarvanghasana**
13. **Matsyasana**
14. **Paschimottansasana**
15. **Badha Konasana**
16. **Janu Sirsasana** on both sides
17. **Ustrasana**
18. **Ardha Matsyendrasana** on both sides
19. **Savasana**

B 60-minute practice plan

1. Complete 2 full rounds of **Surya Namaskara**

2. Perform **step 2** from **Section A**

3. Step the right foot forward and perform **Virabhadrasana I and II** and twist to the right and perform **Parivrtta Parsvakonasana**, then **Uttan Pristhasana.** Step the right foot back and perform **Vasisthasana** on the left hand and foot

4. Lower the right hand to the floor and perform **Chaturanga Dandasana**, then **Urdhva Mukha Svanasana** and **Adho Mukha Svanasana**

5. Step the left foot forward and repeat **steps 3** and **4** on the left side

6. Peform **step 6** from **section A**

Now perform the following poses:

7. **Vrikshasana** or **Ardha Badha Padma Paddotanasana** on both sides
8. **Kakasana** or **Parsva Kakasana** on both sides
9. **Gomukhasana** on both sides
10. **Sirsasana***
11. **Sarvanghasana***
12. **Matsyasana***
13. **Urdhva Dhanurasana**
14. **Upavistha Konasana**
15. **Badha Konasana**
16. **Marichyasana** on both sides
17. **Ustrasana** or **Dhanurasana**
18. **Pincha Mayurasana**
19. **Mayurasana**
20. **Ardha Matsyendrasana** on both sides
21. **Savasana**

* Practise **Padmasana** variations

C 90-minute practice plan

1. Complete 2 full rounds of **Surya Namaskara**

2. From **Pranamasana**, inhale and raise the arms, **Hasta Uttanasana,** exhale, bend forward and perform **Kakasana,** then **Chaturanga Dandasana,** inhale **Urdhva Mukha Svanasana** and exhale **Adho Mukha Svanasana**

3. Step the right foot forward and perform **Kapyasana**, then **Parivrtta Parsvakonasana**, then **Uttan Pristhasana**

4. Step the right foot back and perform **Chaturanga Dandasana**, then **Urdhva Mukha Svanasana** and **Adho Mukha Svanasana**

5. Repeat **steps 3**, then **4** on left side

6. Step the right foot forward and perform **Virabhadrasana I and II**, then **Ardha Chandrasana**, then return to **Virabhadrasana II** and perform **Prasarita Padottanasana**, then return to **Virabhadrasana II.** Place both hands to the floor and repeat **step 4**, then perform **step 6** on the left foot. Bring the hands to the floor and repeat **step 6** from **Section A**

Now perform the following poses:

8. **Svarga Dvijasana** on both sides
9. **Uttitha Tittibhasana**
10. **Tittibhasana**
11. **Bharadvajasana**
12. **Sirsasana***
13. **Sarvanghasana***
14. **Matsyasana***
15. **Urdhva Dhanurasana**
16. **Kurmasana**
17. **Eka Pada Sirsasana** – both sides
18. **Ustrasana** or **Dhanurasana**
19. **Pincha Mayurasana** or **Adho Mukha Vrikshasana**
20. **Mayurasana**
21. **Ardha Matsyendrasana** on both sides

If you have time, conclude your practice with the following breathing and meditation exercises or set aside a time of the day when you can practice these separately:

Pranayama – Nadi Sodhana – 5–10 minutes

Meditation – Dhyana – 5–10 minutes

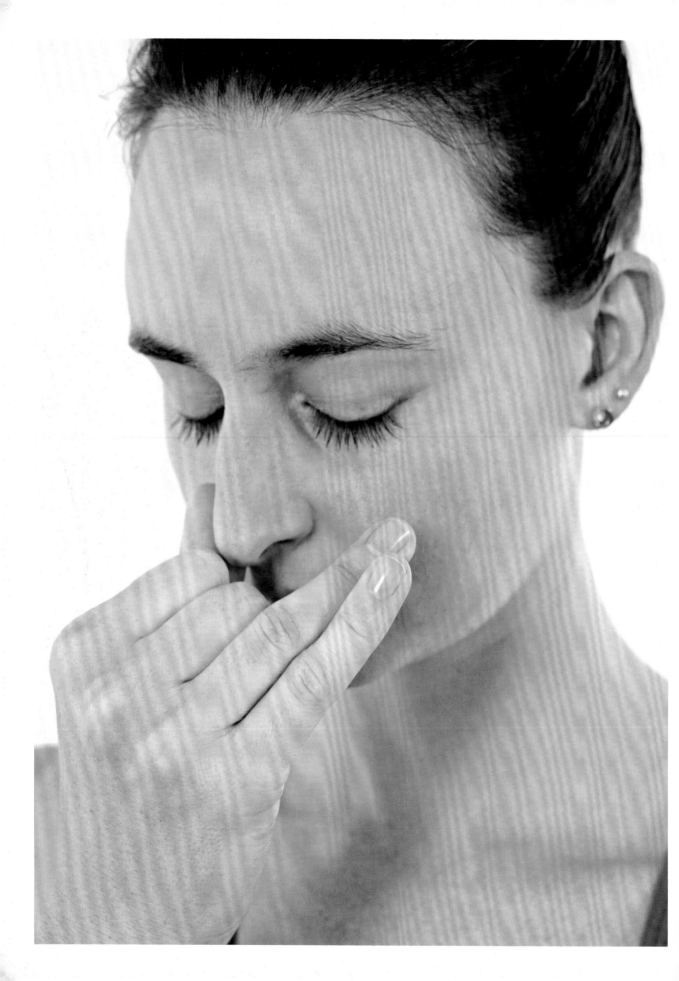

The Art of Breathing

The Hatha yoga we practise today was developed as part of the Tantric civilization that existed in India and other parts of the world more than ten thousand years ago. Two thousand years ago *asanas* consisted of a few seated poses, such as the Lotus, *Padmasana* and *Siddhasana*. The term *asana*, meaning seat, was derived from these poses. They have evolved and expanded over time so that today there is a myriad of postures that stretch, bend, twist and invert us, with the purpose of strengthening the body and increasing our flexibility, taking us on a journey from the physical to the more subtle realms of our being.

Pranayama	216
Bandhas	222
Mudras	224
Meditation	228

Pranayama

There is an intimate connection between the breath, nerve currents and control of the inner *prana* or vital forces. *Pranayama* is the means by which a yogi tries to realize within his individual body the whole cosmic nature, and attempts to achieve perfection by attaining all the powers of the universe. **Swami Sivananda**

The word *pranayama* is composed of two elements: *prana* is the vital energy or life force that exists in all things; *ayama* is defined as expansion or ascension. So *pranayama* means the expansion or ascension of the life force: regulating the *prana* in order to transcend our normal limitations. It involves the conscious control of the inhalation, retention and exhalation of the breath. Through the practice of *pranayama* we harness and direct the *prana* in order to restore and maintain optimal health, and to gain control over the mind.

The purpose of *pranayama* is to improve the function of the respiratory system, which is the gateway to purifying the body, mind and intellect and is essential for sustaining all forms of animal life. Without food or water, we can survive for a few days, but when respiration stops, so does life. The breath influences the activities of every cell in the body, and more importantly is intimately linked with the brain's performance, promoting vitality, perception and sharpening the intellect. Efficient respiration improves the circulatory system, without which the processes of digestion and elimination would suffer, toxins accumulate and diseases spread through the body. Regular practice of *pranayama* also helps to maintain the flow of blood, which tones the nerves, brain, spinal cord and cardiac muscles, maintaining their efficiency.

The respiratory system is a bridge between the conscious and subconscious minds, and there is a distinct relationship between the state of mind and the breath. The breath quickens when we are excited or stressed and becomes deeper and quieter when we relax. By controlling the breath, we are able to control our state of being. The regular practice of *pranayama* strengthens the lungs, increasing breathing capacity and oxygen intake.

On average, humans breathe about 15 times per minute. Each inhalation draws oxygen into the body and triggers the transformation of nutrients into fuel. The freshly oxygenated blood is then carried by the arteries from the left side of the heart, which beats at an average of 70 times per minute, pumping blood to every cell in the body, replenishing their source of life-giving oxygen. Each exhalation discharges carbon dioxide and other toxins in the venous blood. The lungs play an integral part in this disposal, and *pranayama* keeps the lungs free from bacterial disease and increases the circulation of blood and lymph.

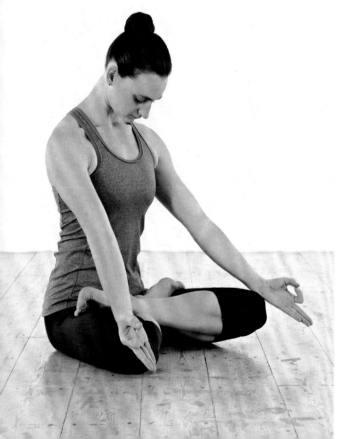

Many people first come to yoga through *asana* practice, but the inclusion of *pranayama* – channelling the pranic energy in the body – is at the core of a rounded Hatha yoga practice.

Pranayama helps to eradicate pain, tension and illness. The rhythmic nature of the breathing exercises improves glandular function. Respiration fuels the burning of oxygen and glucose, producing the energy to power each muscular contraction, glandular secretion and mental process. The exercises also calm the mind and thus balance the heart. This in turn assures good health and purifies the nervous system. Once the nervous system and senses are harmonized, cravings and desires diminish.

Inhalation should be long, deep, rhythmic and even. The energizing ingredients of the atmosphere percolate into the cells of the lungs and rejuvenate life. By retaining the breath, we absorb energy fully and distribute it to the entire system via the circulation of the blood. Exhalation removes toxins, and retaining the breath on exhalation eliminates stress and tensions.

The most important of these steps is *kumbhaka* – breath retention – but in order to perform it we must regulate the process of breathing. This must be done gradually. In the early stages of *pranayama* practice, in order to prepare the lungs and nervous system for *kumbhaka*, more emphasis is given to inhalation and exhalation.

Pranayama uses breathing to affect the flow of *prana* in the *nadis*, purifying, regulating and stimulating the energy channels of the *pranamaya kosha*, the energy body, leading to physical and mental stability. Lifestyle has a significant effect on the *pranamaya kosha* and its *pranas* (see page 60). Exercise, work, sleep, eating, drinking and sexual relations all affect the movement and distribution of *prana* in the body, as do emotions, stress and poor lifestyle habits. These irregularities in the pranic flow can lead to devitalization of the organs and limbs, and ultimately to disease. *Pranayama* reverses this process, rebalancing and re-energizing the *prana* within the *pranamaya kosha*.

Yogic Breathing Techniques
The techniques basically consist of four parts:
Puraka – an inhalation
Antara kumbhaka – the retention of the breath after inhalation
Rechaka – an exhalation
Bahya kumbhaka – the retention of the breath after exhalation

General Notes for Practice

Breathing
Always breathe through the nose unless instructed otherwise. Practise *jala neti* (see page 69) regularly to clean out the nasal passages.

When to Practise
The best time for *pranayama* practice is early morning, when the body is fresh and the mind is free. Try to practise at the same time and in the same place each day for at least 15 minutes. Traditionally, *pranayama* is practised after *asanas* and before meditation, but some schools practise *pranayama* before *asanas*.

Where to Practise
Choose a quiet, clean and well-ventilated room with no draughts. To avoid over-heating, do not practise in direct sunlight.

Sitting Position
Sit on the floor on a folded blanket or a cushion. Keep the spine erect and perpendicular to the floor. It is important to be comfortable so that the body remains steady and does not disturb the breath. Some recommended positions are *Padmasana* (see page 142), *Siddhasana* and *Sukhasana* (see page 141), or even kneeling or sitting on a chair.

Digestion
Pranayama should be practised on an empty stomach: wait at least two hours after meals. A full stomach places pressure on the diaphragm and can affect the depth of the breath.

Contraindications
Do not practise *pranayama* if you are ill. During pregnancy, avoid those forms that involve long retentions of the breath or deep forceful breaths that contract the abdomen.

As with *asana* practice, it is important not to increase your capacity too soon. Follow the advice of an experienced teacher. Practise breath retention only for as long as is comfortable. The lungs are delicate organs and must not be put under any undue strain. Similarly, any unnecessary force can cause mental and emotional harm.

Pranayama practice

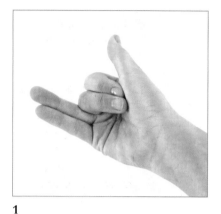

1

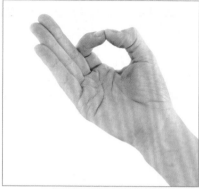

2

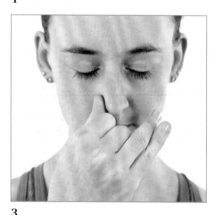

3

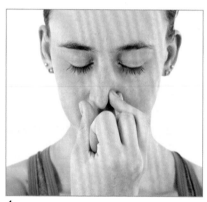

4

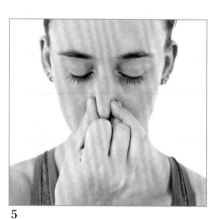

5

During *pranayama* practice, the right hand is in *Vishnu mudra* **(1)** and the left in *Jnana mudra* **(2)**. When *Vishnu mudra* is assumed, the thumb is used to close off the right nostril **(3)** and the ring and little fingers to close off the left nostril **(4)**. During retention, *kumbhaka*, the thumb, ring and little fingers are used to close off both nostrils **(5)**.

Nadi-Sodhana Pranayama without Kumbhaka

Alternate-Nostril Breathing without Retention
Nadi-Sodhana is used to purify the *nadis* and the psychic channels. It involves no breath retention and is therefore *recommended* for those with heart problems and the elderly. With the right hand in *Vishnu mudra* and the left hand in *Jnana mudra*, inhale slowly through the left nostril according to your capacity. Close the left nostril with the ring finger and immediately release the thumb to open the right nostril. Exhale and inhale, then close the right nostril and exhale through the left. This is one complete round.

Nadi-Sodhana Pranayama with Kumbhaka

Alternate Nostril-Breathing with Retention
Place the right hand in *Vishnu mudra* and the left hand in *Jnana mudra*. Close the right nostril with the right

thumb and inhale slowly through the left nostril. Then close the left nostril with the right ring finger and retain the inhaled breath with both nostrils closed. Open the right nostril and exhale slowly. Inhale through the right nostril, then close it with the right thumb, retain the breath, release the right ring finger to open the left nostril and exhale through the left nostril. This is one complete round.

Practise this exercise daily for at least 15 minutes. For the first month, use these ratios: for inhalation (*puraka*) 6 counts, retention (*kumbhaka*) 4 counts and exhalation (*rechaka*) 6 counts. The second month, increase to 8-8-8.

Benefits: This practice nourishes the whole body with oxygen. It purifies the blood and removes toxins, stimulates the brain to function more effectively, improves concentration, relieves stress and increases vitality.
Contraindications: The retention of the breath means that this exercise is not recommended for those suffering from heart disease.

Kapalabhati

Some call this exercise a *pranayama* and some regard it as a *kriya* (see page 68). Take two regular breaths, then inhale slowly, exhale vigorously and pull the abdomen in towards the spine. Exhalations should be two to three times faster than inhalations. Because of the force of the exhalation, the inhalation is passive.

Beginners should start with ten exhalations or three rounds of ten, according to capacity, then gradually build up to (but not exceed) 120 exhalations per minute for up to two minutes. Following *Kapalabhati*, retain the breath for as long as is comfortable. Apply *Jalandhara* and *Mula bandhas* during retention (beginners should practise only *Ashvini mudra*, see page 227).

Benefits: The forced exhalation clears the lower lungs of stale air, making room for fresh oxygen-rich air to cleanse the entire system. This exercise stimulates the mind and creates a feeling of exhilaration; improves concentration; balances and strengthens the nervous system; and tones the digestive organs.

Contraindications: Should not be practised by those suffering from heart disease or high blood pressure, or during pregnancy.

Alternate-Nostril *Kapalabhati*

Like *Kapalabhati*, this exercise requires a forceful exhalation followed immediately by a passive inhalation. Place the right hand in *Vishnu mudra*. Use the right thumb and ring fingers to control the opening and closing of the nostrils. Begin by inhaling through the left nostril and then exhale vigorously through the right. Follow this with a passive inhalation through the right nostril and exhale forcefully through the left. This is one complete round.

Continuously alternate nostrils for 15 seconds or ten slow rounds, then end with an exhalation through the left nostril. Inhale through both nostrils and retain the breath. Apply *Jalandhara* and *Mula bandhas* and hold for as long as is comfortable while concentrating the attention at the navel region. To conclude, slowly exhale through the right nostril.

Note:
For an explanation of *Vishnu mudra* and *Jnana mudra*, used in the following techniques, see *Hasta mudras*, page 224, and for the various *bandhas* see page 222.

Bhastrika

Bellows Breathing

Bhastrika means bellows and in this exercise both out and in breaths are vigorous, like a pair of bellows, creating heat. In all other types of *pranayama*, inhalation sets the rhythm, but in *Bhastrika* exhalation sets the pace. This exercise is similar to *Kapalabhati*, but uses force on both the inhalation and exhalation, expanding and contracting the lungs above and below their resting or basic volume.

Inhale and exhale forcefully through both nostrils at the same speed, gradually increasing the speed. In other words, breathe as fast as you can, like a sniffing dog. (Beginners should do this for 20 seconds, gradually building up to a maximum of two minutes.) Inhale and retain the breath for as long as is comfortable while applying *Jalandhara* and *Mula bandhas*. Release the locks and exhale slowly through both nostrils.

Benefits: The rapid exchange of air in the lungs and the exchange of oxygen and carbon dioxide into and out of the bloodstream stimulate the metabolic rate, which produces heat and flushes out toxins. *Bhastrika* tones the digestive system and balances and strengthens the nervous system, inducing peace and one-pointedness, *ekagrata*.

Contraindications: Should not be practised by those suffering from heart disease or high blood pressure, or during pregnancy.

Chandra-Surya-Kumbhaka Pranayama

Moon-Sun-Holding Breathing Exercise

This form of alternate-nostril breathing is also known as *Anuloma-Viloma*. The left nostril is the path of *ida nadi*, also called *chandra* (moon). The right nostril is the path of pingala *nadi* or *surya* (sun). Hence the name Moon-Sun-Holding *Pranayama*. Through repetition, the practice of *Chandra-Surya-Kumbhaka Pranayama* generates great heat.

Begin and end using the dominant nostril. If both nostrils are equally active, inhale through the left. The left hand should assume Jnana *mudra* and the right hand *Vishnu mudra*. Raise the right hand and bring the thumb beside the right nostril and the ring and little finger beside the left. Inhale through the left nostril to a count of four, closing the right nostril with the thumb. Hold the breath, closing both nostrils to a count of 16. Exhale through the right nostril to a count of eight, closing the left with the ring and little fingers. Then inhale through the right nostril to a count of four, keeping the left nostril closed. Close off both nostrils and hold the breath to a count of 16. Exhale through the left nostril to a count of eight, keeping the right nostril closed. This completes one full round.

For beginners, the count is 4-2-4. For intermediate practitioners, the count is 6-4-6 for the first month and 3-12-6 for the second. For short holds, no locks are employed.

The correct ratio is actually 1-4-2 (the holding is four times longer than the inhalation and the exhalation is two times longer than the inhalation). Once you advance to a ratio of 3-12-6, use *Jalandhara bandha* and *Mula bandha* to seal off the torso. Once you find 3-12-6 easy, increase the count to 4-16-8 and then 5-20-10. With practise, you may reach 6-24-12 and even 7-28-14. Follow your teacher's advice and increase the duration gradually and according to your individual capacity.

Benefits: This exercise restores the natural rhythm of the breath and balances the flow of *prana* in the body. It eventually leads to the ascension of *prana* up the central *nadi, sushumna.*

Sukha-Purvara Pranayama

Easy, Comfortable Breathing Exercise
This simplified variation of *Chandra-Surya-Kumbhaka* is designed to calm and relax. Bring the right hand in to *Vishnu mudra* to open and close the nostrils, inhale through the left nostril, hold as long as you can and mentally repeat *Om*, then breathe out slowly through the right nostril. Breathe in through the right nostril, hold the breath again for as long as you can, then slowly breathe out through the left nostril. It is not necessary to hold the nostrils closed during the retention the hands can rest in the lap. Try to practise this for 15 minutes per session.

Ujjayi

The Sanskrit word *ujjayi* means 'victorious' or 'that which leads to success'. *Ujjayi* is often referred to as the psychic breath, as it leads to subtle states of mind. The heating effects of this *pranayama* soothe the nervous system and calm the mind. The lungs are fully expanded with the chest open. This breathing has a smooth, soft sound in the throat effected by partially closing off the back of the throat with the glottis.

Inhale and lift the chest and hold for two seconds with an anal contraction (*Asvini mudra*). Exhale while consciously constricting the throat a little and squeezing out the air. *Ujjayi* breathing can be practised during most postures, as well as throughout any *Vinyasa* series. After two seconds, repeat the process again up to 12 times.

Benefits: *Ujjayi* aerates the lungs and soothes and tones the nervous system. It reduces phlegm and relieves pain in the chest.
Contraindications: Not recommended for those who are introverted by nature.

Purna Ujjayi

Complete Ujjayi
This *pranayama* involves inhaling through both nostrils while partially closing off the back of the throat with the glottis to make a sound in the throat. During retention, lift the chest and assume *Jalandhara* and *Mula bandhas* with a straight spine. Retain the breath as long as you can without straining. As this is a body-heating *pranayama*, exhalation is confined to the cooling left nostril, with the right hand in *Vishnu mudra* and the right thumb holding the right nostril closed. There is no retention after exhalation.

Benefits: Increases lung capacity and stimulates the lower chakras.
Contraindications: Not recommended for those who are suffering from heart disease, or during pregnancy.

Surya-Bheda-Kumbhaka Pranayama

Bheda means 'that which breaks'. Assume *Vishnu mudra* with the right hand, close the left nostril with the right ring finger and inhale through the right nostril. (In this exercise, you should always inhale through the right nostril and exhale through the left. *Surya*, meaning sun, refers to the right nostril, the path of *pingala nadi*.) Then close both nostrils between the right thumb and ring finger and hold the breath for as long as is comfortable while applying *Jalandhara* and *Mula bandhas*. Move the right ring finger off the left nostril, release the locks and exhale. Beginners should start with two to three rounds and gradually work up to 5–10 minutes.

Benefits: Inhaling solely through the right nostril generates heat, improves the digestive fire (*agni*) and removes impurities that impair the flow of *prana*. This exercise is very stimulating, making the mind more alert and removing lethargy. Recommended for those who suffer from low blood pressure.
Contraindications: Not recommended for those suffering from heart disease or epilepsy, or during pregnancy.

The humming sound produced during *Brahmari* soothes the mind, but be very careful when closing off the ears: do not stick your finger into the ear canal, as it is easily damaged.

Plavini

Plavini means 'to float' and this *pranayama* is of particular help if you are in danger of drowning, as it enables you to float. Swallow small, rapid gulps of air until the stomach is totally filled. *Plavini* is also a *kriya* (see page 68).

Brahmari

Brahmari means 'bee' and this *pranayama* is so called because the sound produced is similar to that of the female honey bee. It induces a meditative state by directing the awareness inwards.

Fold all the fingers except the index fingers into the palms, raise the bent arms with the elbows up and back and gently close off the entrance to the ear canals with the tips of the index fingers (do not push your fingers too far into the ear canals, as this can cause permanent damage. This exercise can also be performed without closing off the entrance to the ear canals). Exhale completely and then inhale and fill the lungs. Exhale through the nose, making a high humming sound with the lips closed. Keep the eyes closed and focus the inner gaze on the space between the eyebrows, behind the forehead. Perform at least three rounds, loud and long, to promote single-pointed concentration.

Benefits: Recommended for anxiety or stress, as the vibrations of the sound have a calming effect on the nervous system. Also improves the voice and helps in the treatment of throat illness.

Contraindications: Not recommended for those suffering from ear infections.

Sitali

This cooling *pranayama* is unlike most others in that the inhalation is through the mouth rather than the nose.

Stick the tongue out a little and curl the sides up; curl the lips around it. Inhale through the mouth, using the tongue like a straw. Then close the mouth, bring the tongue to the upper palate and hold it in place there, concentrating on the coolness held by the tongue. Exhale silently through both nostrils. The moment you feel the sensation of coolness disappear, inhale again through the curled tongue. Repeat 3–5 times or as needed.

Benefits: This exercise cools the body and mind and is believed to control appetite and relieve hunger and thirst. It lowers blood pressure, relaxes the mind and muscles and helps induce sleep.

Contraindications: Not recommended for those suffering from low blood pressure or respiratory disorders. Avoid during the winter months or if you live in a cold climate.

Sitkari

Like *Sitali*, this cooling *pranayama* involves inhalation through the mouth rather than the nose. With the eyes closed and the lips separated, bring the teeth together. Press the tip of the tongue against the palate as you slowly inhale through the mouth, making a hissing sound. Retain the breath for as long as possible and exhale slowly through the nose. Repeat 3–5 times or as needed.

Benefits: This exercise cools the body and mind and is believed to control appetite and relieve hunger and thirst. It lowers blood pressure, relaxes the mind and muscles and helps induce sleep. It is also recommended for keeping gums and teeth healthy.

Contraindications: Not recommended for those suffering from low blood pressure or respiratory disorders. Avoid during the winter months or if you live in a cold climate.

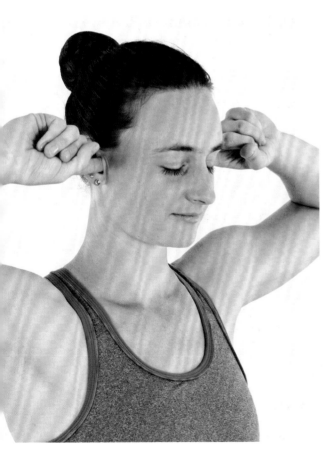

Bandhas

In yoga, a *bandha* or lock is a body manoeuvre designed to confine the life force within the trunk and thereby stimulate it. *Bandhas* increase the cleansing effects of *pranayama* by directing *prana* to those areas where toxins prevent the flow of energy in the body.

Bandha means 'to bind or tie together' or 'to close'. By engaging *bandhas*, you can redirect *prana* to *sushumna nadi* for the purpose of spiritual awakening.

There are in fact four *bandhas*, but only three are usually referred to: *Jalandhara bandha* involves the neck and upper spine, *Uddhiyana bandha* focuses on the area between the diaphragm, stomach and the abdominal organs and *Mula bandha* is concentrated on the area around the floor of the pelvis and the anus. The fourth, *Maha bandha*, is actually a combination of the other three (*maha* means 'great' in Sanskrit). When practised regularly, it can fully awaken the *prana* in all of the main *chakras*.

The Three *Granthis*

Granthis are thought of as psychic knots in the physical, subtle and energetic body. They differ from *chakras* in that they have to be pierced and dissolved to enable the free passage of *prana*. The *granthis* are said to be pierced by the *kundalini* force, so *kundalini* needs to be aroused before the *granthis* are dissolved. These psychic knots also obstruct the activity of the *chakras* and impede the flow of *prana* along the *sushumna nadi*.

The three *bandhas* correspond to the three *granthis*: *Mula bandha* is associated with *Brahma granthi*, *Uddiyana bandha* with *Vishnu granthi* and *Jalandhara bandha* with

Rudra granthi. *Brahma granthi* also corresponds with *muladhara* and *swadisthana chakras*; *Vishnu granthi* with *manipura* and *anahata chakras*; and *Rudra granthi* with *visuddhi* and *ajna chakras*. As each *granthi* is pierced, *kundalini* is able to rise beyond its corresponding *chakras*.

Mula Bandha

This is the principal *bandha* in Hatha yoga. It is performed physically by engaging the muscles in the pelvic floor, but on a subtle level it acts internally to energize and stimulate *muladhara chakra*. It is primarily a contraction of the perineum, but also involves the anal sphincter muscle and the area below the navel. In men, the area of contraction lies between the anus and the testes; in women, behind the cervix. You can perform *Mula bandha* with the lungs full or empty; either way you should feel as if the anus and the navel are going to meet each other. Practise this *bandha* individually at first, as it is difficult to isolate the perineal body; it can then be incorporated with the other *bandhas*, *asanas*, *pranayamas* and *mudras*.

Uddhiyana Bandha

The Sanskrit word *uddiyana* means 'to fly upward', and this lock, which originates in the navel region, is often described as a stomach lift, as it causes the diaphragm to rise up to the chest. It stimulates the solar plexus and *manipura chakra*. This region influences the distribution of energy around the body, and engaging this lock helps direct *prana* into *sushumna nadi*, where it eventually flows to *sahasrara chakra*.

Practise *Uddhiyana bandha* on an empty stomach and with empty bowels, either sitting down or standing up.

Bandhas and Mudras

Ancient texts classified *bandhas* as part of *mudras* (see page 222). In practice, *bandhas* are usually incorporated with *mudras* and with *pranayama* techniques, but because of their locking action they are also effective during *asana* practice. In some schools, *Mula* and *Uddhiyana bandha* are applied to certain *asanas*; so nowadays they are regarded as an important group of practices in their own right.

Caption Three lines of caption text to go here three lines of caption text to go caption text to go here hree lines of caption three lines of caption text to go caption text to go here hree

First, exhale and empty the lungs completely. Then close the throat and, with the abdomen relaxed, inhale and lift the chest and pull the abdominal organs up into the chest cavity. Exhale to release the lock. This creates a strong sensation of suction. This practice stimulates the digestive fire and massages and tones the abdominal organs, increasing blood circulation to the trunk.

Jalandhara Bandha

This lock is performed by contracting the throat. *Jalan* means 'net' and *dhara* means 'flow' or 'stream'. It is suggested that this lock controls the *nadis* or, in physical terms, the blood vessels and nerves in the neck.

Press the chin towards the base of the throat and lift the chest up – eventually, the chin and chest meet. At the same time, rest the tongue against the palate, with the tip behind the upper teeth. Then contract the glottis as if to swallow. There should be no straining when this lock is performed.

Maha Bandha

Maha Bandha regulates the endocrine system, slowing the degenerative processes in the body and increasing cellular renewal. Do not over-practise this *bandha* in the beginning, as it may release too much power and you may not be able to maintain control.

Sit with the legs straight, then bend the left knee and sit on the side of the heel so that it presses against the perineum and the outside of the bent knee rests on the floor to the side. Bend the right knee and place the right foot on the left thigh near the left hip joint (as in the Half Lotus Pose). Place the hands on the knees, straighten and extend the spine, breathing deeply along its length. Inhale to two-thirds capacity and apply *Jalandhara*, *Uddhiyana* and *Mula bandha*. Hold the breath for as long as is comfortable while focusing on the *sushumna nadi*. Then exhale and gently release the posture, straighten the legs and massage the knees. Repeat immediately on the opposite side. Keep the spine straight throughout.

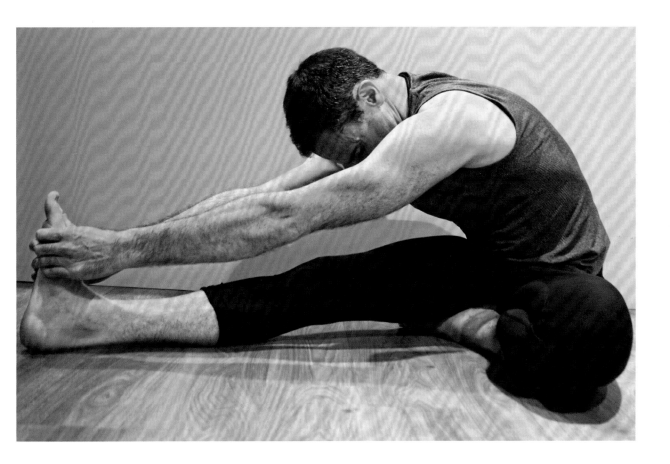

Mudras

While *bandhas* or locks unite the upward force of *prana* and the downward force of *apana* at the navel region, *mudras* act as seals. Together, *mudras* and *bandhas* act like the transformers and switches used when dealing with an electrical current.

Usually translated as 'seal', *mudra* can also mean 'gesture' or 'attitude'. *Mudras* are subtle physical gestures intended to deepen awareness and concentration. There are five categories of *mudra*: *Hasta*, *Mana*, *Kaya*, *Bandha* and *Adhara mudras*. While some *mudras* involve the entire body and are combined with *asanas*, *pranayama* and *bandhas*, most are performed with the hands and fingers.

When *asana*, *pranayama* and *bandha* practices are at a proficient level, the body generates more *prana* through the *nadis* and *chakras*. This usually escapes from the body and dissipates into the atmosphere. The advanced techniques of *mudra* are then introduced: they act like a barrier to redirect the *prana* and prevent it from escaping, inducing deeper states of concentration and increasing the potential for awakening *kundalini*.

Each *mudra* has a different effect on the body, mind and *prana*. The fixed, repetitive nature of these gestures is intended to deconstruct the instinctive and unconscious habitual patterns that originate in the primitive areas of the brain and to establish a more refined consciousness.

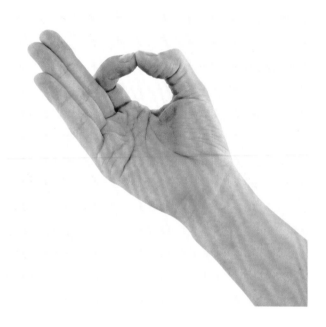

A gesture familiar from many sculptures, *Jnana mudra* is the Seal of Wisdom. When this gesture is performed with the back of the hands resting on the knees, it is known as *Chin mudra*.

Hasta mudras

Hasta or hand *mudras* are meditative, intended to redirect back into the body the *prana* escaping from the hands. Hand *mudras* are also used during *asana* practice. For example, *Kali Mudra* is performed in Crescent Moon Pose (see page 204).

Jnana Mudra
Seal of Wisdom
Make a circle with the tip of the index finger and the tip of the thumb touching and extend the remaining fingers. This *mudra* helps lock in energy and is used in many traditional *asanas* and often for one or both hands when practising *pranayama* (see page 214) or meditation. The last three fingers are believed to represent the three states of consciousness: waking consciousness, sleep with dreams and deep, dreamless sleep. The index finger represents individual consciousness while the thumb represents

supreme consciousness. When the two touch to form a circle, this represents the super-conscious state of self-realization (*Turiya*).

Chin Mudra
Seal of Knowledge
Chin is a derivative of the word *chit*, meaning 'consciousness'. *Chin mudra* is therefore the gesture of consciousness. It is performed like *Jnana mudra* except that the palms face upwards with the back of the hands resting on the knees. This symbolizes ultimate union, leading to yoga. This hand gesture is always an option for both hands during seated concentration or meditation (see page 226).

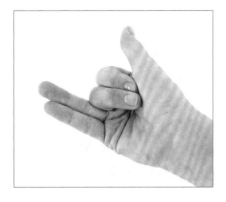

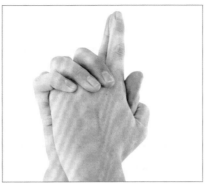

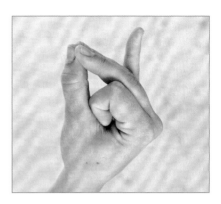

Vishnu mudra

This gesture is usually assumed by the right hand for some of the *pranayamas*. Fold the index and middle fingers into the centre of the palm. Do not let them touch the nose: the index finger represents the ego and the middle finger the intellect; both impede spiritual development. The palm faces the mouth and the thumb is used to close the right nostril, while the ring finger and little finger control the left nostril.

Kali mudra

Kali Ma is the Hindu goddess of destruction and rebirth. In order for new life and ideas to have room to develop and grow, something old must often be destroyed. *Kali mudra* can be applied during *asana* practice to help facilitate the opening and stretching of the shoulders and the chest. Interlace the fingers and thumbs of both hands with the palms together and the arms straight, then straighten and press both index fingers together.

Hridaya mudra
Heart Gesture

This *mudra* redirects the flow of *prana* from the hands back to the heart region. Sit in a comfortable meditation pose with the palms facing upwards on top of the knees. Fold the index fingers into the base of the thumbs as in *Chin* or *Jnana mudra*. Then join the middle and ring fingers to the tips of the thumbs and keep the little fingers straight. The middle and ring fingers correspond with the *nadis* connected to the heart, while the thumbs close the pranic circuit to direct the flow of prana from the hands to these *nadis*. This *mudra* can be practised during times of emotional difficulty to release any pent-up feelings.

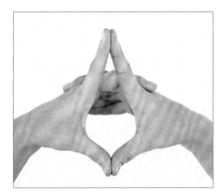

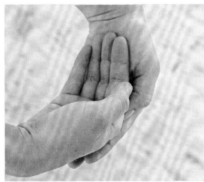

Yoni mudra

Yoni means 'womb', and this *mudra* is believed to invoke the primal energy inherent in the womb of creation. Place the palms together with the fingers pointing away from the body. Interlace the middle, ring and little fingers, but keep the index fingers and thumbs straight. Turn the thumbs towards the body. This develops greater concentration. Placing the tips of the index fingers and thumbs together intensifies the flow of *prana*.

Bhairava / Bhairavi mudra
Fierce or Terrifying Seal

In a comfortable sitting position for meditation, with the palms facing up, place the right hand on top of the left and rest both hands in the lap. This is *Bhairava mudra*, the masculine form. When the left hand is placed on top of the right, this is *Bhairavi mudra* – the feminine counterpart. The two hands represent *ida and pingala nadis* and the union of the individual with the supreme consciousness.

There are five categories of *mudra*:
Hasta or hand *mudras*
Mana or head *mudras*
Kaya or postural *mudras*
Bandha or lock *mudras*
Adhara or perineal *mudras*
There are 23 *mudras* listed in the *Hatha Yoga Pradipika*, the classic treatise written in the 15th century by Swatmarama, which is believed to be the oldest surviving text on Hatha yoga. In this section, we focus on the most commonly used or best-known *mudras*.

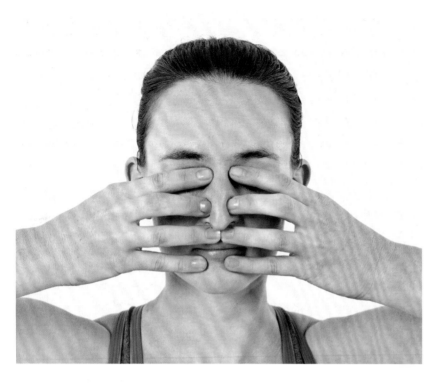

By physically closing off the eyes, ears and nose, practising *Shambavi mudra* leads to *pratyahara* (withdrawal of the senses) and draws the attention inside, resulting in a greater sense of inner perception.

Mana mudras

Mana or head *mudras* use the eyes, ears, nose, tongue and lips.

Shambavi mudra
Great Binding Seal
Close off the ears with the thumbs and close the eyes, resting the index fingers gently on the eyelids. Use the middle fingers to close the nostrils and close the mouth by placing both ring fingers on the upper lip and both little fingers on the bottom lip. Press the lips together, open the nostrils and inhale slowly. This can be done with or without *kumbhaka*, holding the breath for as long as is comfortable. This action shuts the seven gates of the senses – the earholes, eyes, nostrils and mouth. When the hold is no longer comfortable, release the nostrils, exhale and inhale.

Kaya mudras

Kaya or postural *mudras* combine physical postures with breathing and concentration.

Yoga mudra
Sitting in *Padmasana* (full Lotus), interlace the fingers behind the back with the arms straight. Inhale and arch the back, lifting the chest with the chin up. Now exhale and bend forward until the forehead rests on the floor. Lift the arms as high as possible behind you. Inhale, then hold the breath using *Jalandhara bandha* (see page 223), just the throat contraction and the tongue pressed against the palate) and *Mula bandha* (see page 222) for about five seconds. Gradually increase the duration of the hold to 20 seconds. To release, exhale and then inhale as you gradually roll up from the base of the spine. Rest for a few breaths and repeat twice more.

This *mudra* can also be done while assuming *Ardha* or *Sukha Padmasana*.

Viparita Karani mudra
Also known as Sirsasana, Viparita Karani Asana *and the Inverted Psychic Attitude*
This practice is said to raise the *shakti* and lead the aspirant to spiritual bliss. Normally, the power of the sun rests in the solar plexus and that of the moon in the palate, where the nectar of life is released. In Head Stand, *Sirsasana*, this is reversed and the ageing process is suspended. This is enhanced if one visualizes the sun on the palate for 15 seconds, followed by visualizing the moon at the navel region for 15 seconds. On the first day, pursue this process for one minute. Gradually increase to 15 minutes.

After six months of steady practice, wrinkles on the face and grey hair will disappear. Yogis who practise in this manner for three hours daily are believed to conquer death – but there is no evidence to support this claim. As the gastric fire (*agni*) is increased, those who practise this for a long time should relax for ten minutes after coming out of the posture and then take some light refreshment.

Note: Many traditions hold that this mudra *is achieved by combining the visualization with Shoulder Stand. My guru received it from his guru in Head Stand. He teaches that both postures are* Viparita Karani mudra.

Bandha mudras

Bandha or lock *mudras* combine *mudra* with *bandha*.

Maha mudra
Great Seal

Sit with the legs straight, then bend the left knee and sit on the side of the left heel, so it presses against the perineum and the outer edge of the knee rests on the floor out to the side. Lean forward over the right leg and take hold of the big toe with both index fingers. Move the shoulders and head away from the right foot and straighten the spine. Take a few deep breaths, then inhale until the lungs are half full, hold the breath and apply *Jalandhara* and *Mula bandhas* (see pages 222–3). Hold the breath for as long as is comfortable, then exhale gently and release the posture. Repeat on the opposite side, keeping the spine straight throughout.

This *mudra* may also may be done with a retention after exhalation, employing both *Uddhiyana* and *Jalandhara bandhas*. *Maha mudra* may induce sweating. Do not over-practise it in the beginning, as it may release too much power and you may not be able to maintain control.

Maha Vedha
Vedha means penetration of the *chakras* by the *kundalini*. If possible, sit in the Lotus Pose, Half Lotus or *Sukhasana* with the legs crossed (see pages 141–3). Place the hands down on the floor near the hips. Inhale until the lungs are half full. While holding the breath, lift the seat and bounce it rhythmically against the floor for as long as you can hold your breath without any sense of suffocation. This action will shake and stimulate all 72,000 *nadis* and may cause *prana shakti* to enter the *sushumna nadi*.

When you can no longer hold your breath comfortably, stop bouncing, exhale slowly and release the posture.

Adhara mudras

Adhara or perineal *mudras* redirect energy from the lower centres to the brain and are often used to sublimate sexual energy.

Vajroli/Sahajoli mudra
Vajroli for men/Sahajoli for women

Vajroli is derived from the Sanskrit word *vajra*, meaning 'thunderbolt' or 'lightning' and *sahajoli* from *sahaj*, meaning 'spontaneous'. *Vajra* is the *nadi* that connects the reproductive organs to the brain.

Sit in any comfortable meditation posture with the spine straight and the hands on the knees in *Chin* or *Jnana mudra*. Awareness is at the urethra, which is contracted as if to suspend the action of urinating; this will make the testes in men and the labia in women twitch slightly. Hold the contractions for as long as is comfortable and repeat gradually, starting with three contractions and working up to 15. This *mudra* regulates and tones the urino-genital system. In men, it also regulates testosterone levels and sperm count and helps control premature ejaculation.

Ashvini mudra
Horse Seal or Gesture of a Horse

Sitting in any of the meditation postures, bring awareness to the anus, then repeatedly contract the anal sphincter muscle.

Great seal or *Maha mudra* is a one-leg back-stretching posture performed in combination with the *Jalandhara* and *Mula bandhas*, which seal the pelvic and respiratory diaphragms. The aim is to lengthen and extend the spine.

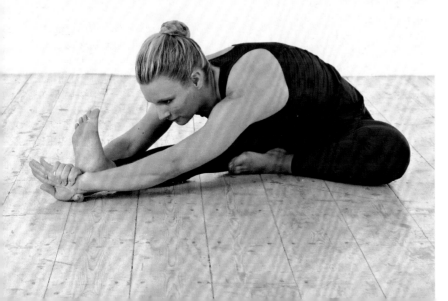

Meditation

Meditation is the most powerful mental and nerve tonic. Divine energy flows freely to the adept during meditation and exerts a benign influence on the mind, nerves, sense organs and body..

Meditation opens the door to intuitive knowledge and realms of eternal bliss. The mind becomes calm and steady, you discover a greater sense of purpose and strength of will and your thinking becomes clearer and more concentrated, affecting all you do. By regular practice of meditation, the mind can be brought under perfect control. If you meditate for half an hour daily, you will be able to face life with peace and spiritual strength.

Meditation and the Eight-fold Path

Patanjali's eight-limbed path takes us on a journey of discovery, which begins by examining our external world. The first two limbs, *yama* and *nyama*, set down guidelines on how to live in society; the third, *asana*, on how to maintain the physical body; the fourth, *pranayama*, on how to regulate the breath; and the fifth, *pratyahara*, on how to subjugate our external senses so that we can begin to explore our inner world. It is at this stage of a yogi's journey that the internalization process really begins and we can examine the practice of meditation, *dhyana*.

What many people regard as meditation begins as concentration or *dharana* – the sixth limb of the eight-fold path. By concentrating on an object, we learn to eliminate any fluctuating thought waves. This leads eventually to the experiential state of meditation, whose principal characteristic is maintaining a continuous flow of concentration on a fixed point or region without intervention or interruption.

Meditation cannot be taught. We can't learn to meditate, any more than we can learn to sleep. Instead we must practise regularly with patience and perseverance. We shouldn't expect to be in a meditative state as soon as we sit and close our eyes. Only by practice can we finally reap the rewards that concentration brings, the unbroken connection between the meditator and the object of his or her meditation. Often the contentment we feel when our minds are fully absorbed on something is less about the activity itself than it is about the fact that, during concentration, we are distracted from our other concerns.

In meditation, we go deep inside the mind; time and space have no meaning. Body consciousness is transcended, leading to the feeling of lightness. The mind is fixed. The flow of cognition towards the object of concentration is smooth and constant, like oil pouring from one vessel into another. This conscious awareness, which begins as one-pointed concentration, leads to a state that has no tangible description.

Meditation is also possible in *asana* and *pranayama*. *Asana* practice is meditation in action, with attention and contemplation steadily sustained. In *pranayama*, observing and measuring the flow of in and out breaths results in total absorption and involvement with the self.

Stilling the Mind

Yoga is the settling of the mind into silence and, by concentration or meditation, we can observe the mind. When the surface of a lake is still, we can see to the bottom very clearly, but if the surface becomes agitated by waves, it's impossible. In the same way, when the mind is still, with no thoughts or desires, then we can see the self.

For many of us, the mind oscillates from one thought to another, wrestling with desires, aversions, emotions and memories, in constant search of happiness. When it achieves its desires, the mind is silenced, but only for

Concentration and meditation are the sixth and seventh of Patanjali's eight limbs. The eighth is *samadhi*, the superconscious state that transcends time, space, body and mind, when the union of individual consciousness with supreme consciousness occurs. This is yoga. According to the ancient *Vedas*, one concentration occurs when we fix the mind on one thought for 12 seconds; one meditation is equal to 12 concentrations – almost two and a half minutes; and *samadhi* is equal to 12 meditations – just under half an hour.

a short while. The whole pattern soon starts over again, because our desire for contentment is always channelled outwards, attaching to external objects that are by nature ephemeral. So the mind itself remains unchanged and the true desire unfulfilled.

In order to achieve a state of lasting happiness and absolute peace, we must first learn to calm the mind, to concentrate and ultimately to transcend the mind. By turning our focus inwards, upon the self, we can deepen that experience of perfect concentration. This is meditation. When we turn our attention inwards, we find that source of joy and wisdom already inside us: an ocean of tranquillity that we can draw from when the mind is still.

An effective tool for controlling the mind is to stop identifying with our emotions, thoughts and actions. Instead, we should take a step back and become the witness, as if we were watching someone else. If we observe ourselves in this way, our thoughts and emotions stop controlling us. We begin to see both mind and body as instruments that we can now control. By detaching from the games of the ego, we learn to take responsibility for ourselves. The closest analogous state to meditation that we can experience is deep sleep, in which there is neither time, space nor causation. Meditation, however, differs from deep sleep, because it works on the psyche by controlling and stilling the oscillations of the mind and leads to mental peace.

On a physical level, meditation helps to prolong the body's anabolic process of growth and repair, and to reduce the catabolic or decaying process. Generally, the anabolic process predominates until the age of 18. From 18 to 35 there is balance between the two, and after 35 the catabolic process takes over.

Every cell in our body is governed by the instinctive subconscious mind. Every cell also has both an individual and a collective consciousness. When thoughts and

desires occur, the cells are activated and the body responds. It has been scientifically proven that positive thoughts have a positive effect on the cells in our body. As meditation brings about a prolonged positive state of mind, it rejuvenates body cells and therefore inhibits the decaying process.

Meditation can take many different forms: the focus of your concentration can be an image, a sound or an abstract idea; you can practise in your home or while walking through nature.

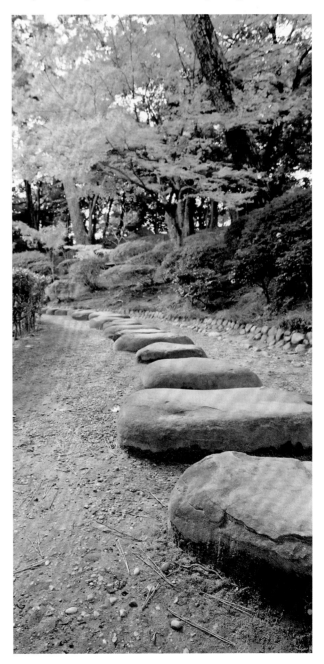

The Benefits of Meditation

- Reduced tension and anxiety
- Increased resistance to stress
- Improved memory and concentration
- Better learning ability
- Increased energy
- Improved health
- Reduced insomnia
- Greater ability to enjoy life
- Increased self-esteem
- Improved relationships
- Reduction of biological ageing

Guidelines to Practising Meditation

- For best results, practise the same meditation daily, at the same time and place.
- If you don't have a spare room for meditation, reserve a part of your home that is clean and free from clutter for your practice. Practising in the same area creates powerful vibrations and generates a peaceful and sattvic atmosphere.
- The best time to practise is between 4 and 6 a.m. This period is known as *Brahmamuhurta*, the Hour of Brahma, when the atmosphere is charged with spiritual force. The mind is calm on waking from its unconscious state and slips easily into meditation. If you can't sit for meditation at this hour, choose a time when you're not likely to be disturbed. Start with five to ten minutes at each sitting.
- If possible, face north or east in order to benefit from the subtle effects of the earth's magnetic field. Sit in a steady, comfortable, cross-legged position with a straight spine. If you can't sit cross-legged, then sit in a chair with a straight back.
- Consciously regulate the breath. Keep the breathing rhythmic, inhaling slowly for three seconds and exhaling for three seconds. Regulating the breath regulates the flow of prana, the vital energy.
- Select a focal point on which your mind can rest. It is usually recommended to focus the attention on the space between the eyebrows, behind the forehead: 'As the physical eyes close, the Spiritual Eye opens and the light of truth shines forth.'
- If the mind is very restless, try focusing on an external object. Choose one that attracts your mind such as a deity or an image of your guru, if you have one. Work with the same object for 30 consecutive days. If you make little or no progress during this time, switch to another object for the next 30 days.
- If you have been given a personal *mantra* by your guru, repeat it mentally and coordinate repetition with the breath. If you don't have a personal *mantra*, use *om*. Although mental repetition is stronger, you can repeat the *mantra* aloud if you become drowsy. Never change your *mantra*.
- With practice, commitment and patience, *samadhi*, the superconscious state, is reached. In *samadhi* one rests in the state of bliss in which the knower, the knowledge and the known become one.

Types of Meditation

These are the two main types of meditation. *Saguna* is meditation on a form, where the attention is fixed on an object, an image or perhaps a *mantra*. *Saguna* meditation is dualistic in character, as the meditator sees himself as separate from his object of meditation. This type of meditation is suitable for everyone, especially those with a more emotional temperament.

Nirguna is meditation without form. The object of attention is an abstract idea, such as the absolute or a concept that is indescribable. Here there is no dualism as the meditator sees himself as one with the object. *Nirguna* is considered more suitable for intellectual types. Most meditation practices begin with *saguna*, since it is much easier to concentrate on something concrete than on an abstract concept.

Meditation Techniques

There are many different meditation techniques to choose from. Some use sound in the form of a *mantra*, others use visual symbols or breathing, but all have one common aim: to fix the mind on a single point and lead the meditator to a state of self-realization.

Third eye meditation

Sitting comfortably, bring your attention to the space between the eyebrows. This area is known as *trikuti*, the third eye or the seat of the mind. You may begin to visualize brilliant light, vibrant colours or mental images. Maintain a steady, inner gaze fixed on the space between the eyebrows. This will stimulate the pituitary gland, which controls the sixth sense, deep inside the brain. Activating this sixth sense will draw you closer to achieving divine perception.

Japa meditation

Japa means 'to repeat in a low voice' and *japa* meditation involves the repetition of a *mantra* or of the name of a celestial being. *Mantras* repeated during meditation bring the individual to a higher state of consciousness. The sound from each *mantra*, when chanted, releases a specific energy, which creates a specific thought pattern in the mind. The energy created by the sounds fuses with the energy created by the thought patterns to purify the mind and the senses and lead to a state of oneness.

So Hum meditation

So hum is Sanskrit for 'I am that, that I am', with 'that' representing the supreme self. This is one of the most powerful and effective of all *mantras*, as it is already contained within the breath of all living creatures. *So* is an integral part of each inhalation and *hum* is an organic part of each exhalation. We humans unconsciously recite it some 21,000 times every day.

Sitting comfortably with the eyes closed, bring your attention to your breath. Imagine during each inhalation you can hear the sound *so*, and with each exhalation the sound *hum*. Another interpretation of the mantra is: 'I am you, you are me.'

Om Japa meditation

For a yogi, *om* is the most powerful symbol and syllable. In the Sanskrit letter, the longer lower curve stands for the dream state and the upper curve represents the waking state; the curve issuing from the centre symbolizes deep, dreamless sleep. The crescent shape stands for *maya,* the veil of illusion; and the dot symbolizes the transcendental state. When the individual spirit in man passes through the veil and rests in the transcendental, he is liberated from the three states and their qualities.

Slowly chant the sound of *om*. This is calling the name of God and employing the sacred, three-part syllable, the *pranava* – the Sanskrit name for the *om*. This is considered to be the highest *mantra* of all: it is the sound vibration that represents God. Begin by chanting as few as three *oms*, and work up to five minutes of sustained recitation. This practice will affect the heart rate and calm the senses.

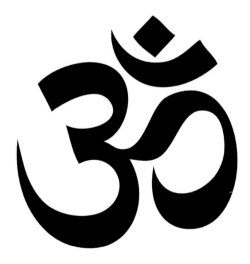

Trataka meditation

Tratak means 'gazing' and in *trataka* meditation the gaze is fixed on an object or point until the image is imprinted on the mind's eye when the eyes are closed. Fixing the gaze on an object brings the restless mind under control. The practice strengthens the powers of concentration, increases memory and leads to greater awareness. *Trataka* is also believed to improve eyesight and stimulate the pineal gland in the brain.

Trataka meditation is most commonly performed on a candle flame, as it is easy to hold the image of the candle flame in your mind with the eyes closed. This form of *trataka* is different from the *kriya* technique described on page 70.

Place a candle 1 m (3 ft) in front of you at eye level. Make sure there are no draughts so that the candle flame will remain steady. Concentrate your gaze on the flame while keeping the eyelids slightly lowered. Stare at the flame for one to two minutes, capturing the image in your mind. Then close your eyes and try to visualize the candle flame in your mind, seeing it at the space between the eyebrows. When the image of the flame fades, open the eyes again and recapture it. Beginners should practise for about five minutes, then build up to ten and later to 15 minutes.

Om symbol *trataka*

Use a picture or a statue of the *om* symbol as the object of contemplation. Allow the eyes to explore it in an anti-clockwise direction, as it imprints itself in the mind; at the same time consider the meaning of the *om* and what it represents. Close your eyes and draw the symbol and its meaning into your mind, then open the eyes and gaze on the object again to cement the image. Close the physical eyes and retain a mental picture of the symbol along with its meaning. This practice will bring bliss-absolute by remembrance of the qualities of the omnipresent, omniscient and omnipotent: the all-prevailing One, God.

Flower *trataka*

This is also a form of *trataka,* but the object concentrated on is a beautiful flower. Observe every detail of the flower: its petals, colours and other distinct qualities. Close your eyes and draw the image of the flower into the mind, to the space between the eyebrows. When the image fades, open the eyes and repeat the practice.

The Sanskrit letter *om* can be the focus of your meditation: you can either chant the sound of *om* or let the symbol itself be the object of your contemplation.

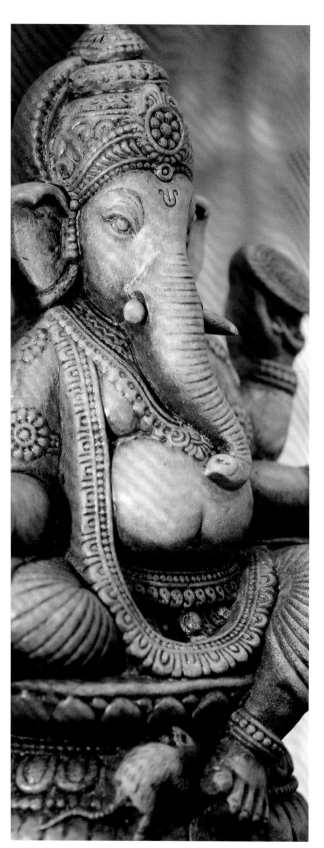

Enlightened being *trataka*

Those who are more spiritually inclined can use the image or statue of a saint as their object of concentration. You can choose Jesus, Lord Shiva, Buddha, Krishna, Moses or an illumined guru who inspires you.

Gaze on the image and try to visualize it in your mind's eye. Then gradually try to feel the qualities of that enlightened being as you concentrate on his or her likeness. In thought and action, visualize or pretend that you are that being with all his or her divine qualities. The aim is to become one with the object of your contemplation and share in his or her wisdom.

Sound meditation

When sound becomes the object of concentration, the mind becomes solely focused on information gathered through the ears, as opposed to the eyes. If you live near a stream or river, sit with the eyes closed and fix the mind on the sounds of nature. Listen for the sounds as they merge into an eternal, unbroken *om*; alternatively, concentrate on the sound of the leaves on the trees rustling in the breeze, or the sound of rain. If it's quiet enough, simply listen to the sound of your own breathing.

You can also practise this form of concentration on any consistent or repetitive sound to which the ear is attracted, for example the music of a tamboura or the sound of Tibetan pipes.

Walking meditation

This practice involves walking a little with the gaze just ahead of the feet, the hands together and the arms straight and loose in front of or behind the torso. Beginning with the left foot, peel it off the ground as slowly and deliberately as possible. The weight shifts to the right foot and the left foot eventually leaves the earth, travelling in slow motion through space, until one part of the foot at a time regains the earth just ahead of the right foot. Without pausing, shift the weight to the right foot and repeat the process on the opposite side. After 10–15 minutes of deliberate, continuous slow motion, bring the feet together and stand with the eyes closed with the breath slow and steady. As the mind becomes fully absorbed, the breathing slows and the thoughts die away.

Remain motionless for a few moments before opening the eyes. This meditation can be practised any time of the day, but early morning is recommended in an area where there is quietude, perhaps in the garden or a nearby park.

Enlightened being trataka involves using an image of a saint, deity or guru as the object of your concentration, like this Indian statue of Ganesha, the Hindu deity associated with beginnings.

Mantra Japa on a *Mala*

The practice of repetition on a *mala* or rosary helps the mind to focus on meditation and prevent any distractions to the steady flow of absorption. In the classical tradition, one recites silently a personal *mantra* given by the guru as a way to honour and connect with the preceptor and gain spiritual benefit. It is also possible to recite a general *mantra*. There are many *mantras* to choose from, such as *Om Nama Shivaya* ('Om and salutations to Shiva') or *Om Namo Narayanaya* ('Om and salutations to Vishnu').

A *mala* necklace has 108 beads, plus one bead which is not counted and sits apart from the rest. This is the head bead or *sumeru* and symbolizes the guru. One hundred and eight is the most sacred number in the Vedic system, as it represents the 108 *Upanishads* and is thought to be the number upon which the entire universe is based. Begin the practice by holding the bead next to the head bead with the thumb and middle finger of the right hand, keeping it above the height of the navel. Mentally repeat one *mantra* for each bead and move the beads towards you, one by one. Move from one bead to the next in rhythm with the *mantra* and the breath. It's important to complete each round of 108 beads, and you can repeat as many rounds as you like – the more, the better.

- **Mala beads** are traditionally made from the wood of three trees with different characteristics:
- **Rudraksha beads** are known as the 'Tears of Shiva'. They are holy seeds from a tree, and come in many varieties with healing properties. The Tears of Shiva are devotional in nature and are used by those who worship Lord Shiva.
- **Sandalwood beads** are made from the wood of the rare sandalwood tree. They are very pure, sattvic and have a pleasant fragrant scent. *Japa* on sandalwood *malas* enhances calmness and a positive state of mind and supports meditation.
- **Tulsi beads** are made from the wood of the holy basil plant, which is chosen for its sattvic nature. *Tulsi* has a purifying and normalizing effect on the nervous system. It is revered as a sacred plant in India, and has been used for thousands of years in Ayurveda. Devotional beads made of *tulsi* wood are perfect for *karma* yogis involved in spiritual practice. The *tulsi mala* is also favoured by devotees of Lord Krishna.

A set of beads can be used to keep count during meditation and as an aid to concentration: a *mantra* is recited or mentally repeated for each of the 108 *mala* beads.

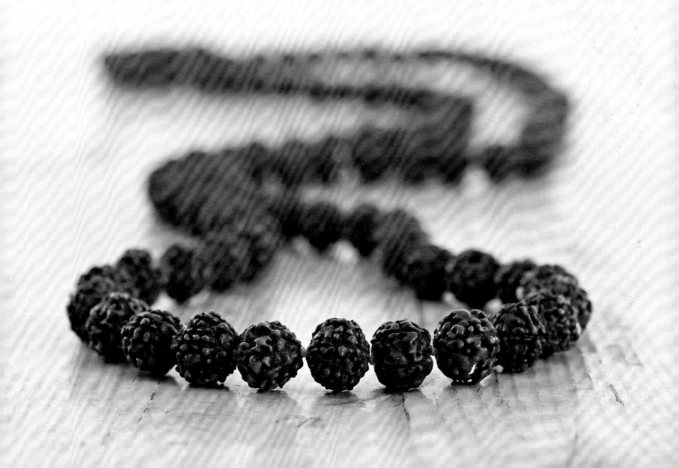

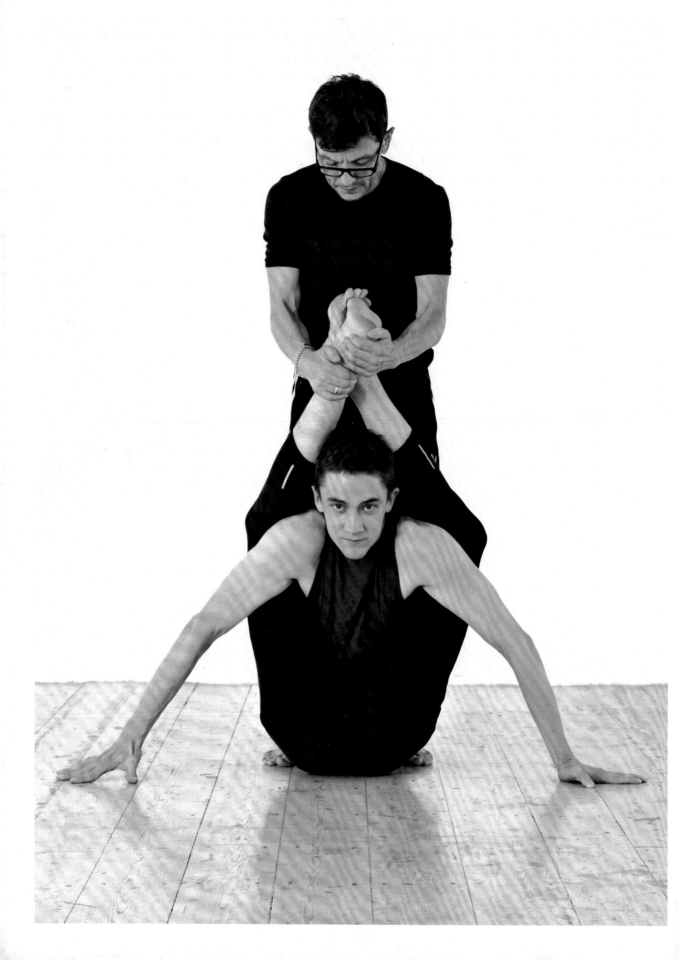

Teaching Yoga

Graduates from teacher-training programmes are given the resources, knowledge and examples of how to live every moment as a true yogi. But applying this knowledge in your classes is when your real training begins.

Being a Yoga Teacher   236
Yoga during Pregnancy   241
Yoga Practice for Older Age Groups   244
Yoga for Children   246
Adjusting Poses   248

Being a Yoga Teacher

As a yoga teacher you have a responsibility towards your students: you are expected to lead by example and embody the qualities associated with a spiritual ambassador.

The first limb of Patanjali's eight-fold path, *yama*, provides us with five ethical disciplines or virtues – non-harming, truthfulness, non-stealing, chastity and greedlessness. Yoga offers us an integrated way of living defined by these virtues, and their observance reflects favourably on the individual and on the lineage he or she represents.

It should be the endeavour of any contemporary yoga teacher to conduct his or her life in accordance with these disciplines. When you adopt the mantle of responsibility required to lead others on the path of self-knowledge, you must cultivate perfection in every thought, word, action and deed in both the public and the private domain.

However, we also have to be realistic about the complexities of modern society, which means adapting these virtues – originally espoused by yogis in pre-modern India – to suit the way we in the West live today. Given the global environmental crisis we are witnessing, we should also be working towards a more sustainable lifestyle.

Teaching Guidelines

The guidelines outlined on these pages are presented to guide you as a teacher. They have been adapted to reflect a contemporary world view, while still being in accordance with the wisdom contained in the heritage of yoga.

These codes of conduct have been put in place to prepare you as a yoga teacher for the obstacles and challenges that will inevitably arise. Your students will look to you for guidance not just on a physical or practical level with regard to their *asana* practice, but also as someone who can guide them along their path of self-discovery. It's no easy task. Remember, in the eyes of your students, you are a role model; your behaviour, your opinions and what you say will suddenly come under a great deal of scrutiny.

Given all of this, teaching yoga is a very rewarding and fulfilling role. It is a great privilege to make a positive contribution to the lives of the students who come to your class. Observing their progress in *asana* as well as subtle changes in their behaviour is a very uplifting experience.

Codes of Conduct

- Yoga teachers are committed to practising yoga as a way of life, observing its moral and ethical guidelines (*yama* and *niyama*) in all areas of their lives; and to sharing this knowledge with their students.
- Yoga teachers understand and appreciate that teaching yoga is a noble and ennobling endeavour that aligns with a long line of honourable teachers.
- Yoga teachers are committed to maintaining the highest standards of professional competence and integrity.
- Yoga teachers dedicate themselves to a thorough and continuing study and practice of yoga, in particular the theoretical and practical aspects of the branch of yoga that they teach.
- Yoga teachers should respect all living creatures and refrain from consuming meat.
- Yoga teachers exemplify honesty, patience and obedience.
- Yoga teachers are committed to being kind and non-judgemental, especially when dealing with students, and abstain from acts of arrogance, cruelty, greediness or harshness.
- Yoga teachers cultivate strength of character, courageousness and forgiveness and avoid cowardly, dependent or unstable behaviour.
- Yoga teachers observe moderation in eating, sleeping, recreation, sexual relations and sensual pleasure.
- Yoga teachers are committed to avoiding drug or alcohol abuse. If, for some reason, they succumb to it, they agree to stop teaching until they are free of this chemical dependency. They will then do everything in their power to remain free of it.

When adjusting a student in a pose, always remember that the student's physical welfare is more important than the pefection of the pose.

- Yoga teachers avoid teaching or living in a casual manner.
- Yoga teachers abstain from giving medical advice or any advice that could be interpreted as such, unless they possess the necessary qualifications.
- Yoga teachers work constantly towards freedom from 'I' and 'mine', growing ever less concerned with name, fame, prestige or personal prosperity.
- Yoga teachers welcome all students irrespective of race, nationality, gender, sexual orientation, social status, financial circumstance or physical disability.
- Yoga teachers accurately and truthfully represent their education, training and experience.
- Yoga teachers are committed to promoting the physical, mental and spiritual wellbeing of their students, as well as themselves.
- Yoga teachers understand the unique student/teacher relationship and will avoid exploiting the trust and potential dependency of any student.
- Yoga teachers will always refer students to other teachers if this is in the student's best interest.
- Yoga teachers avoid any form of sexual harassment of their students.

- Yoga teachers wishing to enter a consensual sexual relationship with a present or former student should seek the counsel of their peers before doing so. This is to ensure that the teacher in question is sufficiently clear about his or her motives.
- Yoga teachers strive not to be critical of any school of yoga, tradition or yoga teacher. When criticism has to be brought, it should be done with fairness and a focus on facts.
- Yoga teachers will never force their own opinions on students, but should respect the fact that every individual is entitled to his or her own world view, ideas and beliefs. At the same time, yoga teachers must communicate to their students that yoga seeks to achieve a deep level of transformation of the human personality, including attitudes and ideas. If a student is not open to change, or if a student's opinions seriously impede the process of communicating yogic teachings to him or her, then yoga teachers are free to decline to work with that individual and, if possible, to find an amicable way of concluding the student/teacher relationship.

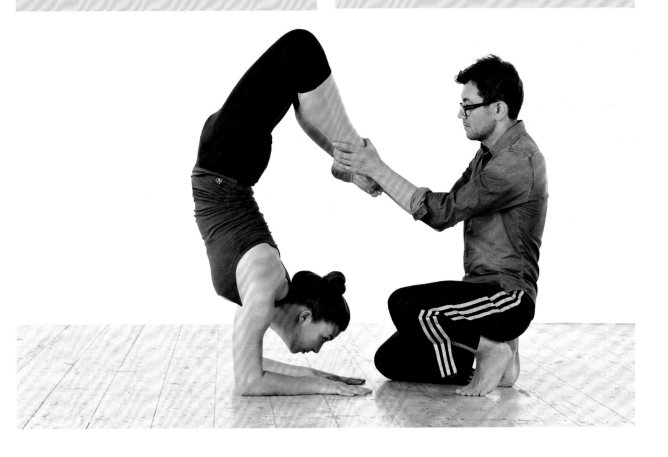

Starting Out

If you have decided to begin a career as a yoga teacher, and have completed your teacher-training, you will know that it is usually a gradual transition. Few teachers find enough classes to make a living from the start, so don't give up the day job: try to negotiate part-time or flexible hours to give yourself time to build up your new career.

It can be difficult to break onto the teaching scene. Few studios are likely to employ a newly qualified teacher, but it is worth sending in your CV and asking to be added to their cover list – covering classes is a great way to build confidence and experience. Social networking sites are a very good way of letting other teachers know that you are available to cover classes. When you do cover a class, make a point of letting the class coordinator know that you enjoyed it and would like to be included on the cover list. Enquire also about any feedback on the class you taught.

Teaching friends is another way to gain experience; if you have space at home, invite a few people over for a class and ask them to comment on your teaching manner and method. If you're still in employment, ask your boss if you may use a meeting room at your office and arrange for some colleagues to practise after work. You could also consider offering free classes at your local community centre. This is a great opportunity to serve your community as well as gain more experience.

Setting Up Your Own Business

Whether you decide to teach at a yoga studio or fitness centre, from home or as a mobile teacher who visits people's homes, there are regulations and insurance matters you need to deal with. In the UK there are at least 17 laws covering health and safety, equipment and the consumer, which need to be adhered to. These apply whether you are working from home or anywhere else.

Opening your own yoga studio is likely to involve substantial financial investment and, until you have established a regular following, there is a risk that this will not yield sufficient returns for your business to succeed. Granted, the set-up costs are comparatively low, as little equipment is required, but there are other issues to consider. If you intend to have your own premises, you need to decide whether you want to rent or own them. You also need to find out about any local regulations and check whether you need to apply for a 'change of use' permit if the space is not already designated as a yoga studio. If you take on a lease, you are likely to be committed for a specific length of time, so find out if you could sublet the premises if you needed to vacate it early.

If you teach from home you must inform your household insurers, which may incur an increase in premium. Similarly, you may need to consider tax implications. In the UK you may be liable for capital gains tax when you sell your house if you have used part of it for business purposes.

Professional insurance and registration

Statutory requirements about insurance vary from region to region, but as a complementary therapy practitioner there is definitely an ethical requirement for you to be insured, even if you teach only one class a week. It is also a requirement from all yoga studios and fitness centres.

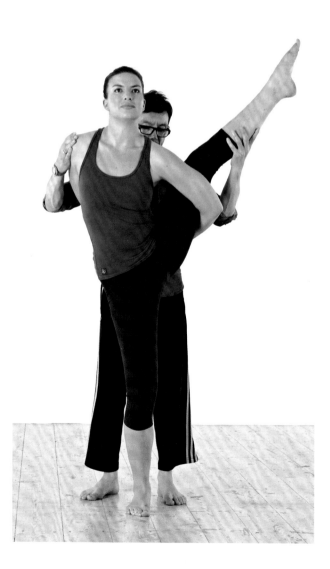

Adjustments should never be forceful. As a yoga teacher, your aim should be to guide your student into a pose rather than push.

Your clients will have more confidence in your professionalism when they see you are fully insured to treat them. In today's litigious climate you need to ensure that you and your clients are adequately protected for professional indemnity and malpractice purposes, as well as for public liability.

- **Professional indemnity and malpractice insurance** Check that your policy covers all the disciplines you carry out in your yoga sessions. Notify your insurers of any changes: for example, a new qualification or if your client base changes – some insurance companies charge a higher premium if a large percentage of your clients are professional sportspeople or dancers.
- **Public liability insurance** covers accidents that may happen off the mat: for example, a client slipping on a wet floor.

Whether you work from home or in a studio, you need both types of insurance. You can also obtain insurance that will cover you while you are a student and can be upgraded once you qualify.

The minimum recommended cover may sound like a very large sum, but you should remember that it would need to cover the high costs of legal fees if a case was brought against you that had to be fought in the courts. Even if you had acted entirely properly, you would have to spend money to prove the fact, so insurance gives you that peace of mind. If a court awarded compensation to the other party, you could lose your home or other personal assets if you weren't adequately insured.

Another type of insurance you might consider is income protection, which provides you with funds if you are unable to work through illness or injury and helps meet rent or mortgage repayments. You also need to insure your vehicle for business use for travelling to and from client or studio.

Opening your own studio may be something you consider for the future, once you are certain that teaching yoga is how you want to make a living. Alternatively, you may wish to hire a space on a weekly or monthly basis. Check with your local church hall or community centre – they often have space available for rent. Many dance studios rent out space for yoga classes too.

In the meantime, if you do teach at fitness centres or yoga studios, it's likely that you will be employed as a freelance contractor and will have to submit an invoice each month for the classes or hours that you have taught. In the UK you will need to register as self-employed with HMRC as a sole trader and will be liable for self-assessment income tax and national insurance.

Marketing

Once you're registered as self-employed and are fully insured, you can begin by building up a client base, targeting either individuals or yoga studios. It might seem inconsistent with the philosophy of yoga to think of it as a business, but you have to be realistic. In the eyes of the law, a business is what it is, and you can't always rely on fate to turn your fortunes around.

Marketing means promoting yourself, letting people know what you do and what is unique about you and the yoga you teach. Spend time planning a marketing strategy. You could start by having a business card printed with your name and contact details. Choose a typeface and colours which you feel represent you as a yoga teacher, and consider listing the school where you trained. On the reverse could be your class schedule if you already have some regular ones.

Website

Websites are easy to design these days and many internet service providers offer packages that include a website template, email address and site name at affordable prices. Make sure you update the site or write blog posts regularly to ensure that people visit it.

Networking

Create your own yoga page on one of the main social network sites and invite people to become your friend. This is a great way to promote your classes. Making use of business networking sites can lead to teaching classes within some of the larger corporations. Many companies are now in favour of having their employees practise yoga on their premises during lunchtime or after work.

If you are certified by the Yoga Alliance or British Wheel of Yoga you can register with them as an approved teacher and have your details added to their websites.

Whenever you teach, leave a notebook out and invite students to write their email addresses down so that you can add them to your contact list and email them about classes and workshops.

Existing clients

Once you have some regular clients, remember to nurture them. Let them know that you appreciate their business as much as they appreciate you teaching them. Include them in your mailings. It can serve as a useful prompt if they haven't been to your class for a while. It's also worth offering private clients a discount if they book a number of classes in advance: give 10 per cent off if they pay for ten classes up front, or make the eleventh class free.

Preparing Your Class

Plan each class in advance, making sure you know what poses you want to teach and in what order and have a back-up plan prepared in case the class is either more or less advanced than you had expected. Have advanced variations ready for the advanced students and easier modifications for the less experienced. Timing is important, too. Make sure you teach at a pace suitable for the level of the class and have enough time to include a variety of *asana*s to ensure a complete practice. Go through the sequence on your own and work out how much time you will need.

Always be punctual, clean and presentable in your appearance. Being late is unprofessional; try to arrive at least ten minutes before your class is due to start. Keep your breath fresh. Avoid coffee or foods such as garlic or spices that will leave an odour on your breath. As you will be in close proximity to your students, also avoid strong perfumes, which can be distracting and misleading.

If you play music in your class, keep the volume lower than the sound of your voice. Music shouldn't distract the students from their practice, so try to keep your choice neutral. Some people turn to yoga after a relationship break-up or if they're suffering from anxiety or depression, so some choices of music may exacerbate their situation.

If you are covering a class, be prepared to face some hostility from students who would prefer their regular teacher. It's not that you are doing anything wrong, you may simply be doing nothing right in the eyes of the student who is attached to his teacher. If this happens, don't be defensive. Remain courteous and professional and concentrate on those who are receptive to you.

First Aid

Occasionally accidents and injuries occur during class, usually as a result of a student being over-ambitious. It is essential that you know what action to take if this happens and have some first-aid experience. There are first-aid courses specifically designed for yoga teachers.

Private Lessons

You may be asked to give somebody a private lesson at their home. Establish what they expect from this so that you can prepare something specific, and check the simplest of things, such as whether they own a yoga mat. When considering how much to charge, take into account the cost of the journey to their home and how long it will take. A class that lasts an hour will usually use up more than two hours of your day, so build this into your fee.

More Training

Learning doesn't stop once you qualify. Few teacher-training programmes cover every aspect of yoga fully: to meet the minimum requirements of a governing body, they may provide little more than a general introduction to the science, philosophy and practice of yoga. It is up to you to take your training further. You could make a more in-depth study of anatomy, deepen your knowledge of the science of yoga or attend workshops given by renowned yogis. The greater your knowledge, the more confidence you will have as a teacher and the more credible you will become in the eyes of your students.

Teaching yoga to children is a very rewarding and joyful experience, so don't restrict yourself to teaching only adults – be open to the idea of teaching students of all ages.

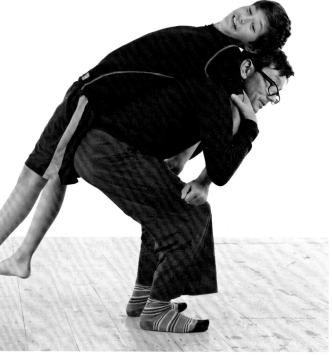

Yoga during Pregnancy

While there are pre-natal yoga classes for pregnant women, some prefer to continue with their regular *asana* practice and modify the poses as their pregnancy progresses.

If you teach regularly, you're likely to have a pregnant student in your class at some point. Yoga can allow a pregnant woman to work on poses that relieve some of the strain on her body and develop the mental focus required for giving birth. Teaching a combination of modified *asana*s, breathing and relaxation techniques will help her face her due date with confidence.

It's important for you as a teacher to determine what is best for the pregnant student – perhaps a regular class or something more gentle and restorative. Once you have assessed the student's general health, the stage of her pregnancy, whether or not it's her first, and her experience with yoga, you can decide which poses are safe for her to practise and which will need to be adapted. For example, a woman who practises yoga regularly and who is in her second pregnancy is capable of a lot more than a first-time mother who has never done yoga, so you should be aware which modifications to apply to both.

Remember, a pregnant woman is not sick or injured. While you need to modify some poses, she is still a strong, capable person. Give her some options and let her do the practice in a way that feels good to her. She is the only one who can really feel what is going on in her body, and she needs to learn to trust her own instincts.

Early Stages of Pregnancy

Although there is little evidence on the outside, in the first three months of pregnancy the body is busy developing a life-support system for the fetus, and all this internal activity can be exhausting.

A woman in the early stages of pregnancy should be able to do most basic yoga poses, but it is important for her to listen to her body and recognize when she needs to exercise and when she should rest. A student might be tempted to push herself, but it's important for her not to practise anything too dynamic.

- Practise basic poses with a few modifications. Build strength and encourage flexibility with familiar poses.
- Have props available in case the student feels unbalanced or tired.

- Avoid inversions, deep twists and back bends. The student shouldn't do anything that might compress the uterus or overstretch the abdominal muscles.
- During pregnancy, the hormone relaxin softens a woman's joints and these are easily dislocated if stretched too far.
- Encourage a long relaxation at the end of class. This is a perfect time to practise focused breathing and to clear the mind.

Even what appear to be the simplest of poses can be challenging for an expectant mother, whose back and abdominal muscles are under a lot of strain. Always exercise caution.

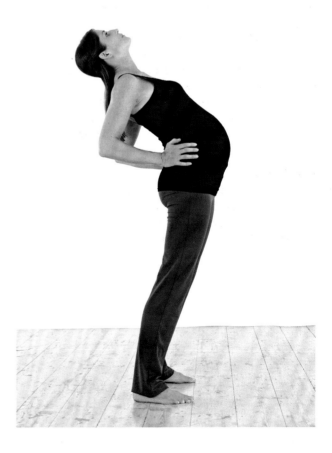

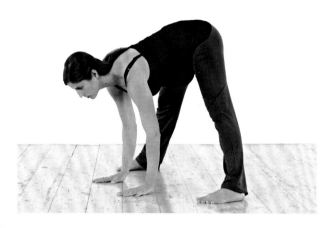

As an alternative to inversions, offer *Prasarita Padottanasana* (Wide-Legged Forward Bend).

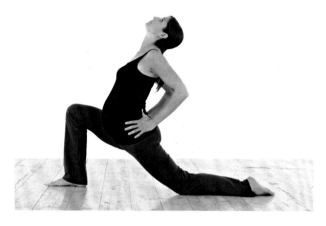

Most back bends stretch the abdominal muscles too much – so stick to Crescent Moon.

Cautions

Inversions should be avoided as they direct circulation away from the uterus. Also, because pregnant women often experience low blood pressure, inversions can cause dizziness. However, *Adho Mukha Svanasana* (Downward Facing Dog) is fine for short periods.

Middle Stages of Pregnancy

In the middle stages of pregnancy a student should no longer lie flat on her back for any extended length of time, due to the weight of the uterus and baby on the vena cava, which moves blood from the lower part of the body to the heart. Poses such as *Malasana* help increase circulation to the legs, open the hips and relieve the back.

This is a also good time to introduce *pranayama* exercises such as *Ujjayi* and *Nadi-Sodhana pranayama* (see pages 218, 220). They teach the pregnant student how to focus on her breath, which helps her relax, and these techniques will also help during labour and delivery. Avoid any *pranayama* that involves retention of the breath (*Anuloma-Viloma*) or changing the flow of air (*Kapalabhati*), as they will affect the delivery of oxygen to the fetus.

As the belly grows, the abdominal muscles and ligaments are stretched, so most strong abdominal poses such as *Navasana* (Boat Pose) or leg raises should be avoided.

The student's changing shape will require further modification to any poses that involve folding or twisting. To avoid compressing the belly in all forward bends, she should spread her legs slightly and fold at the hip joint.

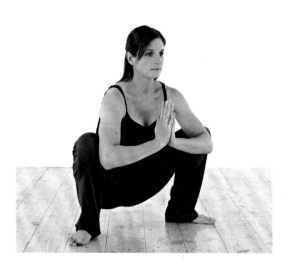

Regular practice of *Malasana* keeps the hips flexible and is good preparation for childbirth, as it opens the pelvic area.

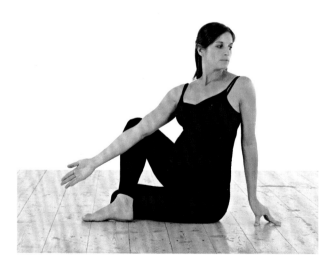

Keep any twists simple during pregnancy to avoid straining the abdominal and back muscles.

Open twists can relieve some of the back pain, but now the twist should not be too deep. Most restrictions will be obvious, because the size of the student's belly will limit much of this activity, but make sure she knows which poses can be modified and which she shouldn't do.

Later Stages of Pregnancy

By the last three months of pregnancy, a mother-to-be is constantly aware of the baby inside her. She has probably gained 10–15 kg (20–30 lb), and this additional weight can cause great discomfort. The pressure of the crowded uterus on the internal organs results in heartburn, frequent urination, lower back pain, cramping in the front and side abdominals, and shortness of breath. The large, unyielding mass of her belly causes interrupted sleep, difficulty moving and clumsiness. The hormone relaxin, which allows her pelvis to widen so that she can deliver, makes her joints unstable. She may also experience dizziness as well as swelling in the hands and feet because of slowed circulation caused by the hormone progesterone.

The main priority with *asana* at this stage is to protect the joints and maintain balance. Even an experienced practitioner will have to adapt to her quick weight gain and unbalanced shape. Throughout the pregnancy, basic standing and balance poses are good for building strength in the legs, re-establishing proper alignment in the spine and encouraging circulation.

Hip-opening postures such as *Upavistha Konasana* (Seated Wide-legged Forward Bend Pose) can help relieve aches in the lower back and create space around the pelvis. They also help release the lumbar spine and open the hip joints and are good positions for the mother during labour.

Because a student in the later stages of her pregnancy has restricted mobility, there should be more emphasis on breathing techniques and less on *asana*. Practising

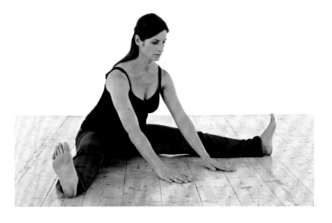

This gentle variation of *Upavistha Konasana* encourages greater hip flexion and relieves lower back pain.

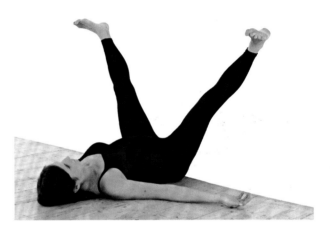

This alternative to the shoulder stand is a great way to relax the veins in the legs.

pranayama not only encourages relaxation, but also helps improve concentration. It can be done on its own or during *asana* practice to encourage focus in preparation for labour.

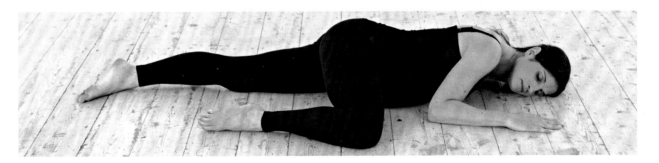

Lay the pregnant student on her left side in *Savasana* (Corpse Pose). All side-lying poses should be on the left side, to avoid pressure on the vena cava.

Yoga Practice for Older Age Groups

Although there are classes specifically for people over 50 or 60,
don't be surprise to see older adults in an open class. Some might
come for a restorative practice, while others hope to fend off
osteoporosis, stiffness and other issues associated with ageing.

As we approach midlife, the body begins to lose its flexibility, and stiffness sets in as the spine compresses. We lose joint mobility and balance, and muscle and bone mass decrease. For most, by the age of 50, a largely sedentary lifestyle and years of bad posture result in neck and back problems. Even the very active cannot always escape the assault of time on their bodies.

Yoga provides a solution to the stiffness that settles into the body as we age. Slow-moving and gentle *asanas* are ideal for older students, helping the mind and body remain young and active, while breathing exercises increase the supply of oxygen to the brain. Some *asanas* can be practised while sitting on a chair, or even in bed. Some counter the effects of gravity by lengthening the spine, improving posture and moving each joint through its full range of movement. Whereas the emphasis for the younger student is on building and challenging the body, by midlife this turns to maintaining optimum health, including the prevention of injury through a yogic lifestyle, for example the study of the activities of the mind, the biomechanics of the body and safe *asanas*, breathing exercises, proper diet, rest and relaxation.

When people start yoga over the age of 50, it's not unusual for them to be suffering from a number of ailments commonly associated with the ageing process, such as stiffness, back pain, arthritis, osteoporosis, knee and hip replacements, heart disease and high blood pressure. We shouldn't assume everyone with greying hair has a bad back or arthritic knees, but it's important for a teacher to understand age-related conditions, whether they're teaching an entire class of older students or trying to integrate a handful of older adults into a younger class. Having some idea of typical changes and health concerns and how these affect movement and strength can help a teacher gauge how much to challenge a student, what to modify and how to help them gain most benefit from yoga.

Moving slowly and gently allows an ageing body to go deeper into a pose, although this can be a challenge in itself. Many older men in particular may try to keep up with what someone younger and more adept in the class is doing. A lot of younger students come to yoga for the external benefits, to improve their physique. But for the older student, the focus should move inwards. Fluidity of movement and creating space in the joints is more important than the external nature of yoga. Having said that, the threshold for when to slow down varies. It usually depends on when you started yoga and what shape you're in. Some 60-year-olds may be stronger or more flexible than a 30-year-old who has never practised yoga before.

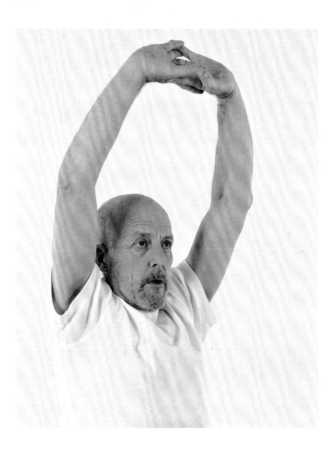

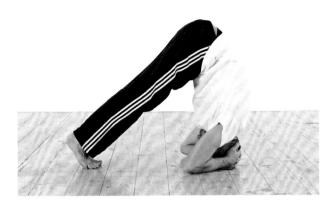

In the half headstand, the internal organs are inverted and massaged and there is a renewed supply of blood to the brain.

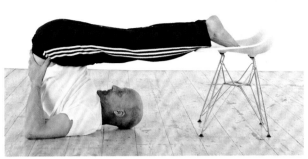

To avoid straining the neck or shoulders, the legs are placed on a chair in this shoulder stand variation.

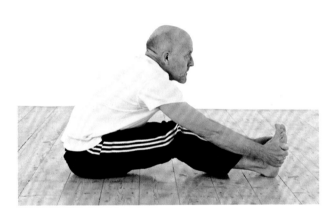

In this gentle forward bend, the back and the legs are stretched as the sides of the feet are held and pushed forward.

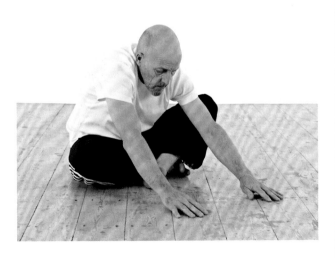

This posture gently opens the hips, massages the abdominal organs and also relieves lower back pain.

Points to Consider when Teaching Older Students

- Inverted postures are a must for ageing bodies, so get the head below the level of the heart. Encourage students to practise an inversion – the head stand or shoulder stand can be modified to suit all abilities.
- Practise in a way that is appropriate and healing. Be patient and never use force.
- Avoid teaching poses that bear weight directly on the neck and head. People with kyphosis or osteoperosis should only practice inverted poses under supervision until they have built strength in the upper body strengthening poses, such as Downward- and Upward-facing Dog, and Plank.
- Always have modifications for challenging *asanas*. When teaching more difficult poses, make it clear that students can repeat the basic pose that usually precedes the more challenging one, and that using props to help them is perfectly acceptable.
- Focus on lengthening the spine and opening the chest in all categories of poses, including forward bends, twists and back bends.
- Encourage students to move from the hip joint, keeping the upper body in one unit and the spine elongated. If the hamstrings are tight, it's difficult to bend sideways or forward without rounding and shortening the spine. Using a wall or chair can help someone bend from the hip joint while keeping length in the spine.
- Encourage older students to practice *pranayama* and meditation daily. Proper breathing is important in later life and meditation can dispel fear and loneliness.

Yoga for Children

Yoga at an early age is an excellent foundation for children. It leads to greater self-esteem and body awareness through a physical activity that is non-competitive.

Encouraging children to learn techniques that can improve their physical wellbeing, help them relax and increase their confidence will enable them to cope more effectively with life's challenges. Cultivating cooperation and compassion through yoga is a great gift to the young.

Physically, yoga increases children's flexibility, strength and coordination and also improves their concentration. They are naturally more flexible than adults and find many of the poses much easier to adopt than we do.

During a yoga class children can exercise and play. The names of the postures enable them to develop a closer relationship with their environment. When the ancient yogis developed the *asanas*, they lived close to the natural world and used animals and nature as inspiration for poses such as the Cobra, Tree and Fish. When children imitate the movements and sounds of nature, they have a chance to inhabit another being and embody its characteristics.

Children are more likely to interact and enjoy a yoga class when the emphasis is placed on playful expression rather than physical concerns regarding alignment and breathing.

When they assume the pose of the lion (*Simhasana*), for example, they experience not only the power of the lion, but also their own sense of power. The physical movements introduce children to the meaning of yoga: union and understanding their own nature.

Yoga with children offers many possibilities to exchange wisdom, share good times and lay the foundation for a lifelong practice. It should be kept fun and experimental. The poses can be a springboard for exploring many other areas – animal adaptations and behaviour, playing musical instruments and storytelling.

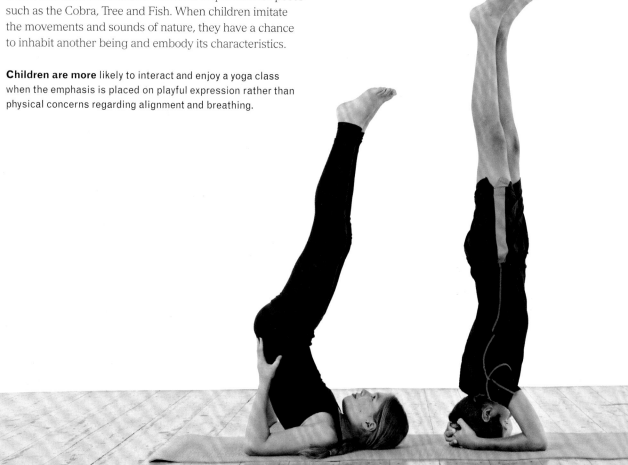

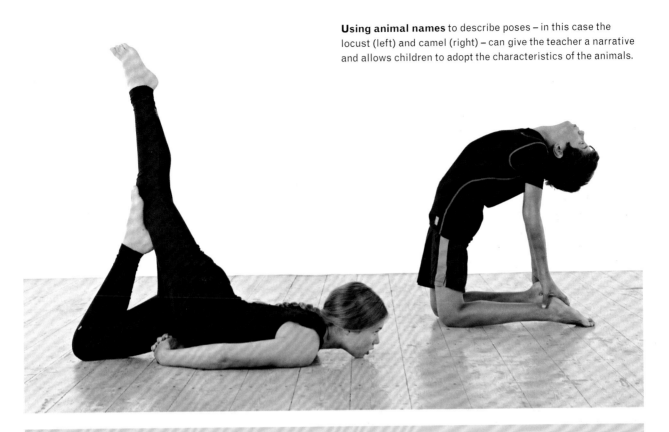

Using animal names to describe poses – in this case the locust (left) and camel (right) – can give the teacher a narrative and allows children to adopt the characteristics of the animals.

Points to Consider when Teaching Children

- Children will jump at the chance to assume the role of animals, trees, flowers, warriors. Take a step back and allow them to bark in the dog pose, hiss like a cobra and roar like a lion. They can also recite the alphabet or numbers as they are holding poses. Sound is a great release for children and adds an auditory dimension to the physical experience of yoga.
- Children need to discover the world on their own. Telling them to think harder, do it better or be a certain way because it's good for them can undermine their sense of who they are. Instead, provide a loving, responsive, creative environment in which they can uncover their own truths. As they perform the various animal and nature *asanas*, engage their minds to deepen their awareness. Use your own imagination to encourage the child's learning: for example, you could teach the head stand to a group of children as if each of them were a skyscraper, joining together to form a city skyline.
- Breathing correctly is as important with children as with adults. Try teaching a child abdominal breathing

while he is lying on his back: place a rubber duck or toy boat on his tummy, then ask him to observe how it floats on the water as he breathes in and out.
- Meditation can also increase a child's powers of concentration. In schools where this is taught, improvements in class work and group interaction have been recognized.
- The greatest challenge with children is to hold their attention long enough to teach them the benefits of yoga: stillness, balance, flexibility, focus, peace, grace, connection, health and wellbeing. Luckily, most children love to talk and to move, both of which can happen in yoga.
- When they stretch like a cat, balance like a crow or stand strong and tall like a tree, they are making a connection between the macrocosm of their environment and the microcosm of their minds and bodies. The importance of respect for all life and the principle of interdependence becomes apparent. Children soon begin to understand that we are all the same, but exist in different forms.

Adjusting Poses

When it comes to adjusting a student in a yoga pose, one size does not fit all. Self practice brings a greater awareness of the body and any limitations, which can be an effective means of helping someone else in a pose without the need for force.

Learning how to adjust or assist students safely and correctly in a yoga pose is now on the curriculum of many yoga teacher-training programmes. But this is a relatively recent addition, and may be linked to an increase in the number of reported injuries that are alleged to have occurred as a result of using too much force when adjusting, particularly in some of the popular styles such as Ashtanga yoga and other more dynamic practices.

As a teacher and practitioner, I've usually found assisting (and being assisted) in poses to be a very effective means of increasing flexibility and exploring my own and the student's awareness of the pose.

There are different ways to assist someone in a pose. While some traditions offer a more physical, hands-on approach, others rely on verbal cues that enable students to explore their own physical potential in a pose. There are also some schools of yoga that offer the use of props and blocks to help a student advance in a pose.

The purpose of an adjustment should be to correctly align the student in a way that will bring optimum physical and mental benefits and give full expression to the pose. Experience has taught me only to give assistance when it seems appropriate, and with the student's safety at the forefront. Most adjustments can be made verbally, by giving clear and precise instructions, such as telling a student to change the position of a hand or a foot. Often it's neither necessary nor in the student's best interest to make a physical adjustment, as the student may already have reached his or her physical limit. There are, however, occasions when the only way a student can attempt or experience a pose is by means of you physically assisting them – this is often the case with inversions.

The interplay between you as a teacher and your student is never more apparent than when you adjust them in a pose, so it is important to be clear about your objectives. Will it benefit the student? What you might consider to be helpful the student might interpret as a criticism, so it is always good to clarify your objectives from the outset.

Learning to read body language will help you understand what's happening on a psycho-energetic level. The expression on your student's face is usually an indication of how they are feeling in the pose. If they look uncomfortable, then they're probably feeling uncomfortable and could be using too much force in the pose. Use verbal instructions to get them to relax their facial features. When offering verbal adjustments, your voice and tone should be encouraging and nurturing. Never bark commands at your students and never humiliate them by pointing out their weaknesses. Always try to build on their strengths.

How you adjust someone is transmitted directly to the recipient. Your student should feel secure and supported. Any uncertainty on your part will usually be detected by the student, and may lead them to become more tense in the pose, in which case your attempts to improve their pose will be in vain. So, approach the student with confidence, but never arrogance, and never use too much force. Often a light touch is all that is needed to guide the student deeper into a pose.

Your own breathing should be calm, smooth and steady, to reassure the student. This will enable you to approach the adjustment of the pose with greater awareness and sensitivity. When your breath is regulated and synchronized with your movements during an adjustment, the student will often respond by synchronizing his or her breath with yours and this will facilitate greater depth and awareness in, and of, the pose.

Adjusting often depends on how receptive and comfortable with being touched your student are. Remember, the adjustment is for the benefit of the student and you should always respect their wishes, in spite of the pose and your ego.

On a more cautionary note, I have noticed that some students come to rely on adjustments rather than striving to achieve the pose on their own. Be careful how much help you give. It can make a student too dependent on you – and on occasions it could also be misinterpreted.

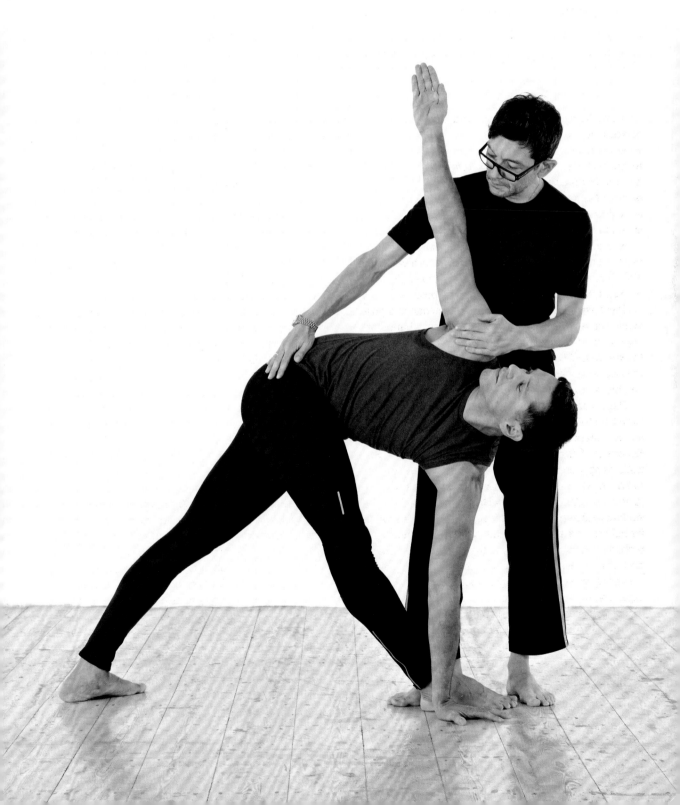

Index

abdominal cavity 30, 31, 222

abdominal muscles 30–1, 47, 51–2, 70, 222–3; strenthening 136, 140, 160, 162, 164, 166, 168, 171, 172, 175, 177, 192; stretching 148, 151, 158, 178, 196, 198, 200, 202, 208

Adept's Pose (Siddhasana) 141

adjusting poses 236, 241, 242, 245, 248

adrenal gland 35, 70

ageing 8, 24, 41, 48, 226, 229, 244–5

alternate nostril-breathing 71, 218–20, 225

anatomy 27–54

ankle 48, 49, 54; beneficial poses 139, 141, 143, 151, 195, 196, 202; problems 106, 107, 141, 143, 151, 198, 200

Anuloma-Viloma 71, 219, 252

anxiety, reducing 94, 221, 229

apana 60, 61, 62, 224

appetite 60, 70, 221

Ardha Baddha Padmottanasana (Half-bound Lotus Forward Bend) 101, 213

Ardha Chandrasana (Half Moon Pose) 55, 108–9, 213

Ardha Matsyendrasana (Half Spinal Twist) 51, 122–3, 212, 213

Ardho Mukha Svanasana (Downward-facing Dog) 179, 210, 213, 242, 245

Ardho Mukha Vrikshasana (Downward Facing Tree Pose) 158–9, 213

arms 47, 50, 51, 52, 53, 54, 139; strengthening 87, 114, 155, 158, 160, 162, 164, 166, 168, 171, 172, 175, 176, 177, 178, 183, 184, 192, 204, 206

arteries 32–3, 34

asanas 11; benefits of 28, 37, 41, 79–81; cardiovascular system 32, 33; counter poses 212; development 7, 8, 11, 22, 23, 25; digestive system 37; endocrine system 35; joints 48; lymphatic system 34; meditation 228; movement planes 50–1; musculoskeletal system 42, 45, 46; nervous system 39; practice 80–1, 82, 212–13; preparation for 209; respiratory system 30

Ashtanga Namaskara 211

Ashva Sanchalanasana (Equestrian Pose) 210, 211

Ashva Sanchalasana (Crescent Moon Pose) 204–5, 224, 242

Astavakrasana (Eight-limbed Pose) 176–7

asthma 118, 124, 152, 179, 188

astral body 58–9, 64

atman 14, 21, 22, 66, 67

attachment 7, 17, 19, 20, 21, 75

austerity 19, 80

awareness 66, 79, 80, 82, 155, 209, 228

back 47; balancing poses 156, 158, 160, 162, 164, 166, 171, 175, 178; inverted poses 183, 184, 188; pain relief 90, 122, 135, 243, 245; seated poses 126, 135, 136, 140, 141; standing poses 87, 94, 103, 110–11; supine poses 148, 152

back-bending poses 191–208, 212, 241, 242

back problems: back-bending poses 192, 195, 196, 198, 200, 202, 204, 206, 208; balancing poses 145, 168, 171; causes 45,

244; inverted poses 183; seated poses 118, 122, 126, 131, 132, 138; standing poses 90, 94, 97, 103, 104, 106, 107, 111; supine poses 148, 151

Back-stretch Forward Bend (Paschimottanasana) 37, 69, 118–19, 212, 213

Badha Padmasana (Bound Lotus Variation) 143

Badhha Konasana (Bound Angle Pose) 128–9, 213

balance, improving 80; balancing poses 155, 168, 172; standing poses 95, 98, 100, 106, 107, 109, 110

balancing poses 155–79, 243

Balasana (Child's Pose) 52, 115

Ballet Pose (Natyasana) 50

bandhas (body locks) 22, 23, 29, 62–3, 71, 219, 222–3, 227

basti 68–9

Beerasana (Dragonfly Pose) 160–1

Bellows breathing (Bhastrika) 219

Bhagavad Gita 14–15, 16, 21

Bhakti yoga 15, 22

Bharadvajasana (Bound Half-Lotus Spinal Twist) 134–5, 213

Bhastrika (bellows breathing) 219

Bhujanghasana (Cobra Pose) 53, 208, 210; see also Upward-facing Dog

Bird of Paradise Pose (Svarga Dvijasana) 107, 213

blood 33, 35; cells and tissues 40, 41, 42; digestive system 37; inverted poses 181; lymphatic system 34; respiratory system 31, 218, 219; transport 32, 81; vessels 32–3

blood pressure 29, 32, 38

blood pressure, high:
  poses to avoid: back-bending 195, 196, 202; balancing 156, 158; breathing 219; inverted 156, 158, 183, 186, 188; standing 87, 88, 89, 92, 95, 110, 111; supine 148
  therapeutic exercises 71, 120, 179, 221

blood pressure, low:
  poses to avoid: back-bending 195, 196, 202; breathing 221; seated 140; standing 86, 90, 92, 95, 96, 100, 109, 110, 112; supine 148
  therapeutic exercises 220

Boat Pose (Paripurana Navasana) 53, 140, 242

body: anatomy 28–9; annamaya kosha 66, 67; cells and tissues 41; Hatha yoga 23; movement planes 50–1; nutritional needs 76; pranic 61; pressure in 28, 29; temperature 31, 35, 39, 40; unity with mind 20, 25, 80, 82

body locks see bandhas

bones 35, 41, 42–3, 80, 155

Bound Angle Pose (Badhha Konasana) 128–9, 213

Bound Fish Pose 149

Bound Half-Lotus Spinal Twist (Bharadvajasana) 134–5, 213

Bound Lotus Variation (Badha Padmasana) 143

Bow Pose (Dhanurasana) 202–3, 212, 213; Upward-facing 192–3

brahman 13, 14, 21, 22

brahma nadi see sushumna nadi

Brahmari 221

brain 38–9, 41, 42; ajna chakra 65; nadis 62; pranayama benefits 71, 218

breathing 28, 30–1, 32, 60, 215; body and mind 80, 155, 217; Savasana (Corpse Pose) 153; So hum meditation 230–1; teaching children 247; see also pranayama; respiratory system

calming 143, 153, 217, 220, 231

Camel Pose (Ustrasana) 194–5, 213

candle flame 70, 231

carbon dioxide 30, 31, 71, 219

cardiovascular system 29, 32–3, 60, 62

carpal tunnel sundrome 161, 162, 178, 179, 192

cartilage 41, 42, 44, 48

cells and tissues 40, 229

central nervous system (CNS) 38, 39, 62

Chair Pose (Utkatasana) 96, 213

chakras 20, 64–5, 192, 222, 227; bandhas 222; Hatha yoga 23, 24, 25, 58, 63; and the nadis 62, 63

Chakrasana (Wheel Pose) 192–3

Chandra-Surya-Kumbhaka Pranayama 219–20

Chaturanga Dandasana (Four-limb Staff Pose) 177, 213

chest 30, 31, 47, 50, 148; breathing exercises 220; older age groups 245; stretching 139, 147, 156, 178, 192, 196, 198, 200, 202, 204, 208

children 246–7

Child's Pose (Balasana) 52, 115

Chin Lock (Uddiyana Bandha) 30, 69, 70, 71, 222–3, 227

circulatory system 28, 29, 31, 32, 33, 36; beneficial poses 128, 181, 216; pranas 60, 66, 67

class: attending 80, 240; covering 238, 240; preparing your 240

Classical Yoga 16–20

cleansing 24, 68–71, 77, 212, 217

clients, finding/keeping 239

Cobra Pose (Bhujanghasana) 53, 208, 210; see also Upward-facing Dog

codes of conduct 236–7

colon 37, 68–9, 76

Compass Pose (Parivrtta Surya Yantrasana) 138

concentration 25, 155, 246; dharana 14, 18, 20, 228; and meditation 228, 229, 231; pranayama effect 218, 219, 243; shatkarmas 68

connective tissue 41, 42, 48

consciousness: awakening 20, 22, 23, 25, 63, 228; and chakras 64, 65; Chin mudra 224; dhyana 14, 18, 20, 213, 228; inhibiting 20; karma 72; practising asanas 80; pure 17, 65, 67; self-realization 57, 60; universal 8, 14, 20, 22

constipation 37, 69, 70, 131, 132

contentment 19, 228–9

cooling exercises 221

Corpse Pose (Savasana) 153, 212, 213, 243

coveting 19, 236

Cow Face Pose (Gomukhasana) 52, 139, 213

cramp 88

Crescent Moon Pose (Ashva Sanchalasana) 204–5, 224, 242

Crow Pose (Kakasana) 162–3, 164, 212, 213

cycle of birth/death/rebirth 14, 72

daily practice 81, 212–13, 217

Dancer Pose (Natarajasana) 112–13

deities 12, 13, 14–15, 22, 24, 65, 232, 233

depression 75, 118, 183, 192

Dhanurasana (Bow Pose) 202–3, 212, 213

dharana 14, 18, 20, 228

dhyana 14, 18, 20, 213, 228

diaphragm 30, 31, 70, 222

diet 48, 61, 74–7, 240

digestive system 28, 35, 36–8, 40, 80; balancing poses 166; cleansing kriyas 68–9, 70, 71; diet 75, 76; fasting 77; pranamaya kosha 66; pranayama practice 217, 219; pranic energies 60; seated poses 118, 120, 122, 124, 130, 132; standing poses 92, 94, 101; supine poses 151, 152; Uddiyana Bandha 30, 69, 70, 71, 222–3

disease 61, 76, 216, 217; protection 31, 33, 34, 40, 122, 143

divine 15, 19, 22, 23, 64, 232

Downward-facing Dog (Ardho Mukha Svanasana) 179, 210, 213, 242, 245

Downward Facing Tree Pose (Ardho Mukha Vrikshasana) 158–9, 213

Dragonfly Pose (Beerasana) 160–1

drinking 75, 76, 77

dualism 16, 17, 21, 22, 23, 230

Dwi Pada Sirsasana (Two-Legs or Feet-Behind-the-Head) 132–3

Dwi Pada Viparita Dandasana 193

Eagle Pose (Garudasana) 50, 98

Easy Pose (Sukkhasana) 141

ego 7, 14, 17, 20, 229, 237

Eight-limbed Pose (Astavakrasana) 176–7

Eka Pada Raja Kapotasana I/II (King Pigeon Pose) 51, 52, 198–9, 200–1

Eka Pada Sirsasana (One-Foot-Behind-the-Head) 130–1, 213

elbow: joint 48, 49, 52, 53; problems 104, 166, 168, 172, 176

elements 65, 66, 67

elimination processes: beneficial asanas 92, 101, 166; fasting 77; muladhara chakra 65; prana 60, 61; pranamaya kosha 66; pranayama 71, 216, 218, 219, 220; shatkarmas 68–9, 70; waste products 31, 32, 33, 34, 36, 39

emotions: anahata chakra 65; and anatomy 35, 38; and diet 75; Hridaya mudra 225; manomaya kosha 66, 67; nauli 70; pranic body 61

endocrine system 28, 29, 31, 32, 35, 42; beneficial poses 181, 222, 223; pranamaya kosha 66

energy, pranic 60, 61, 209, 217

energy centres see chakras

Equestrian Pose (Ashva Sanchalanasana) 210, 211

Eternal Etheric Records 7

excretion see elimination processes

exhalation 60, 71, 217, 218, 219

Extended Hand to Toe Pose (Uttitha Hasta Padangusthasana) 106

Extended Side Angle Pose (Utthita Parsvakonasana) 53

Extended Side Angle Twist (Parivrita Parsvakonasana) 51, 213

Extended Triangle Pose (Uttitha Trikonasana) 51, 90–1

eyes 60, 70, 231

face 29, 60, 226, 248

fasting 77

fatigue 94, 115, 122, 186, 188, 229

Feathered Peacock Pose (Pincha Mayurasana) 156–7, 213

feet 48, 49, 54; beneficial poses 85, 100, 151, 179; walking meditation 232

Firefly Pose (Tittibhasana) 168–9, 213

First Aid 240

Fish Pose (Matsyasana) 148–9, 212, 213

flexibility 28, 85, 244, 246

fluid, in body 31, 32–3, 34

food: and diet 48, 74–6; digestion 36–7; manipura chakra 65; three gunas 19, 74, 75

Forward Bends: daily practice 212, 213; Maha mudra 227; older age groups 245; seated 37, 69, 118–19, 120, 126–7, 212, 213; standing 52, 69, 94, 101, 102–3, 210, 213

Four-limb Staff Pose (Chaturanga Dandasana) 177, 213

Front Splits (Hanumanasana) 144–5

Galavasana (Pose of the Sage Galava) 170–1

gallbladder 36, 37

Garland Pose (Malasana) 97, 242

Garudasana (Eagle Pose) 50, 98

gastrointestinal system 29

gestures, symbolic see mudras

glands see endocrine system

gluteus muscles 47, 50, 53

Gomukhasana (Cow Face Pose) 52, 139, 213

Granthis, Three 222

groin, beneficial poses: back-bending 195, 196, 198, 200, 202; balancing 160, 162, 168, 175; seated 120, 126, 128, 144; standing 97, 104, 112

gunas, three 17, 74–5

Halasana (Plough Pose) 188–9

Half-bound Lotus Forward Bend (Ardha Baddha Padmottanasana) 101, 213

Half Moon Pose (Ardha Chandrasana) 55, 108–9, 213

Half Spinal Twist (Ardha Matsyendrasana) 51, 122–3, 212, 213

hamstrings 47, 51, 52, 53; problems 114, 138, 144; stretching 138, 144, 179

hands 49, 54; binding 93, 107, 123, 125, 200; mudras 218, 224–5; swadisthana chakra 65

handstand 95, 158–9

Hanumanasana (Front Splits) 144–5

happiness 19, 228–9

Hasta Uttanasana 210, 211, 213

Hatha yoga 11, 23–4, 25, 27–9, 58

Hatha Yoga Pradipika 23, 25, 60, 68

head 43, 51, 55, 60, 226

headaches, poses to avoid 148, 156, 158, 192, 195, 196, 202, 206

Head Stand Pose (Sirsasana) 33, 35, 182–3, 184–5, 212, 213, 226, 245

Head-to-Knee Pose (Janu Sirsasana) 120–1, 212, 213

health benefits 7, 8, 23, 28; breathing 31, 216–17; children 246; and diet 75, 76; meditation 229; older age groups 244

health and safety 4, 9, 238

heart 32–3, 40, 46; beneficial poses 128, 196, 231; chakra 64, 65; and diet 76; heart rate 32, 38, 63; Hridaya mudra 225; nadis 62;

problems 88, 156, 183, 192, 218, 219, 220; purification 64; samana 60

hernia, poses to avoid 131, 132

hips 48, 49, 50, 52, 53; back-bending poses 195, 196, 198, 200, 202; older age groups 244, 245; problems 114, 198, 200, 244; seated poses 128, 135, 139, 140; standing poses 97, 99, 101, 111, 114; supine poses 148

history/origins of yoga: Classical Yoga 16–20; Post-classical period 21–4; Vedic/Pre-classical period 12–15; yoga today 25

home, working from 238, 239

hormonal system 28, 29, 31, 32, 35, 42, 70

Horse Pose (Vatyanasana) 99

Hummingbird Pose (Beerasana) 160–1

hypothalamus 35, 38, 39

ida nadi 24, 60, 62, 219

immune system 28, 29, 34, 40

in breath/inhalation 60, 71, 217

indigestion 37, 70

injury 81, 82, 239, 240

inner focus 7, 13, 20, 81, 229

Insect Pose (Utthita Tittibhasana) 104–5, 213

insurance 238–9

intelligence 65, 66

Intense Side-stretch Pose (Parsvottanasana) 111

inverted poses 29, 33, 181–9, 226; during pregnancy 241, 242; older age groups 245

jalandhara bandha 219, 220, 222, 223, 226, 227

Janu Sirsasana (Head-to-Knee Pose) 120–1, 212, 213

Japa meditation 230

Jnana yoga 14, 15, 16, 21

joints 41, 46, 48–56, 241, 243, 244

Kakasana (Crow Pose) 162–3, 212, 213

kapalabhati 30, 33, 69, 71, 219, 242

Kapotasana (Pigeon Pose) 196–7

karma 14, 72–3

Karma yoga 14, 15, 16, 21

kidneys 94, 118, 120, 122, 124, 128, 140, 152

King Pigeon Pose I/II (Eka Pada Raja Kapotasana) 51, 52, 198–9, 200–1

knee 46, 48, 49, 52, 53; beneficial poses 101, 141, 143, 151; problems 97, 98, 99, 101, 115, 120, 128, 141, 143, 151, 198, 200, 244

knowledge 14, 16, 224

koshas 66–7, 217

kriyas 68–71, 219, 221

kumbhaka 217, 218, 226

kundalini 23, 24, 25, 39; awakening 58, 60, 63, 68, 122, 143; and chakras 64, 65; and granthis 222; sushumna shakti 62

Kurmasana (Tortoise Pose) 136–7, 213

legs 46, 47, 50, 51, 53, 55, 85

liberation 15–25, 62, 65

life force see prana

ligaments 41, 42, 44, 45, 48

liver 37, 70, 76, 94, 118, 120, 122, 124, 152

Lizard Pose (Uttan Pristhasana) 114, 213
Locust Pose (Salabhasana) 30, 53, 206–7
Lotus Pose (Padmanasana) 142–3
lunging poses: Ashva Sanchalanasana 210, 211; Ashva Sancha lasana 204–5, 224, 242; Virabhadrasana 50, 87, 88, 89, 213
lungs 30–1, 32, 70, 71; pranayama effect 216, 219, 220; stretching 92, 178, 204, 208
lymphatic system 29, 34

mala, mantra repetition 233
Malasana (Garland/Squatting Pose) 97, 242
mantras 13, 22, 23, 64, 65; meditation 230–1; om 65, 220, 231; Sun Salutation 209; using mala 233
Marichyasana (Pose of the Sage Marichi) 124–5, 213
marketing 238, 239
Matsyasana (Fish Pose) 148–9, 212, 213
Mayurasana (Peacock Pose) 30, 166–7, 213
meat eating 75, 76, 236
meditation 228–33; and chakras 64; children 247; daily practice 212, 213; dhyana 14, 18, 20, 213, 228; historic yoga 14, 15, 16, 18, 22; manomaya kosha 66; older age groups 245; posture 20, 23, 79, 82, 141, 142–3, 209, 221; shatkarmas 68; see also mantras
membranes 40, 41
menopause 186
menstruation: beneficial poses 122, 143, 151; poses to avoid 158, 183, 186, 188
mental powers 7, 8, 18
metabolism 35, 63
migraine 148, 195, 196, 202
mind: -body unity 20, 25, 28, 80, 82; calming 143, 153, 217, 220; and diet 76; five sheaths/koshas 66, 67; inverted poses 181; meditation 228–9, 231; pranayama effect 216, 217, 219
Mittra, Sri Dharma 7, 25
mood 20, 35
Moon-Sun-Holding Breathing Exercise 219–20
moral restraints 18, 19, 236
Mountain Pose (Tadasana) 86
mouth 68, 221
mudras 22, 23, 24, 25, 103, 218, 224–7; Asvini Mudra 69, 219, 220, 227; Jnana mudra 142, 218, 224, 227; Vishnu mudra 218, 219, 220, 225; Yoga Mudra 35, 226
Mula bandha 71, 219, 220, 222, 226
muscular system 29, 30, 31, 42, 46–7, 80
musculoskeletal system 28, 42–5; cells and tissues 40, 41; musculoskeletal pump 29; nervous system 38; skeletal muscles 34, 46; synovial fluid 41; thyroid function 35
music 240

nadis 24, 25, 58, 60, 62–3, 75, 217, 218, 223, 227
nadi sodhana pranayama 71, 213, 218, 242
Natarajasana (Dancer Pose) 112–13
Natyasana (Ballet Pose) 50
nauli 30, 33, 37, 69, 70, 212
neck 47, 51; beneficial poses 135, 148, 186, 198, 200; Jalandhara bandha 219, 220, 222, 223, 226, 227; pranic energy (udana) 60; problems: back-bending poses 195, 196, 206; balancing poses 156, 158; inverted poses 183, 186, 188; seated poses 139; standing poses 88, 92, 109; supine poses 148

relaxation 29
nervous system 28, 29, 32, 35, 36, 38–9, 41, 80; pranayama 71, 217, 219, 220, 221
neti 69, 212, 217
networking 238, 239
nirguna meditation 230
non-violence 19, 76, 236
nose 30, 62, 69, 71, 212, 217, 218–21
nutrients 60, 75, 76, 216; transport 28, 30, 31, 32, 33
nyama 19, 20, 22, 23, 228

Om mantra 65, 230, 231
One-Foot-Behind-the-Head (Eka Pada Sirsasana) 130–1, 213
One Leg Raised Up (Urdhva Prasarita Eka Padasana) 95
out breath 60, 71, 217, 218, 219
ovaries 35
oxygen 28, 29, 30–1, 32–3, 38, 71, 181, 216–17, 218

Padma Mayurasana 167
Padmanasana (Lotus Pose) 142–3; alternative poses 141
pain 80, 81, 82, 217, 220, 245
pancreatic gland 35, 37, 70
parasympathetic nervous system (PSNS) 38, 39, 62
parathyroid gland 35
Paripurana Navasana (Boat Pose) 53, 140, 242
Parivrtta Parsvakonasana (Revolving Side Angle Twist) 51, 92–3, 213
Parivrtta Surya Yantrasana (Compass Pose) 138
Parivrtta Trikonasana (Revolving Triangle Pose) 51, 91
Parsva Kakasana (Side Crow Pose) 164–5, 213
Parsvottanasana (Intense Side-stretch Pose) 111
Paschimottanasana (Back-stretch Forward Bend) 37, 69, 118–19, 212, 213
Patanjali, Maharishi 7, 14, 16, 18–20, 80, 228
Patan Vrikshasana (Wobbling Tree Pose) 110
Peacock Pose (Mayurasana) 30, 166–7, 213
pelvic-floor muscles 31, 71, 219, 220, 222, 226
perineum 65, 222, 227
peripheral nervous system (PNS) 38
Phalakasana 211
Pigeon Pose (Kapotasana) 196–7, 213; see also King Pigeon Pose
Pincha Mayurasana (Feathered Peacock Pose) 156–7, 213
pineal gland 35, 183, 184, 231
pingala nadi 24, 60, 62, 209, 219, 220
pituitary gland 35, 39, 65, 81, 183, 184, 192, 230
Plank Pose 177, 245
Plavini breathing 221
Plough Pose (Halasana) 188–9
Pose of the Sage Galava (Galavasana) 170–1
Pose of the Sage Marichi (Marichyasana I) 124–5, 213
Pose of the Sage Vishvamitra (Vishvamittrasana) 174–5
Post-classical period 21–4
posture 42, 86, 202, 206, 244
postures see asanas
prakriti 16, 17, 21, 22
prana: currents/pathways 58, 62; directing 20, 23, 62–3, 81, 222; five pranas 60, 61; and food 74, 75; manipura chakra 65;

pranamaya kosha 66, 67, 217

Pranamasana (Prayer Pose) 210, 211, 213

pranayama (breath control) 216–21; alternate nostril breathing 71, 218–20, 225; breath retention 60–3, 71, 217, 218, 226; and chakras 64; daily practice 212, 213, 217; during pregnancy 242, 243; effects of 29, 30, 63, 216–17; historic yoga 13, 14, 15, 22, 23, 24; meditation 228; modern yoga 25; older age groups 244, 245; recommended poses 141, 142–3; shatkarmas 68; Sun Salutation 209; Yoga sutras 18, 20

pranic energy 60, 61, 209, 217

Prasarita Padottanasana (Wide-legged Forward Bend) 102–3, 213, 242

pratyahara 14, 15, 18, 20, 22, 228

Prayer Pose (Pranamasana) 210, 211, 213

Pre-classical period 12–15

pregnancy 241–3; beneficial poses 128, 143, 183, 186, 188; poses to avoid 115, 124, 136, 140, 152, 160, 162, 164, 179, 208, 217, 219, 220, 241, 242–3

private lessons 240

props 241, 245, 248

prostate gland 128, 140, 186

purification 24, 68–9, 71, 77, 212, 217

purity 17, 19, 65, 75

purusha 16, 17, 21, 22

rajas 17, 74, 75

raw foods 74, 75, 76

reality 15, 16–17, 21, 22, 63

Reclining Hero Pose (Supta Virasana) 150–1

relaxation 23, 28, 29; breathing 220, 221; Corpse Pose 153, 212, 213, 243; pregnancy 241, 242, 243

renunciation 14, 16, 19

reproductive system 29, 60, 65, 66, 70, 118, 128, 131, 132, 217

respiratory system 28, 29, 30–1, 32, 38; anahata chakra 65; nauli 70; pingala nadi 62; prana 60; pranamaya kosha 66; pranayama effect 216, 217

resting poses: Balasana (Child's Pose) 52, 115; Savasana (Corpse Pose) 153, 212, 213, 243; Uttanasana (Standing Forward Bend) 52, 69, 94

Revolving Side Angle Twist (Parivrtta Parsvakonasana) 51, 92–3

Revolving Triangle Pose (Parivrtta Trikonasana) 51, 91

root lock (mula bandha) 71, 219, 220, 222, 226

rotation 46, 51, 54, 55

saguna meditation 230

Salabhasana (Locust Pose) 30, 53, 206–7

samadhi 14, 18, 20, 22, 24, 65, 228

samana 60, 61

Samasthiti 86

Sanskrit 13–14, 58, 64, 72

Sarvangasana (Shoulder Stand Pose) 33, 186–7, 212, 213, 226

sattva 17, 19, 74, 75

Savasana (Corpse Pose) 153, 212, 213, 243

sciatica 100, 122, 131, 132, 135, 143, 179

science of yoga 58–77

scripture, study 66

Seated Forward Bend (Paschimottanasana) 37, 69, 212

seated poses 82, 117–45, 217

self: absorbtion of 14, 18, 20; atman 14, 21; self-discipline 19;

study of 19, 229

self-realization 8, 15, 17, 25, 57, 60; five sheaths 66, 67; Jnana mudra 224; karma 72; meditation 230

senses: chakras 65; koshas 67; nervous system 38; Shambavi mudra 226; three gunas 17; udana 60; withdrawal of 14, 15, 18, 19, 20, 22

sexual abstinence 19, 227

sexual organs 35, 65, 227

sexual practices 22, 61, 70, 237

shakti 22, 58, 63, 65, 226, 227

shamkini 62

shatkarma 24, 25, 37, 68–71

sheaths, five 66–7

shiva 22, 58, 65

shoulders 47, 48, 49, 50, 51; back-bending poses 198, 200, 204, 208; balancing poses 156, 158, 178, 179; inverted poses 186, 188; problems 88, 104, 139, 156, 158, 168, 172, 176, 177, 204; seated poses 135, 139; standing poses 87, 96, 110–11, 112, 114; supine pose 152

Shoulder Stand Pose (Sarvanghasana) 33, 186–7, 212, 213, 226; alternatives 243, 245

Siddah Siddhanta Paddhati 23

Siddhasana (Adept's Pose) 141

Side Crow Pose (Parsva Kakasana) 164–5, 213

Side Plank Pose (Vasisthasana) 172–3, 213, 245

Sirsasana (Head Stand Pose) 33, 35, 182–3, 184–5, 212, 213, 226, 245

Sitali breathing 221

Sitkari breathing 221

skeletal system see musculoskeletal system

skin 41

sleep 35, 60, 61, 186, 221, 229

Sleeping Yogi Pose (Yoga Nidrasana) 152

So hum meditation 230–1

solar plexus 65, 222, 226

soul 14, 16, 20, 22, 66, 67, 72

sounds 64, 65, 221, 230, 231, 232, 247

spine 42–5, 49, 51, 52, 53, 85; chakras 64; Hatha yoga 23, 24; Jalandhara bandha 219, 220, 222, 223, 226, 227; nadis 62–3; nervous system 38, 39, 41; sushumna nadi 24, 60, 62; see also back; back problems

spiritual aspects: karma 72; spiritual body 66; spiritual power 7, 8, 13, 18, 58; spiritual practice (sadhana) 81; vishuddha chakra 64, 65

Splits (Hanumanasana) 144–5

Squatting Pose (Malasana) 97, 242

stamina 155

Standing Forward Bend (Uttanasana) 52, 69, 94, 210, 211, 212, 213

standing poses 85–115

steadiness 23, 25, 106, 155

stealing 19, 236

Stork Pose 105

strength 28

stress 29, 35, 38, 39, 61, 229; relieving 115, 118, 153, 183, 188, 218, 221

students: adjusting poses 236, 241, 242, 245, 248; advising 28, 236, 237

studio, opening 238, 239

subtle body 58, 60, 61, 62, 222
suffering 15, 16, 17, 21
Sukha-Purvara Pranayama 220
Sukkhasana (Easy Pose) 141
Sun Salutation (Surya Namaskara) 209–11, 212, 213
supine poses 147–53
Supta Kurmasana 137
Supta Virasana (Reclining Hero Pose) 150–1
Surya-Bheda-Kumbhaka Pranayama 220
Surya Namaskara (Sun Salutation) 209–11, 212, 213
sushumna nadi 24, 60, 62, 63, 64, 65, 220, 222, 223, 227
Svarga Dvijasana (Bird of Paradise Pose) 107, 213
sweat glands 31
sympathetic nervous system (SNS) 38, 39, 62, 66
synovial fluid/joints 41, 48, 49

Tadasana (Mountain Pose) 86
tamas 17, 74, 75
Tantra yoga 11, 22–3
taxation 239
teaching yoga 235–49
telepathy 65
tendons 42, 46, 48
testes 35
thalamus 39
thighs, stretching 128, 139, 144, 151, 195, 196, 198, 200, 202
third eye 65, 81, 230
thoracic cavity 30, 31, 60
throat: Brahmari 221; chakras 64, 65; Jalandhara bandha 219, 220, 222, 223, 226, 227; stretching 148, 196, 202
thymus 34
thyroid gland 35, 140, 186, 188, 192
Tittibhasana (Firefly Pose) 168–9, 213
Tortoise Pose (Kurmasana) 136–7, 213
transcendence 64, 65, 66
trataka 70, 231, 232
Tree Pose (Vrikshasana) 100, 212, 213
Triangle Poses 51, 90–3
trikuti (third eye) 65, 81, 230
truth 19, 67, 236
twisting poses: balancing 164–5, 176; daily practice 212, 213; during pregnancy 241, 242, 243; joints 51; seated 122, 125, 134–5, 212, 213; standing 91, 92–3
Two-Legs or Feet-Behind-the-Head (Dwi Pada Sirsasana) 132–3

udana 60, 61, 67
Uddiyana Bandha 30, 69, 70, 71, 222–3, 227
Ujjayi breathing 220, 242
the Upanishads 13–15, 16, 62, 233
Upavistha Konasana (Wide-angle Seated Forward-bend Pose) 126–7, 213, 243
Urdhva Dhanurasana (Upward-facing Bow Pose) 192–3, 213
Urdhva Mukha Svanasana (Upward-facing Dog) 178, 213, 245
Urdhva Prasarita Eka Padasana (One Leg Raised Up) 95
urinary system 29, 31, 65, 70; beneficial poses 128, 141, 143, 227
Ustrasana (Camel Pose) 194–5, 213
Utkatasana (Chair Pose) 96, 213
Uttanasana (Standing Forward Bend) 52, 69, 94, 210, 211, 213

Uttan Pristhasana (Lizard Pose) 114, 213
Utthita Parsvakonasana (Extended Side Angle Pose) 53
Utthita Tittibhasana (Insect Pose) 104–5, 213
Uttitha Hasta Padangusthasana (Extended Hand to Toe Pose) 106
Uttitha Trikonasana (Extended Triangle Pose) 51, 90–1

vahnisara exercise 71
Vasisthasana (Side Plank Pose) 172–3, 213, 245
vasti 68–9
Vatyanasana (Horse Pose) 99
Vedanta 13, 16, 21–2
the Vedas 12, 13, 16, 72, 228
Vedic/Pre-classical period 12–15
vegetarian diet 74, 75, 76–7
veins 33, 34
vertebrae 44
Vinyasa 29, 212, 220
Virabhadrasana I-III (Warrior) 50, 87, 88, 89, 213
Vishvamittrasana (Pose of the Sage Vishvamitra) 174–5
visualization 230
Vrikshasana (Tree Pose) 100, 212, 213
vyana 60, 61

walking meditation 232
warming up 209
Warrior I-III (Virabhadrasana) 50, 87, 88, 89, 213
waste products see elimination processes
Wheel Pose (Chakrasana) 192–3
Wide-angle Seated Forward-bend Pose (Upavistha Konasana) 126–7, 213, 243
Wide-legged Forward Bend (Prasarita Padottanasana) 102–3, 213, 242
willpower 68, 72
wind 37, 68, 70
wisdom 14, 15, 67, 224, 229, 236
Wobbling Tree Pose (Patan Vrikshasana) 110
wrist 48, 49, 54; beneficial poses 111, 158, 160, 162, 164, 166, 171, 172, 175, 176, 177, 178, 192; problems 99, 104, 158, 162, 166, 168, 171, 172, 176, 177

yama 18, 19, 20, 22, 228, 236
yoga: benefits 7, 8, 28, 37, 41, 79–81; daily practice 81, 212–13; definition 7, 8, 13; eight-fold path 14, 16, 18, 21, 80, 228; history/ origins 11–25; modern 18, 25; six-fold path 14, 23; teaching 235–49; three-fold path 15
Yoga Mudra 35, 226
Yoga Nidrasana (Sleeping Yogi Pose) 152
Yoga Sutras 7, 16, 18–20, 80

Picture Credits

Main photography: Octopus Publishing Group/Russell Sadur

Other Photography:
akg-images/Nimatallah 13; R. u. S. Michaud 14, 15, 22, 59. Alamy/Art Directors & TRIP 73; Francois Werli 23; World History Archive 18.
Bridgeman Art Library/© British Library Board. All Rights Reserved 17.
Fotolia/surabhi25 64.
Getty Images/Anshu 77; Hulton Archive 44; Ingram Publishing 47 left, 47 right; Jasmina 74; Juergen Sack 229, 232; James L. Stanfield 12.
Thinkstock/Hemera 231; iStockphoto 65.
TopFoto/ullsteinbild 21.
Wellcome Library, London 63.

Acknowledgements

Executive Editor: Liz Dean
Editor: Alex Stetter
Copy Editor: Caroline Taggart
Picture Researcher: Jen Veall
Deputy Art Director: Yasia Williams-Leedham
Design: Mark Kan
Photography: Russell Sadur
Production Controller: Sarah Kramer

Author's Acknowledgements

This book is dedicated to the memory of David Kan.

There are many people I would like to thank for helping me bring this book together. Firstly the teachers who have inspired me since I set off on this wonderful path: Ashley Gregory, Martin McDougall and Leila Miller. You played a pivotal role in my transformation, providing classes that inspired me, wisdom to guide me and the desire for knowledge and improvement that led me to Sri Dharma Mittra. For this I will always be grateful. From my first teacher training in India, Swami Govindananda, your dedication to the teachings of Swami Sivananda and your knowledge of the science and philosophy of yoga is matched only by your enthusiasm to share it with others.

To Sri Dharma Mittra. It is an honour to have your wisdom as the foreword for this book. You are a beacon of light in the lives of all who know and love you. Through your own experience you have taught us how to live with humility and compassion in a challenging world. Thank you for sharing your knowledge and for the Shiva Namaskara Vinyasa - a practice which I am privileged to share with so many on this side of the pond.

To my family, especially Ann and Susan, always there to listen and offer support when I've needed it. To my dearest friends, old and new, thank you for your support, encouragement and patience while I put the book together.

To the many of you who have attended my classes over the years – thank you for your loyalty and commitment, in particular Steve Hardman and Paul Anderson – this journey would have been very different without you both.

Special thanks to Julia Woodford for your valued and careful scrutiny when I wrote the book, and to Alex Stetter for making sense of it all; Yasia Wiliams for making it look like a book worth reading and to Liz Dean for trusting me to write it.

Finally, a massive thank you to those who gave their time and inspiring poses to the book: Steve Hardman, Paul Anderson, Eleanor Brumfitt, Alexandre Matias, Michael Eley, Esther Hielckert, Kirsty Stuart, Minna Skirgard, Nicole Kuepper, Brett Lamb-Shine, Alexandra Slattery and Angelika and Noah Imber and Mia Carlisle.